THE
INDEPENDENT MEDICAL
TRANSCRIPTIONIST
Third Edition

Donna Avila-Weil, CMT
and
Mary Glaccum, CMT

Rayve Productions

Rayve Productions Inc.
Box 726 Windsor CA 95492

Senior Editor: Barbara F. Ray
Cover Design: Leeann Schy

First printing, 1991
Second printing, 1992
Third printing, revised, 1994
Fourth printing, 1996
Fifth printing, 1996
Sixth printing, revised, 1998
Seventh printing, 1998
Eighth printing, 1999

Printed in the United States of America

Library of Congress Cataloging-in-Publication Data
Avila-Weil, Donna, 1945-
    The independent medical transcriptionist / by Donna Avila-Weil and Mary Glaccum. -- 3rd ed.
    p.   cm.
Includes bibliographical references and index.
    ISBN 1-877810-23-1 (alk. paper)

    1. Medical transcription. I. Glaccum, Mary. II. Title.
    R728.8.A98   1997
    653'.18--dc21   97-31753
                                                            CIP

The authors and publisher have attempted to ensure accuracy and completeness of information in this book. Any errors, inaccuracies, omissions, inconsistencies or slights against people or organizations are unintentional.

Dedication

To Vera Pyle, CMT, dear friend and colleague . . .
remarkable and inspiring human being.

Mary Glaccum and Donna Avila-Weil

Mary Glaccum, CMT, has been a medical transcriptionist for 27 years. She was an active member of the American Association for Medical Transcription (AAMT) from 1981-93, and the California Association for Medical Transcription (CAMT), serving as a delegate and chairing many committees. Mary founded the Central Coast Chapter, AAMT, serving as President from 1981-82, and as Newsletter Editor and Scholarship Committee Chair. She is currently a member of Beach Cities Chapter, AAMT.

Mary taught medical terminology and transcription at Allan Hancock College in Santa Maria, California for five years, and she worked in a variety of transcription settings before embarking on her career as a self-employed medical transcriptionist ten years ago. Mary is the owner/manager of The Dictation Station in the greater Los Angeles area, and is a popular keynote speaker and workshop presenter.

Mary has been working with disadvantaged youth for the past six years, first as a professional clown and more recently, as a mentor. Her spare-time passions include antique swap meets, collecting old dolls and toys, and "countryfying" her home.

Donna Avila-Weil, CMT, has been a transcriptionist since 1968. She received her ART credential in 1977 and has worked as an independent for 19 years. Donna was a founding member of the Central Valley Medical Transcribers Association, from which the American Association for Medical Transcription was born, and has served as a delegate of the California Association for Medical Transcription (CAMT) and as CAMT President. In 1991 Donna was honored as CAMT Member-of-the-Year.

Donna has worked extensively in the acute care setting and as an independent medical transcriptionist and consultant, and continues to do so. She is a popular keynote speaker, workshop presenter, and mentor for novice transcriptionists.

Donna and her family enjoy a quiet country life in Northern California, where Donna is active in community activities and pursues creative writing in her free time.

Together . . . Since writing *The Independent Medical Transcriptionist*, Mary and Donna have coedited and published a newsletter, *The Independent*, and have traveled widely in the United States, promoting the medical transcription profession at speaking engagements and workshop presentations.

Acknowledgments from
Donna Avila-Weil

To my family, for believing in me and for their help, patience and support through the years. I love you all very much.

Deepest appreciation to our many colleagues and clients from whom we have learned so much over the years and who inspired us to put our experiences into writing.

To all of you who have the courage, ambition, and motivation to make the move to independence — it is an exciting time.

And finally, to Mary Glaccum, CMT, for this "excellent adventure" again. It's time to gas up that motor home!

Acknowledgments from Mary Glaccum

Since the first printing of *The Independent Medical Transcriptionist*, I have had the privilege and honor of speaking to many, many medical transcriptionists about becoming self-employed and have been able to share in their many successes as well as their occasional stumbles. Each and every one of them has shown such great determination and ingenuity that they have been and continue to be a real inspiration to me. Thank you for sharing your stories.

Of course without my IMT buddies such as Kathryn Hunter-Dyer, Abby Toulson, Doreen Jamieson, Sheila Kelly and Doris Anderson, I would have felt very isolated and alone in this big city. Thank you for always being there and sharing your wisdom.

To my family, John, Linda, Katy, "Little John" and Breanna, Gordon, Chris, Wendy, Sana and Jasmin, thank you for reminding me not to take this thing called life — and myself — too seriously.

To Miranda, my "daughter" this past year, thank you for the privilege of allowing me into your life.

To my dear friend of 31 years and one of my mentors, Grace Bach, thank you for showing me the meaning of true grit and courage, Gradie Sue.

Last but not least, to Donna Avila-Weil, my coauthor. Thank you, dear friend, for the opportunity to again experience the exhilaration of flight. I'm ready for the motor home, how about you?

"Trifles make perfection and perfection is no trifle."
—Michelangelo

Contents

Introduction

Even though there has been a deluge of material published about working independently, this has only managed to whet the appetite of those seeking more comprehensive information. Because of the rapid changes taking place in the medical transcription industry and more emphasis being placed on the home office as an alternative workplace, it became apparent that an even more comprehensive book addressing these issues was needed.

We have continued to promote working independently and in our travels throughout the country have had the pleasure of networking with many people. These experiences have aided our research and work on this edition and reinforced our commitment to helping meet the need for a comprehensive and up-to-date resource for working independently as a medical transcriptionist.

Our backgrounds have changed little since we wrote the first edition. Our experiences are based on two perspectives: "Country Mouse" (Donna Avila-Weil) and "City Mouse" (Mary Glaccum). Donna is from a rural community in Northern California, and Mary hails from the Greater Los Angeles area. During our many years as medical transcriptionists — sometimes employed by others, sometimes independently employed — we have experienced diverse and exciting careers. Professionally, we have also taught, lectured, conducted seminars, served as mentors, written articles, developed our own IMT newsletter, and advised hundreds regarding details of self-employment and the how-to's of establishing a medical transcription business.

Through years of trial and error, we planned, studied, and endured numerous frustrations as we traveled the circuitous road to independent transcription success.

No straighter road was available at the time. Few resource materials existed. Until this book there were few, if any, comprehensive sources to educate or refer to if questions or difficulties arose.

On the following pages we share with you our knowledge about the medical transcription field and the requirements, benefits, pitfalls, and methods of becoming an independent transcriptionist. The facts, figures, and vignettes are provided as guidelines for those interested in pursuing careers as medical transcriptionists and independent medical transcriptionists.

Through the years we have enjoyed assisting intelligent and talented transcriptionists as they pursued successful careers. We wish you the greatest success, too.

What Is Medical Transcription?

*"The future belongs to those who believe
in the beauty of their dreams. "*

— Eleanor Roosevelt

Medical Transcription

The translation of sound into organized,
well-expressed written statements that
communicate medical meaning.

Medical transcription has existed since the dawn of civilization and the beginning of experimentation. Rudimentary medical record keeping in the form of drawings was scratched onto prehistoric cave walls, evolving to clay tablet records, hieroglyphics, papyrus, parchment, and finally paper.

In mid-fifth century B.C. Greece, during the time of Hippocrates, often referred to as "The Father of Medicine," physicians' notes established new heights in rational, empirical medical reporting. They served not only as a written record of current medical actions, but also provided reference information for future patient care. Comparisons, conclusions and research were developed from medical record reviews, and medical information was shared to nurture medical education. Over the centuries, medical records have become increasingly important. With expanding medical specialization, new developments in technology, and government and health care regulations, accurate documentation is critical. The medical record has expanded voluminously to meet these demands.

Until the twentieth century, physicians were both providers of medical service and scribes for medical communities. In the 1900s, medical stenographers began to take dictation in shorthand directly from physicians. Soon, a succession of voice recording machines evolved. The invention of magnetic tape storage in the form of cassette tapes launched medical stenographers into medical transcription careers.

Today, medical transcription is a vital link in the health care industry, a highly respected profession, and one of the most fascinating and rewarding of allied health careers.

THE HEALTH CARE INDUSTRY

Health care is one of the most technologically diversified industries of this decade. The expanding scope and specialization of health care has created a growing demand for processing, coordinating, and communicating accurate documentation of clinical information. Now more than ever, timely, reliable, accessible, accurate health care information is needed to facilitate quality patient care, and this need has increased the demand for experienced, well-qualified medical transcriptionists.

The upkeep of the medical record has been called the "invisible profession." As the upcoming decade advances toward the "paperless record," the increasing challenge will be how to maintain quality, accuracy, and information integrity in the patient record.

In yesteryear's health care setting, when medical procedures were less sophisticated, state and federal regulations minimal, and malpractice lawsuits practically unheard of, physicians routinely documented patient progress in longhand. Today, however, handwritten reports are increasingly inappropriate.

INFORMATION MANAGEMENT

In the current environment, health care is focused on caring for "populations," not individual patients. To meet the information requirements needed for this paradigm shift, the effective and efficient delivery of patient care requires organized information management (IM). Health care organizations require organized systems information management to avoid scattered data bases (e.g., duplication of data gathering, inconsistent reports and inefficiencies in the use of economic resources).

The following are generally accepted objectives of health care information management.

1. Identify the information needs of the organization in providing patient care services.

2. Evaluate the existing data for accuracy, availability, accessibility, security, necessity, and performance.

3. Develop action plans to enhance and improve organizational performance in patient care, governance, management and support processes to meet the goals of the organization.

4. Improve turnaround time of results.

5. Reduce unnecessary duplication of data entries.

6. Provide timely access to information throughout the organization.

7. Provide patient-centered information systems and technology.

8. Provide for the collection, generation and analysis of data.

All of the above apply to the transcribed medical documentation provided through services inside or outside of the organization.

The demand for more detailed and accurate medical records will increase in direct proportion to the growing complexity of our health care system.

THE IMPORTANCE OF TRANSCRIBED REPORTS IN HEALTH CARE TODAY

Documentation is an integral and necessary part of health care with content and format influenced by legislation, compensation mechanisms, and liability exposure. As a result, today's health care records must be accurate, detailed, legible, and easily duplicated.

All health care providers face increasing demands to provide quality patient care as quickly as possible, documented by ever-more-thorough records. To meet these demands, reliance is placed on skilled physicians and other medical team members, state-of-the-art technology, and well-trained transcriptionists for accurate recording of patient care and treatment.

Transcriptionists are medical language specialists. The reports they produce are indispensable to modern health care because handwritten reports — especially quickly written reports that may contain illegible phrases or errors — not only waste time, but also present serious potential problems in quality assurance, risk management, professional recertification and licensing, and third party reimbursement.

When dictating reports to be transcribed, physicians tend to record more detail about exams, conversations with the patient, medical decisions, advice dispensed, and laboratory and pharmacy information. In addition, it is easy for doctors to send copies of transcribed reports to associates, which improves patient care and reduces physician correspondence.

Transcribed reports are less likely to be misinterpreted by clinicians, referring physicians, attorneys, and others who make decisions based on information in the medical record. As a result, the health care provider experiences fewer interruptions of his or her work, spends less time in review and response, and faces fewer requests to appear in court to interpret handwritten reports.

The litigation crisis that has developed in recent years compels doctors and health care administrators to focus on accurate, comprehensive patient records. These superior medical records — in conjunction with other quality control measures — improve patient care, reduce risk exposure, lower insurance costs, and bring greater peace-of-mind to patients and health care providers.

THE MEDICAL RECORD AND QUALITY ASSURANCE

The quality of patient care is directly related to the quality of the medical record. Whether in an acute-care facility, convalescent hospital, physician group practice, or other medical setting, the many caregivers who attend the individual patient refer to, and depend on, accurate medical records to provide quality continuity in patient care.

Although doctors, nurses, and other members of the hands-on-health care team bear the primary responsibility for immediate, handwritten patient-care documentation, the medical transcriptionist also plays an important role as transcribed reports become a legal part of the medical record.

Medical records provide the means by which standards of care are evaluated. The quality and accuracy of the information in the health care record is continuously examined, and physicians are legally required to attest to the accuracy of the recorded diagnoses and procedures in patients' records.

At the administrative level, health care facilities depend on accurate medical records to meet ethical and legal standards of patient care and to provide accurate documentation of patient-care history for future reference during accreditation or medical/legal situations.

The medical record documents the facts of a patient's illness, symptoms, diagnosis, and treatment. This includes the daily care and treatment of that patient. Health care facilities, in accordance with accepted professional standards and practices, are required to maintain a medical record for each patient These records must be complete, accurate, current, readily accessible and systematically organized. Where patient care is concerned, the medical record is the principal means of communication between health care professionals. The medical record is an important patient-care planning tool which accomplishes the following:

1. Records the course of the patient's treatment and changes in the patient's condition.

2. Documents communications between the practitioner responsible for the patient and any other health professional who contributes to the patient's care.

3. Assists in protecting the legal interests of the patient, the organization and the practitioner.

4. Provides a data base for use in statistical reporting, continuing education and research.

5. Provides information necessary for third-party billing and regulatory agencies.

ILLEGIBLE ENTRIES — WHY TRANSCRIBED DOCUMENTATION IS IMPORTANT

Handwriting has long been a major problem in interpreting the events surrounding the care of patients, but illegible handwriting can no longer be tolerated in the modern health care environment. The American Medical Association (AMA) urges physicians to print, type or computerize prescriptions. A Harvard study found that " . . . penmanship was among the causes of 220 prescription errors out of 30,000 cases."

Today it is essential that medical record entries be legible, clear, and meaningful to each patient's course of treatment. Illegible medical records may have adverse effects on the performance of other health professionals who read the record and act on what they read. Illegible records may also make it difficult or impossible for caregivers or facilities to defend themselves.

Licensure rules and regulations contained in state statutes generally describe requirements and standards for the maintenance, handling, signing, filing and retention of medical records.

The failure of a medical facility or physician to maintain a complete and accurate medical record may affect the ability of that facility or physician to obtain third-party reimbursement (e.g., from Medicare, Medicaid, or Blue Cross). Under federal and state laws, the medical record must accurately reflect the treatment for which the facility or physician seeks payment. Third-party payers rely on timely and accurately dictated and transcribed documents in the record for determining reimbursement. Thus, the medical record is important to health care facilities and physicians for medical, legal and financial reasons.

It is important to remember that just as though it were set in stone, the medical record is a document that cannot be erased once a recording has been made.

LEGAL PROCEEDINGS AND THE MEDICAL RECORD

The importance of complete, accurate, and timely medical records as an evidentiary tool in legal proceedings cannot be overemphasized. The integrity and completeness of the medical record is extremely important in reconstructing the events surrounding any alleged negligence in the care of the patient.

Medical records aid police investigations in providing information for determining the cause of injury or death, and the extent of injury in workers' compensation or personal injury proceedings.

When health professionals are called as witnesses in legal proceedings, they are permitted to refresh their recollections of the facts and circumstances of particular cases by referring to the medical records. Under such circumstances, a complete, accurate and timely medical record is vitally important for accurate testimony. Furthermore, if medical records are proved to be inaccurate or incomplete or made long after the event they purport to record, they may be used as damaging evidence against health care facilities and medical caregivers.

CONFIDENTIALITY OF THE PATIENT RECORD

All health care professionals who have access to medical records have a clear legal, ethical, and moral obligation to protect the confidentiality of the information in the records. The communications between a physician and his or her patient and the information generated during the course of the patient's illness are generally accorded the protection of confidentiality. Thus, the information in the medical record must be dealt with in a confidential manner; otherwise, a medical facility or organization could incur liability.

NEW TECHNOLOGY DEMANDED

The importance and value of the medical record will be even greater in the future. With increasing numbers of individuals receiving medical care, and as patient information systems continue to merge with patient financial systems, the information demands of users of medical record information will increase. Technology must be continually developed to meet these demands.

According to the U.S. Department of Labor, by the year 2000, the need for technicians skilled in database and information technology may increase by as much as 75 percent. In this rapidly emerging and ever changing industry, medical transcriptionists will continue to play a vital role.

THE COMPUTERIZED PATIENT RECORD (CPR)

Although the health care industry lagged behind most other fields in becoming computerized, today's health care professionals depend on computers. They are found in the admitting office, business office, operating room, nursing unit, pharmacy, laboratory, medical imaging, satellite unit and medical records departments.

Computers are efficient, offer great flexibility and have unlimited capacity to store data. They are definitely here to stay! The medical record is no longer a conglomeration of handwritten entries but includes fetal monitoring strips, electrocardiogram strips, electroencephalogram strips, electronic output from the laboratory, pharmacy and radiology services, nursing documentation, medication administration, etc.

The computerized patient record has been introduced in an effort to improve productivity and quality of patient information, and to provide the economic benefit of reducing costs. In addition, the CPR can support clinical research, be interactive, and facilitate computer-assisted diagnosis.

The CPR is used in telecommunications around the world on a real-time basis to transport picture graphics between nations. For instance, radiographic images that may have been taken in a hospital in Saudi Arabia at 3 a.m. can be reviewed on a real-time basis in the United States.

Critical lab values can immediately be communicated electronically. Via software, a physician can be notified when he or she has ordered medications; about risks, benefits, complications; and when to renew orders. Transcribed medical documents are an integral part of the CPR.

There are some disadvantages to the CPR. Although computers are becoming a necessity in modern health care, they are not infallible. Several problems have been identified including lack of technical knowledge and support to integrate systems; loss of confidentiality and unauthorized disclosure of information, which have necessitated the development of sophisticated security systems; equipment unreliability; and concerns regarding the accuracy and reliability of data input by computer operators.

Another major problem slowing down health care's leap forward into the CPR age is the lack of system responsiveness. For peak efficiency, a system must respond quickly to any request for information. Some do not.

Often, computer communication and response time is negatively impacted by the operator's lack of ability to use the hardware effectively. Many health care organizations attempting to undergo computerization have underestimated the size and design of the system required to integrate effectively. Not only is the selection of adequate hardware and software needs essential, but the technical training required to operate these systems and keep them up and running has been a huge problem. It is wonderful to have technology at your fingertips, but if you don't know how to use it, what good is it?

CONFIDENTIALITY AND THE COMPUTERIZED PATIENT RECORD (CPR)

Critics say that computer security and existing laws cannot protect medical information. Although there are a variety of federal laws that protect credit information, there are very few laws protecting the computerized medical record.

Is Independent Medical Transcription the Profession for You?

"I do not know anyone who has got to the top
without hard work. That is the recipe.
It will not always get you to the top
but should get you pretty near."

—Margaret Thatcher

You are intrigued with the idea of self-employment and have decided to investigate freelancing. We look forward to helping you reach your goal. In this book we focus on the medical transcription profession, but the general information we provide, and the methods we recommend, may also be utilized as research and marketing tools for other personal service specialties.

THE ENTREPRENEURIAL PERSONALITY

According to the Small Business Administration, research indicates that successful small business entrepreneurs have a number of characteristics in common. The following questions will help you evaluate your personality and entreprenuerial potential. How do you measure up?

_____ I have a strong desire to be my own boss.

_____ Win, lose, or draw, I want to be master of my own financial destiny.

_____ I have significant specialized business ability based on both my education and my experience.

_____ I have an ability to conceptualize the whole of a business; not just its individual parts, but how they relate to each other.

_____ I develop an inherent sense of what is "right" for a business and have the courage to pursue it.

_____ One or both of my parents were entrepreneurs; calculated risk-taking runs in my family.

_____ My life is characterized by a willingness and capacity to persevere.

_____ I possess a high level of energy, sustainable over long periods, to make my business successful.

While not every successful home-based business owner starts with a "yes" answer to all of these questions, three or four "nos" and "undecideds" should be sufficient reason for you to stop and think twice before going it alone.

EXPERIENCE

Do you have the necessary tools to be a successful independent transcriptionist? Independents are generally paid by production — by the line, page or character count. If you are highly productive, capable of transcribing accurately and quickly, your earnings might be excellent. On the other hand, if you are a low volume producer, you should carefully consider whether self-employment is the right career move for you.

How much medical transcription work experience do you have? If you have been employed specifically for medical offices, clinics, or other specialties and feel you are well qualified, it is probably best to concentrate your independent transcription work within your field of expertise.

RURAL VERSUS CITY TRANSCRIPTION

Some transcriptionists are more comfortable in a rural setting; others prefer the city. In more rural locales, your clients will probably be close to your home. You will become familiar with physicians in your area, their styles of dictating, and their idiosyncrasies, especially if you work for small clinics or one doctor's office. On the other hand, if you work in a large metropolitan area, the chances that you will be transcribing for doctors located near your home are slim, and you will probably experience a greater variety of dictation.

In either setting, you also have the option to market your services to clients outside your geographical area through telecommuting.

DIALECT DIFFICULTIES

Dialects present great difficulty for many transcriptionists. Some find dialects totally impossible, and even transcriptionists with an ear for languages generally find dialects challenging. This writer still shudders from the vivid memory of hearing her first "ezofeygous" for "esophagus" and wondering if she was ever going to make it through the day.

Hospitals and medical offices frequently send dictation they do not wish to deal with to outside services (e.g., self-employed transcriptionists). This dictation usually includes a variety of different dialects. On average, if your account is a large facility, many dictating doctors will be foreign-born. If you do not have an ear and an aptitude for dialects, you may find it difficult or impossible to service these accounts.

HOSPITAL VERSUS MEDICAL OFFICE TRANSCRIPTION

There is a great difference between hospital transcription and doctors' office transcription. Doctors' office transcription generally focuses on histories and physical examinations, patient chart notes, and referral letters. Hospital transcription covers many specialties, extensive procedures, operative reports, radiology, pathology, and many other subspecialties.

Hospital work can be an exciting and rewarding market, but do not assume you will succeed with hospital transcription if you have had no hospital transcription experience. Only an experienced hospital transcriptionist, or certified medical transcriptionist, should attempt hospital accounts.

If you have not been trained and do not have experience in hospital specialties, it would be a disastrous mistake for you to accept hospital accounts under the assumption you could transcribe the dictation adequately. Gain hospital transcription experience first, gradually increasing your knowledge of each specialty. We have seen many people attempt self-employment only to fail because they did not have adequate training and experience. Wise transcriptionists learn as much as possible and allow additional time for the seasoning of experience.

OPPORTUNITIES FOR THE VISUALLY IMPAIRED TRANSCRIPTIONIST

There are many visually impaired transcriptionists working in the health care field. For reference materials, they depend on books such as Dorland's *Medical Dictionary in Braille*. This comes in approximately 49 volumes and each volume is about three inches thick. Another reference is Dorland's *Medical Speller*, which is seven volumes in Braille. Braille references are expensive, about $400 or more for the full dictionary, but they are essential resources for visually impaired transcriptionists.

Transcription equipment for the visually impaired transcriptionist can also be very costly. One helpful device is an Opticon. This converts printed letters to a tactile display and costs approximately $5000. The Opticon is not ideal for every visually impaired transcriptionist, however. It requires patience. Although it does make print and computer screens accessible, it is **slow**.

Visually impaired medical transcription students usually do well using adaptive devices for their work. In some locales, vocational rehabilitation departments have adapted headsets for transcribing machines. Using this headset, the visually impaired transcriptionist hears dictation played in one ear and the voice synthesizer in the other ear.

There are also medical textbooks available for the visually impaired. For more information, contact the following:

- **Recordings for the Blind**
  800-221-4792 or 609-452-0606

For information on opportunities for visually impaired transcriptionists, contact:

- **National Association of Blind Secretaries and Transcriptionists**
  816-444-5918

- **American Association for Medical Transcription (AAMT)**
  800-982-2182

If available in your area, also contact the Commission for the Blind, which will provide assistance in locating training programs.

SPEECH SYNTHESIS TECHNOLOGY

For the visually impaired medical transcriptionist's home transcription system, a speech synthesizer is utilized, dedicated text-to-speech and software to make the synthesizer operate. This enables the MT to hear what she is typing, listen to what she has already typed, and read anything sent to her via computer or on computer diskette. In this mode the transcriptionist can read about 300-500 words per minute.

One drawback of this system is spelling errors that can creep in if one is not careful; and some words are saved strangely. It takes patience and diligence to adapt to a synthesizer, but transcriptionists who do adapt find it very helpful. Prices for quality speech synthesis and software range from $1200-$2000.

Another exciting aspect of speech synthesis technology is that it can access and use online bulletin boards like GEnie. This allows visually impaired transcriptionists excellent opportunities to network with their peers, learn more about their profession, and broaden their personal horizons.

OPPORTUNITIES FOR COURT REPORTERS IN MEDICAL TRANSCRIPTION

Court reporters and medical transcriptionists do very different types of work, but they use similar skills, and it is possible for a court reporter to make a successful transition from court reporting to medical transcription. Some individuals even combine court reporting and medical transcription. Success rates, of course, vary from person to person.

The average court reporter spends three or more years in training. They learn keystroke, response to the spoken word, and grammar; and they work hard to develop the dramatically high speeds required to be successful court reporters. For many, however, the desired speed is not attained — the goal is not reached. Generally, however, the speed they have attained is adequate for medical transcription.

Speed is not enough, however, to be a successful medical transcriptionist. In fact, court reporters who move into medical transcription have to accept and implement different transcription parameters that are not based on speed if they are to be successful.

While SPEED of production is paramount in court reporting, QUALITY of the finished product is the focus of medical transcription.

Court reporters are trained to respond to the spoken word, to keystroke the spoken word instantaneously, verbatim, without stopping. At the time they are transcribing, they pay little attention to details like punctuation and spelling. This is done at a later time (away from the actual recording setting) by the reporter or by a "scopist."

The scopist, who is knowledgeable in legal terminology and proceedings, proofs and corrects the court reporter's computer generated transcription, often relying on dictation to aid in the proofing. The scopist will scan the document and correct punctuation, but the *verbatim* dictation remains the same. Working as a scopist is an excellent background for someone wanting to become a legal or medical transcriptionist.

Medical transcriptionists must pay close attention to detail as they are transcribing, and they do not necessarily transcribe verbatim. They edit as they progress through their reports, which must be grammatically correct, with format and content completely accurate. Medical transcriptionists use a tape and transcribing machine to do their transcription, allowing them to stop, back up and listen again to what the dictator is saying. They may reformat material, spending additional time on details of sentence composition, adding or deleting unnecessary punctuation.

Court reporters who do not already have a medical transcription background will face considerable training if they are to make a successful transition into medical transcription. They will need solid skills in grammar, medical terminology, and anatomy/physiology, and they may need training or retraining on medical transcription technology and transcription practice using tapes of actual physician dictation.

COURT REPORTING EQUIPMENT FOR MEDICAL TRANSCRIPTION

The equipment court reporters utilize costs approximately three times as much (sometimes $10,000 and up) as the equipment required for medical transcription (approximately $3000). Can court reporters use their technology to do medical transcription? Yes. There are court reporters who successfully generate court documents and medical transcription using their court reporting technology.

Some court reporting equipment, such as the *RAPIDTEXT*® steno captioner, has been successfully adapted for use in medical transcription. This piece of stenographic equipment is very effective. RAPIDTEXT entry is the method of using a steno machine to input data or information into a computer at speeds of 120-200 or more words per minute. Although the concept of using this technology for general industry use is fairly new, the court reporting industry has successfully applied a similar technology to produce "legal documents" for the past decade. RAPIDTEXT utilizes the same theory of writing steno, but has the added capabilities of instant display of translated English and word processing functions and capabilities available from the steno keyboard. The equipment required is an IBM compatible computer with a hard disk and 640K or greater memory, a computer compatible steno machine, and the RAPIDTEXT software package.

StenEd® is another type of real-time machine shorthand using the Stenotype keyboard. This keyboard allows one to enter text and commands much more quickly than with a standard QWERTY keyboard, doubling or even tripling the rate at which text is entered. The *Stenotype Text Entry*®(STE) marries real-time

19

translation to online word processing. It is a real-time Computer Aided Transcription (CAT) system.

StenEd also offers a very good reference called *Medical Terminology and Advanced Medical Topics*, which was written for stenotypists. It has an excellent anatomy and physiology section.

Other educational products are available, as well as an entire home study program. For information, contact the following company:

- **Health Professions Institute (HPI)** — Training
  P.O. Box 801
  Modesto, CA 95353
  209-551-2112

Establishing an Independent Medical Transcription Business

"Whatever your goal in life, be proud of every day
that you are able to work in that direction."

— Chris Evert

The key word here is "business." You need to plan for, and take action regarding, all aspects of organizing and running a business. That means developing your marketing strategy, your business operations strategy, and your financial strategy. You need to set goals and put systems in place to achieve those goals. And you must make a personal commitment to work hard to make it all happen.

According to the Robert Half firm, 47% of those who voluntarily leave their jobs (some of which become self-employed) do so because they believe their jobs offer limited opportunity for advancement; 26% leave because they feel they suffered a lack of recognition; and the remainder leave for other causes, including dissatisfaction with their salaries and benefit packages.

Our motivation for working at home is the pleasure of independence and flexibility. Your motivation may be something different — a desire for greater income, career growth, prestige, recognition in the business world. Whatever, you must be motivated to succeed in order to withstand the monumental challenges that occur in business management.

THE INDEPENDENT TRANSCRIPTIONIST'S WORKSITE

We live in a highly mobile, competitive, ambitious society in which enterprising entrepreneurs often seek rewarding self-employment when it is a feasible alternative to traditional workplace jobs. In the medical transcription profession, there are various worksite alternatives, and working at home has been a viable option for many years.

The number of home-based workers is on the rise. In the past five years, fewer than 50% of the 5.6 million displaced workers have found full-time replacement jobs. But more than 440,000 of those 5.6 million have gone into business for themselves. Over the last decade in some areas of the country, home-based independents grew by 122%, while all other workers grew only about 22%. Forecasters are predicting that by the year 2000, 58% of the work-force will be working from home and will be part of the information superhighway now under construction.

ADVANTAGES OF SELF-EMPLOYMENT

The home-based career has definite advantages. It offers freedom, flexibility, and best of all, professional respect and unlimited opportunity for success and fulfillment. The independent medical transcriptionist establishes personal goals, sets a schedule, and manages daily life. She or he is in control.

As an independent, duties are performed with little or no supervision, and decisions are made without a great deal of red tape or waiting indefinitely for someone higher on the management chain-of-command to approve a task that could have been accomplished immediately.

The independent transcriptionist determines the work schedule, work pace, and work hours — day or night.

Office colors and styles are personal favorites. Business equipment and furniture are rearranged whenever and however desired.

The program of work is designed to allow time for other interests — creative projects, professional and community organizations, classes, sports, friends, and family.

Each day's schedule determines work attire — casual, classic, sporty — and bare feet are acceptable on the home-front. The independent is free to wear bold perfume, bright jewelry, listen to classical, country or rock music, snuggle a pet, laugh out loud, whistle, sing, talk to friends or family on the phone, and generally enjoy life with no fear of disturbing co-workers or being scolded for wasting company time.

The independent medical transcriptionist does not have to pay for expensive day care for children, arise before dawn and arrive home after dark, fight daily commute traffic, scramble for parking spaces, tolerate an uncomfortable office setting, endure office politics, withstand autocratic supervision, avoid low-producing co-workers or suffer through intolerable working hours!

If "home-based" sounds good to you, as it does to so many, consider the following important factors.

THE MULTI-TALENTED TRANSCRIPTIONIST

Becoming self-employed requires many talents beyond those that propelled you into business in the first place. First and foremost, you must be seriously committed to your career as an independent. In addition, advanced planning and preparation will be essential if you are to succeed.

Evaluate your professional knowledge and skills proficiency. Rate yourself as objectively and as honestly as possible, and don't be tempted to rationalize about areas where knowledge is lacking or skills are weak. If you are not certain you are completely prepared to accomplish the goals you have outlined, take additional classes to improve your skills and increase your confidence.

DOING YOUR HOMEWORK BEFORE
GOING INTO BUSINESS

Don't reinvent the wheel . . . or medical transcription. Learning basic information, ways to be more efficient, and how to avoid professional pitfalls from someone who has already been there will save you time, money, and prevent headaches.

Do your homework before attempting to establish a business. Gather as much information as you can from a variety of sources, including your competition.

However, be cautious when opinions are offered. Good advice can be invaluable, but beware of naysayers with negative attitudes, who may never have taken a risk or were stymied by adverse experiences. Learn to differentiate fact from fantasy. Sit down and make a list of the benefits and drawbacks of being self-employed. Then make your own educated decisions.

JOINING PROFESSIONAL ORGANIZATIONS

Join local medical transcription organizations and participate in professional activities that will inform and inspire you. Networking with transcriptionists offers you important professional exposure, visibility, and encouragement. In addition, you will maintain a competitive edge as current professional information is shared, and you will enjoy opportunities for state and national networking as your career progresses.

Consider joining other professional organizations, too. Your local chamber of commerce, word processing and secretarial groups, home-based workers groups, and other business-oriented groups offer excellent opportunities for personal and career development, interaction with a variety of professionals, and community involvement. You will discover that extra hours invested in organizational meetings and community participation can yield exciting rewards.

There is an association for most every group, cause, idea or occupation now in existence. They all have membership lists and a good many of them publish newsletters. Investigate the various associations in your area and consider joining some of them. This is where you'll meet your community's "movers and shakers," learn valuable business tips from individuals and newsletters, and you may even pick up some referrals.

Professional organizations also hold conventions, and if you think conventions are designed just to meet annual organizational requirements and take care of board of directors' business, think again. The main reason conventions are held is to provide optimum opportunity for the dissemination of information and for interaction with other professionals. In one or two hours at a convention, you can make more GOOD CONTACTS than in two weeks of cold-calling.

Every major city has a convention bureau because convention business represents a sizable share of a city's revenue. Find out who's holding what and where, or get convention resource information from the convention bureau. To attend a convention, you will generally only have to pay a registration fee. For this, you will receive a program, sometimes a list of attendees, and you will have access to numerous vendors, products, workshop presentations, and professionals in your field.

BUSINESS ALLIANCES

National Association for the Self-Employed (NASE) — If you are in business for yourself, there are many associations and organization that would be of benefit to you in your day-to-day working environment. One of the most well-known is the National Association for the Self-Employed (NASE).

Not only is this organization very active in promoting legislation that will help and empower the self-employed, it also offers many benefits such as health insurance, discounts on business services, products and travel, and business legal advice. NASE also publishes a bimonthly newsletter that reports details of recent legislation affecting our businesses, new products and available services as well as asking for feedback. The thing we like most about this organization is that its leaders welcome feedback from members — suggestions and new ideas — and encourage members to be proactive in their personal and professional lives. Having a strong membership base, NASE is able to greatly influence positive changes for the self-employed. For more information, contact NASE.

- **National Association for the Self-Employed (NASE)**
  800-232-NASE

Women Incorporated (WIC) — Women Incorporated is located in Sacramento, California. WIC welcomes all self-employed entrepreneurs, including men. During the past few years, Women Incorporated has been instrumental in forming alliances with the Money Store Investment Company and the Small Business Administration to procure start-up financing for new businesses as well as financing to expand member businesses. Before WIC's involvement, it was difficult for women business owners to get financial backing, but with WIC's help, that has changed throughout the country. WIC also offers group rates for health insurance, discounts, a quarterly magazine, and sponsors the annual National Conference for Women in Business. For more data, contact WIC.

- **Women Incorporated (WIC)**
  800-930-3993

BUSINESS PUBLICATIONS FOR INDEPENDENTS

There are a multitude of publications that are extremely helpful to the self-employed. Some of our favorites are the following:

- *The Self-Employed Professional*
  Business Media Group
  800-366-7857

- *Home Office Computing*
  800-288-7812

- *MT Monthly*
  800-951-5559

- *Advance for Health Information Professionals* (which is free)
  800-355-1088

Being home-based and disconnected from the outside world for the most part, it is very important that we become involved with business groups that will not only enhance the way we run our businesses, but also will fight for the changes necessary to compete successfully.

WHEN IN DOUBT, CONFER WITH AN EXPERT

Don't hesitate to consult experts for help in areas where your knowledge and experience are limited. Smart entrepreneurs seek guidance and support, and build a stronger business by including accountants, bankers, attorneys and other skilled professionals in their management team. Access to the Internet has also opened up many opportunities to network with these professionals through e-mail, chat rooms, newsgroups, Web pages, etc.

TELEPHONE QUERIES FROM NOVICES

There is great misunderstanding about the medical transcription field and what is required to be a competent transcriptionist. Many believe that anyone who can type and knows a few medical terms can transcribe medical reports. However, medical transcription is a language skill and not a typing/keyboarding skill.

Each week we are contacted by individuals interested in becoming home-based transcriptionists. Unfortunately, the large majority of these people do not have the education and skills necessary to succeed. Some have had experience as medical office receptionists, insurance billers, or hospital admission clerks. One physician's wife explained that although she lacked some technical training, she did know how to type and her husband was willing to help her decipher the medical terms.

During our years as transcriptionists, we have encountered people who dreamed of rewarding medical transcription careers but entered the field ill-equipped for the job. It was a painful experience for them and their employers or clients.

Many of these transcriptionist hopefuls had never seen a transcribing machine and didn't know how to use a headset. Others couldn't use a foot pedal, preferring instead to stop and start the tape by hand.

Some had poor grammar skills and were unable to spell correctly or punctuate sentences. Many did not understand the necessity of, and were not interested in, taking courses in medical terminology, anatomy, and physiology to develop transcription competence.

To be a skilled medical transcriptionist, one should know something about the basic elements of language because medical terminology is a mix of Latin and Greek word parts, roots, prefixes, suffixes, English, and a smattering of miscellaneous other foreign terms. A working knowledge of biology, human anatomy and physiology is also necessary to understand dictation. And excellent grammar, spelling, and punctuation are essential for creating a document that is correct, professional looking and interpretable to others.

Word processing skills are important, too. Gone are the days when transcriptionists used manual typewriters and got by typing 60 wpm. Today, the minimum acceptable typing speed for medical transcription work is over 80 wpm, and well-trained MTs efficiently use computers, a variety of software programs, and other technological devices that give them a competitive edge. For the new medical transcriptionist, technical training is a necessity, usually in the form of vocational or technical college, medical transcription programs, or an accredited medical transcription home-study program.

Most of us "old-timers" learned transcribing "OTJ" (on-the-job training). Unfortunately, that option is rarely open to new transcriptionists today. Hospitals and clinics, faced with budget cutbacks, limited staff, and pressures to produce transcribed records as quickly as possible, seldom hire trainees.

BREAKING INTO THE FIELD THE RIGHT WAY

There are tried and true paths to success. Many colleges offer courses in medical transcription and terminology. There are also home study programs available, which are discussed in this book. Find the path that's right for you, make a commitment to excellence, and a bright future awaits.

Today, transcriptionists take a more realistic view of career communication, are more confident and assertive in the workplace, and are reaping the professional benefits of this new attitude. Increasingly, formally educated individuals are coming into the medical transcription field as crossovers from other career fields like finance, education, marketing, communication and other health care professions, to name a few. For reasons that are financial, economic or even just to change careers, they are seeking self-employment as MTs, and they are bringing with them skills from their former professions, putting them well ahead of the game in many respects.

THE COMPETENT HOME-BASED MEDICAL TRANSCRIPTIONIST

As a home-based medical transcriptionist, you will face daily challenges. You will be responsible for transcribing many different types of medical reports, dictated by a variety of practitioners, with an assortment of accents that will require a good ear for deciphering dialects. You will have to be a stickler for detail and learn new terms on a daily basis.

You will have to remain focused, concentrating on individual projects over long periods of time. You will be "plugged into a machine," typing for eight or more hours a day.

A quick mind, solid basic skills and fingers that fly across the keyboard are independent transcription essentials, for you will be paid by production. Correctly transcribed production. Quantity combined with quality.

While building your business, you may need to forego vacations, sick days, and weekend leisure. Health insurance and retirement benefits may be unaffordable luxuries for an indefinite period of time.

As an independent business person you will be responsible for marketing, public relations, quality control, troubleshooting equipment problems, delivering and picking up work, and general bookkeeping and billing. Simply stated, YOU will be the business!

Until the advent of the computer, very few medical transcriptionists enjoyed the option of working independently. Technology, however, has opened new doors for medical transcription entrepreneurs.

Businesses are outsourcing everything these days. Contract employment has never seen such a boom as companies look to outside expertise to get the job done. After a decade of seeing the rise and fall of many large medical transcription services, the health care industry is discovering what independent transcriptionists have always known — that small is better. Small is more flexible, small is closer to the customer, small means quality, small means speed and SMALL IS SMART.

Independent medical transcription services are establishing their own niche in the medical transcription industry, each focusing on a microslice of the market, which enables them to provide maximum service to their clients. These smaller, livelier companies are creating significant pressure in a once large-service-dominated industry and the competitive battles are shifting. As information technology gets better, independent services are finding it easier to provide excellent service and compete with large services.

Global telecommunication has reached the medical transcription industry and is redefining the meaning of "BIG." According to Link Resources of New York, there are 9.5 million telecommuters using technology at home. It just keeps getting "smaller" out there. With a PC, FAX, desktop publishing, and data base management software one person can do the job it took several people to do fifteen years ago. If you add telecommunication to this, an independent entrepreneur can do things that used to require a huge organization.

The key words here are *responsiveness*, *flexibility* and *independence*. Independent services are enormously successful in today's competitive marketplace because 1) they thoroughly understand every aspect of their business and its position in the marketplace, and 2) they understand the need for, and are willing to make, immediate business transitions to provide continuing excellent service and to remain competitive. Indeed, independent services eagerly anticipate opportunities for positive change, and because of their small size, often have a distinct advantage over large, monolithic businesses.

Successful independents know there is always room for improvement and take personal responsibility for bringing about that improvement. They don't depend on or wait for directives from industry "experts," who are often out of touch with independent career variables, are content with the status quo or are slow to react to market issues. Independents waste no time. They read, study, and evaluate facts and alternatives and, based on their unique business situation and location, make sound decisions that move their business forward. They control their destiny. They take the risks and they get the rewards.

Before walking across the threshold of entrepreneurial independence, commit yourself to excellence and develop your potential. Obtain an appropriate education and practice your skills. At the end of that time, evaluate your skill level, and if you feel you are ready for the challenging world of self-employment, by all means, proceed.

This book was designed to be an informative and helpful guide, taking you step-by-step through the complicated maze of establishing yourself as an independent medical transcriptionist. Success and respect await those with excellent skills, diligence, integrity, and a passion for their profession. May success be yours!

TESTING THE WATERS

Evaluate your lifestyle and your goals for the future. How far do you want to go, and how big do you want to become? Will it be feasible for you to be self-employed? Are you doing it for the income, because you want to be your own boss, to be independent, have flexible working time, work at home, or other reasons?

If you are not completely sure of the answers, you may want to "test the waters" before plunging completely into self-employment.

> *"Before walking across the threshold of entrepreneurial independence, commit yourself to excellence and develop your potential."*

CONSIDER MOONLIGHTING

Moonlighting has launched many businesses and may be the ideal way for you to try out a new career path. Assuming that you are employed, we advise you to **hang onto that job while determining whether you want to be independent**. Regular salary checks can alleviate that sink-or-swim feeling while you experience the real world of independence, allowing your business to develop while you continue to feed the family.

It is possible, of course, to earn a fine wage if you are an industrious individual and a high-volume producer, but few entrepreneurs start out at such a comfort level. And if you discover that you are a low volume producer — which may occur for a variety of personal and professional reasons — you may decide that self-employment will not be suitable for you.

WORKING FOR A SERVICE

Another alternative to consider is working for a transcription service that uses the talents of home-based medical transcriptionists. A transcription service will give you greater flexibility, allowing you to decide how much work you wish to take each day.

Transcription work can be mailed, picked up and delivered by hand or transmitted via modem. Larger services often provide pickup and delivery to home-based transcriptionists unless they are using a digital dictation system. In that case, the finished product is modemed to either the service or the institution where the work originated. If you work for a smaller service, however, you will probably have to pick up and deliver the work to the service yourself. Services generally provide necessary formats, physician lists and stationery. The independent transcriptionist provides the labor.

Working for a service of any size is a great learning experience. You will see how a service functions, giving you an edge over less experienced persons just entering the field of medical transcription. Some services utilize their own dictation equipment and have 800 numbers that make it convenient for medical transcriptionists to call in and download dictation. Most services use state-of-the-art technology so you may be required to have a high-tech computer setup to interact with their systems.

PRODUCTIVITY PAYS

Independents are generally paid by production, and a low-volume producer may not be as successful as an independent. For instance, if a transcriptionist earns more working at an hourly rate for an employer than she earns by the line, character count, etc., as an independent, she is probably a low-volume producer and may not succeed self-employed.

In addition to covering living expenses, the self-employed independent must also cover business expenses such as office equipment, supplies, insurance, twice the amount of FICA an employer would withhold, and allow for health, accident and other benefits normally provided by an employer. Self-employment may not be practical unless there is another stable income to fall back on.

HOURS IN YOUR WORK WEEK

Successful self-employed transcriptionists are those who are aware of and prepare for the more difficult side of independence. The profession is not all fun and games, and not everyone is suited to the challenge. Individuals must examine their goals, skills, schedule, and lifestyle carefully to determine whether or not they are likely candidates for an independent transcriptionist career.

Will your working commitment be a part-time venture, two, four, or six hours a day, a few days a week, or are you planning to do this full-time, perhaps at least 40 hours per week? This may be difficult to judge at first, if you are completely new at freelancing.

Much depends on knowing your own transcription production limits by hour, line, character, minute, tape, etc. There are many variables. To plan ahead and make accurate projections, it is important to know your professional capabilities. As your service grows and your management responsibilities increase, these will be very important revenue production factors.

DETERMINING YOUR PRODUCTION CAPABILITIES

If you are not sure of your production capabilities, begin slowly with a few hours and gradually increase as you become comfortable with your output. This may take a few weeks or months depending on the type of accounts you assume.

Generally, production can be determined on minutes of dictation and lines transcribed. With new equipment technology on the market today, it is quick and easy to monitor production rates accurately and you should do this on a regular basis.

RATE OF PRODUCTION FORMULAS

There are several simple formulas for determining the rate of production: Minutes of dictation, lines transcribed, hours worked.

Minutes of dictation divided by hours worked = minutes transcribed per hour, divided by total hours = lines transcribed per hour. In monetary terms, charging by the line, lines transcribed x $ per line = $ earned, by hour, and by job (total lines). This is a simple formula for determining production by minutes, lines, and of course, dollars earned.

If you are choosing physician office dictation, it may take more than one account to reach a volume that is comfortable for you. If, on the other hand, there are three physicians in the practice, the volume from that single office may be sufficient. To be on the safe side, work with new accounts, determining average time commitment and volume (which generally increases in a positive working relationship) before soliciting more transcription clients.

Over the last six years since the first edition of this book was released, we have answered many questions about medical transcription. One question frequently asked has been: "How can I net $40,000 per year in my business?"

The good news is that it is possible to net that amount; the bad news for new people entering the field is that in order to do so you will probably have to work anywhere from 17-31 hours per day!

If you intend to **net** $40,000 per year, you must first **gross** approximately $80,000 per year. In other words, your revenue received from billing your services should be $80,000 if you want to end up with $40,000 net income from your business. You determine taxable income by subtracting your business expenses ("tax deductions") from your revenue. (See example on pages 353-355.)

The following table demonstrates what it takes to achieve about $80,000 per year in billings according to lines transcribed per day, line rate charged, and working five days a week.

LINE RATE BILLED	LINES BILLED PER DAY	GROSS YEARLY BILLINGS
10 cents	3100	$80,600
12 cents	2550	$79,560
13 cents	2350	$79,430
14 cents	2200	$80,080
15 cents	2050	$79,950
16 cents	1900	$79,040
17 cents	1800	$79,560
18 cents	1700	$79,560

The following three tables show you how many billable hours you need to work per day at various billing rates in order to achieve your $80,000 annual billings goal if your typing speed is 200, 300, or 400 lines per hour.

200 LINES/HOUR	LINE RATE
15.5 hrs/day	10 cents
12.75 hrs/day	12 cents
11.75 hrs/day	13 cents
11 hrs/day	14 cents
10.25 hrs/day	15 cents
9.5 hrs/day	16 cents
9 hrs/day	17 cents
8.5 hrs/day	18 cents

300 LINES/HOUR	LINE RATE
10.3 hrs/day	10 cents
8.5 hrs/day	12 cents
7.8 hrs/day	13 cents
7.3 hrs/day	14 cents
6.8 hrs/day	15 cents
6.3 hrs/day	16 cents
6 hrs/day	17 cents
5.6 hrs/day	18 cents

400 LINES/HOUR	LINE RATE
7.75 hrs/day	10 cents
6.3 hrs/day	12 cents
5.8 hrs/day	13 cents
5.5 hrs/day	14 cents
5.1 hrs/day	15 cents
4.7 hrs/day	16 cents
4.5 hrs/day	17 cents
4.2 hrs/day	18 cents

NOTE

If your billing is based on character count instead of gross line count, you should reduce the above tables by 10% to 15%.

Most experienced medical transcriptionists using the latest computer technology including macro abbreviation programs can average between 300-400 lines per hour or higher, depending on the type of dictation. As stated earlier, if you are new to the field and only typing 100 lines per hour, your expectations must be scaled down realistically.

Also take into account that the above formula is just for hours transcribed, not for the one to two additional hours per day (unless your work is modemed) you will spend printing, logging and delivering the work. Those extra hours must also be factored into your work day, billable hours available, and billing line rate chosen.

Medical Transcription Education

*"Education is a private matter between the person
and the world of knowledge and experience,
and has little to do with school or college."*

— Lillian Smith

Do you know what skills and training are necessary to be a competent and successful medical transcriptionist? Are your education and skills sufficient for professional success? Affirmative answers to these questions are essential. Solid educational preparation is the basic foundation underlying every successful transcriptionist's career.

I know several medical transcriptionists who have learned transcription through extensive training in independent study or community college classes and a couple of years hospital internship. After only four or five years, they are making almost as much as I do after twenty-five years as a medical transcriptionist. I should point out, however, that I learned on the job and took college courses in my spare time over the years, boot-strapping my way up.

A bright, industrious student can make it big in medical transcription work — with hospital training, after extensive book learning and transcription of **authentic** physician dictated reports. However, this takes a tremendous amount of effort and does not happen with a six-week-crash-course.

Generally speaking, you will not find training programs within the work setting today. In our modern health care era, hospitals, clinics, and most doctors' offices do not have the time nor the personnel necessary to educate inexperienced trainees in the complexities of medical transcription. Transcriptionists must seek basic training elsewhere.

AAMT'S COMPRO

To better evaluate your medical transcription qualifications, the American Association for Medical Transcription offers a competency profile, COMPRO, which lists competencies necessary for medical transcription professionals.

BEYOND THE BASICS

To build a more solid foundation for working in the medical transcription field, we recommend including a college level anatomy and/or physiology course.

An extensive medical terminology class (more than eight weeks) is essential. There is an excellent study guide for medical terminology published by W.B. Saunders, *The Language of Medicine*, by Davi-Ellen Chabner, B.A., M.A.T. This guide is particularly helpful when used in conjunction with a medical terminology class or simply as an independent study guide. Audio tapes are also available, with Davi-Ellen pronouncing the medical terms. If the guide is used without the audio tapes, you will lose the advantage of learning the correct pronunciation of each medical term, which is crucial in transcribing medical reports.

JUNIOR COLLEGE COURSES

If your education consists of one eight-week medical transcription course at the local junior college, you probably need more education. Although junior college medical transcription courses can be helpful, usually offering general information about transcription equipment, as well as some medical terminology, they are often limited in scope and do not provide adequate medical transcription training. Frequently, such classes are designed for medical assisting students, not medical transcriptionists.

In one college we evaluated, the dictation courses employed dictators whose diction was perfect. They also used perfect sentence structure, indicated correct placement of all punctuation marks, and spelled all uncommon words. Let us assure you that this is not the real world of medical transcription!

FOR-PROFIT TRANSCRIPTION SCHOOLS

We are not opposed to for-profit schools that provide what they promise, but we have no patience with those that do not. Beware of these! In recent years, a number of ethically questionable medical transcription schools have sprung up. Like fast food restaurants, they promise to instantaneously satisfy the appetites of career-hungry people.

These schools extol the virtues of their training programs and ensure unsuspecting and eager students that in just eight to sixteen weeks they will be able to work as home-based transcriptionists, earning generous incomes. When that rosy scenario does not occur, few students are confident enough to protest.

The tuition for such schools is usually high, ranging from $2000-$7000. Some schools offer government sponsored student loans, which are paid directly to the school. Students must repay these loans.

> "I cna tpye 200 wrods per mniute! oHw fsat cna ouy tpy?e"

HOME STUDY COURSES

The end of the 1980s found us in a time of self-discovery and suffering from the I-want-it-now-syndrome. Schools sprang up offering to teach medical transcription in a short three to six month home-study program. These schools marketed themselves aggressively, even advertising in *TV Guide* and *The Enquirer*. (You know the old saying, "If it's in *The Enquirer*, it has to be true.") The ads claimed that after completing their course, one could earn the grandiose salary of $35,000 a year. One school promised free job placement at the end of training, which consisted of nothing more than a two-year-old list of physicians.

Before selecting a transcription training program, make sure it is accredited. Ask other transcriptionists for their thoughts and advice when choosing a program. Remember, "If it looks too good to be true, it probably is."

SUM Program — Training like that provided by the SUM Program for Medical Transcription Training offered by Health Professions Institute is a very good educational reference that can be used in a course setting or as independent study material. The course utilizes actual physician dictation and was developed by certified medical transcriptionists.

As a medical transcriptionist, you will be required to produce quality work. However, this will be impossible if you have not had a solid medical transcription education.

When evaluating education programs for quality, be sure to cover all the bases. Ask to see the course syllabus, which will give you the description, objectives and intended outcome of the course. Ask to see what subjects are taught and what textbooks are provided or are needed. Are textbooks well-written and thorough? How many are there? Is authentic physician dictation provided?

The course should include, but not be limited to, the following:

- anatomy & physiology

- computer training

- grammar, punctuation, editing and proofreading skills

- basic medical principles: laboratory values & procedures, drugs/pharmacology

- professionalism, ethics and medicolegal issues

- disease processes

- specialty courses

- transcription equipment

- reference books

- medical transcription practice

- externship/available networks

Ask about the teaching staff. What are their credentials, and what type of technical support can a student rely upon?

How long is the course? Is the course accredited? Is there college credit or a certificate-of-completion awarded?

Medical transcription is not easy, and to be a successful medical transcriptionist, your education must be thorough and well-rounded. You will also have to work hard to develop the skills necessary in this highly skilled profession. All of this takes time, so don't expect to learn the basics and develop your skills overnight.

LESSONS AFTER SCHOOL

If you are ambitious and have recently completed a qualified course in medical transcription, you may have a burning desire to work as an independent transcriptionist.

With little or no experience as a transcriptionist, it will probably be difficult to break into the transcription field. However, there are several steps that may help you achieve your goal.

- Join the American Association for Medical Transcription (AAMT). Student membership category (available to nonemployed students enrolled in medical transcription courses at accredited schools) is a nominal fee. Fees for working transcriptionists are somewhat higher.

  AAMT membership provides you with excellent resource material, newsletters, meeting, seminar and convention information that you can use for networking with other transcriptionists and industry supporters. In addition, AAMT has local chapters that offer student membership.

- Find a mentor from the above sources. You will find this a valuable resource for information about techniques, skills, and trends in transcription practices.

- Review reference materials promoted in AAMT publications and other sources. Mentors are generally eager to share information and advise you regarding resource materials.

- Pursue continuing education through medical lectures, transcription practices seminars, and other related sources.

If you show your eagerness to listen and learn, you will find others willing to help and provide the information and support you seek.

MEDICAL TRANSCRIPTION STUDENT NETWORK

Health Professions Institute has formed the Medical Transcription Student Network (MTSN). This medical transcription network is open to all students in classroom study, home study or in self-directed programs. For $25 per year, the student receives a one-year subscription to *Perspectives on the Medical Transcription Profession* magazine, 10% discount on all books from HPI and Williams and Wilkins. For more information contact HPI.

- **Health Professions Institute (HPI)**
  209-551-2112

CERTIFICATION OF HEALTH PROFESSIONALS

The certification of health professionals is the recognition by a governmental or professional association that an individual's expertise meets the standards of that group. The standards established by professional associations generally exceed those required by government agencies. Some professional groups establish their own minimum standards for certification in those professions that are not licensed by a particular state. Certification by an association or group is a self-regulation credentialing process.

The Medical Transcription Certification Program (MTCP) is a nationally recognized, voluntary recertification program for medical transcriptionists, designed "to promote professional standards and improve the practice of medical transcription by giving special recognition to those professionals who demonstrate requisite knowledge, expertise, and performance through successful completion of the exam and who maintain certification through the fulfillment of stated requirements." According to the MTCP *Cert Alert*, there are more than 3000 medical transcriptionists certified.

Many dedicated and experienced medical transcriptionists seek this personal achievement. The certification examination consists of two parts, which are given separately.

Part I — The Written Exam — The written exam consists of 120 multiple-choice questions covering:

- medical terminology

- English language usage

- anatomy and physiology

- disease processes

- health care record

- professional development

Part II — The Practical Exam — Candidates must pass the written exam to be eligible for the practical exam. The practical exam requires transcription of original physician dictation in a wide variety of specialty areas and report types. Candidates who successfully pass the certification exam may then place the initials CMT (Certified Medical Transcriptionist) after their names.

To request information about the certification program contact MTCP.

- **MTCP**
  209-551-0833
  Fax: 209-551-1722

MAINTAINING CERTIFICATION

After becoming certified, a transcriptionist must acquire continuing education credits to maintain certification, which is standard procedure in credentialed professions. Read the continuing education guidelines that accompany your certification information to learn about creditworthy activities that will allow you to receive continuing education credits (CECs). Keep track of your CECs on an ongoing basis and pay close attention to paperwork and any updates on information regarding recertification guidelines.

Currently, to maintain certification, the transcriptionist must pay an administration fee of $20 per year. Recertification cycles are three years, and in a three-year period, the CMT must accumulate 30 CEC credits.

OTHER CERTIFICATION EXAMINATIONS

There are two other associations that offer certification examinations for medical transcriptionists:

- **American Association of Medical Assistants, Inc. (AAMA)** offers certification as a medical assistant (CMA), administrative (CMA-A), or clinical (CMA-C).

- **American Medical Technologists (AMT)** organization awards the Registered Medical Assistant (RMA).

For more information, contact AAMT, AAMA and AMT.

- **American Association for Medical Transcription (AAMT)**
  P.O. Box 57617
  Modesto, CA 95357-6187

- **American Association of Medical Assistants, Inc.**
  20 North Wacker Street, Suite 1575
  Chicago, IL 60606

- **Registered Medical Assistants of AMT**
  710 Higgins Road
  Park Ridge, IL 60068

NOTE

A medical transcriptionist does not have to belong to a professional organization to become certified or to maintain certification status. However, professional organizations can provide many opportunities and resources that will aid the transcriptionist in maintaining continuing education credits (CECs) for ongoing certification.

Building a Successful Home-based Business

"Confidence is an important part of any business venture.
If you don't think you can, you won't."

—Beatrice Gage

According to many leading journals and business magazines, the number of home-based businesses is growing and will continue to increase during the 1990s and beyond. This trend is occurring for a variety of reasons. Two significant factors are 1) the accelerating movement within this country toward a service-based economy and 2) the rapidly advancing technology that is continually creating new home-based career opportunities.

In the medical transcription profession, working at home has been an option for many years. Today, business consultants list home-based transcription as one of the top entrepreneurial career opportunities in the nation. That's good news for those with excellent medical transcription skills.

The Small Business Administration predicts that women will own half of all small businesses in the United States by the year 2000. Unfortunately, many of those businesses will not be successful. Statistics show that of all new businesses launched, 13% will fail within the first year. Why?

Businesses ultimately fail for many different reasons, but the basic element found in most failures is a significant lack of preparation prior to business start-up. The successful entrepreneur knows not only the skills of trade but the basics of business management, too.

Those who are not prepared establish businesses without a business plan and adequate analysis of their market. When they actually face the realities of a competitive marketplace, they are unable to resolve the multiplicity of unanticipated problems confronting them. Many fall by the wayside almost immediately, a few hang on for a time before giving up, and a minute number survive. But most unplanned businesses fail sooner or later.

Business success cannot be guaranteed. Even with preparation, and under the best circumstances, business is a day-to-day challenge. The road to independence is full of sharp curves, detours and potholes, but if you prepare yourself realistically for the future, you increase your chances of succeeding.

BEFORE GOING SOLO

Before embarking on a freelance career, ask yourself the following questions:

- Can I earn an adequate income freelancing?

- Am I capable of managing my own business?

- Will I be working at what I like best?

- Am I willing to take on additional responsibilities, including other essential, but less glamorous, tasks such as sales, accounting and paper work?

If the answer to all of the above is "yes," then ask yourself these questions:

1. Am I ready to make a COMMITMENT?

2. Am I SELF-DISCIPLINED?

3. Do I have enough EXPERIENCE?

FACING INDEPENDENT REALITY

In the early stages of your home-based career, be prepared to sacrifice much in order to give your business your all. Expect to do without a high quality personal life, free time, socializing with family and friends, and evenings out. This period of self-sacrifice won't last forever, it will be worth the effort, and it is actually not so bad if you are prepared for it.

Anticipate initial long days that do not end after eight hours. For a time, every day may seem like a Monday. You won't be able to call in sick and vacations will be out of the question.

You will discover that building your new business requires days and/or nights filled with mundane organizational tasks and responsibilities. And you will face daily distractions that interrupt your work schedule — nonbusiness telephone calls, salesmen, and friendly neighbors.

We know from experience that it takes drive and stamina to survive this period. Some transcriptionists find the pressure too great and decide that being independent is not their cup of tea. It takes a great deal of fortitude and self-discipline to follow through on commitments, especially when you are unsupervised. It may sound like fun to be your own boss, but without adequate self-discipline, it is very tempting to "kick back," put off the work, and miss deadlines.

You can do what you want! You will not punch a time-clock or have a time-conscious supervisor peering over your shoulder. You will decide your priorities and establish your work schedule. And it will be you, and you alone, who will determine your success or failure.

ESTABLISHING PRIORITIES

Do you have your priorities straight? Are you able to set up a work schedule for yourself and not deviate? You may find it tempting to put off working until the last minute, thereby jeopardizing your delivery and pickup times.

Schedule a specific set of hours in which you do nothing but work. Prioritize your time and have a set schedule or block of hours in which to transcribe.

THE EMPLOYER MENTALITY

It is imperative to step away from the employee mentality and get into the employer mentality. Remember that you are the owner of this business, therefore the boss, and that you must provide yourself with all the things that you have come to expect from an employer, i.e., health insurance, disability insurance, retirement benefits, sick days, vacation days, a five-day work week, setting up an accounting system, and paying estimated taxes.

MANAGING FAMILY LIFE

Being your own boss and working out of your home offers wonderful flexibility for home and community activities. Being home-based, you can spend more time with family and attend school and after-school functions with your children, participating more fully in their lives. It does take planning, however, to find the ideal balance between family and profession.

It is nearly impossible to maintain a set work schedule with children racing through the house, demanding attention, arguing over television programs, dancing to the boom box, answering doors or phones, and generally just being children! To eliminate this type of stress, it is imperative that you reduce noise, avoid interruptions, provide adequate child care, and maintain good communication with family members, particularly children.

It is essential to establish rules in the beginning. Ask your spouse to respect your work schedule by avoiding unnecessary telephone calls during your work hours, especially if the questions are, "What's for dinner?" or "Did you pick up my clothes at the dry cleaners?"

CHILD CARE

The most difficult issue to deal with is child care. After all, if you choose to work at home in order to be near your children, what have you accomplished if you send them away to be taken care of?

If your children are preschoolers or young enough to require supervision after school, you may be faced with hiring at least part-time care for them. You may choose to have that childcare in your home or outside your home, depending on family members' personalities and your work setup. Either way, you will still be able to spend more time with your children.

Some home-based professionals find it convenient and satisfying to work in one part of the house while the children are cared for in another part of the house. This offers more parent/child contact during breaks and lunch and provides flexibility to answer your caregiver's questions and respond to emergencies.

If your children are at school full-time during the day, it isn't difficult to work around their schedule, hiring someone to come in for a few hours after school, if necessary.

Whether the children are in-house or out, the home-based professional can readily leave her office and adjust work hours to accommodate family and personal priorities.

FAMILY COMMUNICATION

Communication with your family is crucial, especially when the business is located in the home and is a new experience for everyone. Suddenly, household rules have changed. Certain rooms are off-limits. Mother (or Dad) is home but not home. The new regimen can be frustrating for all concerned.

Give your children as much information as possible about when and where you will be working, when you will and won't be available, who will be available when you can't be, and exactly what is expected of them. This will help to allay many fears and questions they may have.

Without the cooperation and support of the family, home-based self-employment is impossible. It takes family team work, and even then, it will be challenging in the beginning. By working together, your family members will soon wonder how you ever lived and worked any other way.

Marketing

"No one can arrive from being talented alone.
God gives talent, work transforms
talent into genius."

—Anna Pavlova

You have made the decision to freelance, and are moving ahead. You have studied hard, learned medical terminology, and honed your keyboarding skills. Now you must have a plan. Work is not likely to simply fall into your lap. You will have to go after it. You can work, you want work, but how do you go about getting it?

MARKET AND COMPETITION ANALYSIS

One of the first steps you should take is to do a market and competition analysis, which is not necessarily complex. In fact, it is essentially logical. It can be as simple as one, two three.

1. Research adequate facts/information

2. Organize and study the facts

3. Develop a business plan

INNOVATIVE MARKETING — YOUR BLUEPRINT FOR SUCCESS

Resources state that 80% of new businesses that fail do so because they do not have enough clients. Determining the probability of success for your medical transcribing service, which will really determine the probability of success for the business, takes planning. Planning is the root for developing a successful business. Granted, many businesses succeed without planning; however, most businesses that do not plan do not succeed. Planning for business success is very much like planning for your vacation. In order to make sure that you can find your vacation destination, a map is secured and followed. The business plan is a tool to map your path towards success. There are various components of a business plan, however. Here we will focus on innovative and inexpensive ways of marketing your service. Within each business plan, there should be a marketing plan.

THE MARKETING PLAN

The marketing plan should take care of many aspects within the business plan. It should concern itself with the following:

• Who are the potential clients in my market?

• How many potential clients are in my market?

• What are the needs of those potential clients?

• How well will my product or service meet clients' needs?

• What is the price of my product or service?

• How will my service be delivered to clients?

• Who are my competitors and what benefits do they offer?

• What promotional vehicles will I use to promote services to potential clients?

By organizing the information listed above and committing to it on paper, a business can get a much clearer perspective regarding a service's potential for success.

Your market research should clearly answer the following questions:

• Who will buy my services?

• Why will they buy it?

• What do I need to charge to ensure a healthy profit?

• What services will mine be competing with?

• Am I positioning a service correctly? In other words, if there is much competition, you might want to look for a specialized market niche.

• What government regulations will my service be subject to?

Once your analysis shows that the service has a good probability for success, the promotional program is set into motion. Deciding where best to commit your advertising dollars will be determined in large part by who your clients will be.

BUSINESS PROMOTION AND ADVERTISING

By looking at the list of potential clients, you will discover logical groupings. Those groupings will determine how you will advertise and promote your services. For instance, if potential clients belong to associations and read professional journals, it might be beneficial to advertise your business there. Or if clients will be actively shopping for your services, perhaps a yellow-page ad will be best. Only by writing down who your clients might be, can you get a handle on what might work best for promotion.

> "Within each business plan, there should be a marketing plan."

PRICING

Pricing is an item that seems simple but can be the most complex issue of all. Small-business owners too often overlook factors that are essential in determining their total costs accurately. Most everything that you do to bring your services to market involve some cost. The cost for your equipment, utilities, insurance premiums, gas in your car, advertising and the time spent picking up tapes are all costs related to conducting business. Unless you enjoy giving money away in the form of those cost items, you should include those items in the price of your services.

Now that you have determined your target market, found the best promotional strategy to reach it and the distribution channels for getting to it, you need to make the sale.

SELLING YOUR SERVICES

Sales are rarely made without some type of human contact. Services do not sell themselves; people sell them. As a small business owner, be prepared to be your lead salesperson. To be a successful salesperson, it is necessary to be client-focused. To be client-focused, the clients' needs will become your needs. When clients can see that you have solutions that meet or exceed their needs, you have the opportunity for sales. By becoming a partner in satisfying your clients' requirements, you are well on the way to success.

Other factors in making the sale include price, delivery schedule, etc., but those details can usually be ironed out later. By assessing the needs of your client and being actively involved in satisfying those needs, you can develop the type of trust that is necessary to do business today.

Clients are becoming more concerned with value than with price. If your services are exactly like your competitor's services, then price, obviously, is extremely important. However, if you can distinguish your services from your competitor's, then it is up to you to sell the value of what you have to offer. Be creative in analyzing your services, and be prepared to offer what others do not. In short, develop a competitive advantage over your competitors. By having a competitive advantage, price will not be the central issue.

SIX SUGGESTIONS FOR SUCCESS

Here are some suggestions for doing business in the '90s:

1. Focus on a smaller market

For every trend, there is at least one countertrend. It is sometimes better to focus on a smaller market — one nobody is serving because they are all catering to a bigger trend.

If you are setting up a one-person medical transcription service, don't go after the large hospital accounts or even large clinic accounts. Let the bigger companies compete for those markets. Target local physicians and smaller clinics (four doctors or less).

Ancillary departments in hospitals are an excellent resource for the smaller business. Most hospitals have emergency rooms, cardiac catheterization laboratories, gastroenterology labs, radiology and pathology departments, which are excellent sources of income for the smaller business, since most of that work is now being outsourced.

2. Beware of the negative

Make sure you deal with all your clients in good faith and with integrity. Negative word-of-mouth, especially on computer bulletin boards and systems like the Internet, can cripple your business even more than positive public relations can help. Remember, physicians talk to one another. If a physician is pleased with your service, word-of-mouth referrals will follow.

3. Be ready for change

Medical transcription technology changes on a monthly basis. Be adaptable. If your client wants a faster turnaround time than your competitors, consider installing a modem and sending all completed work back to the client's office to be printed. You might even consider buying a call-in-line system for faster turnaround times. Always think ahead and research business methods that will save you and your client time and money.

4. Get on the ball.

Be ready to be *where* your client wants you, *when* your client wants you, with *what* your client wants. Just-in-time marketing is critical as people become spoiled by 24-hour, seven-day-a-week customized products and services. Of course, you must set boundaries with accounts at the beginning of your relationship or some may treat you like a doormat. Under all circumstances, keep the lines of communication open at all times. Always listen carefully to what clients have to say, evaluate their comments and, if appropriate, do your best to meet their needs.

5. Keep your clients.

Keeping clients is far more cost effective than finding new ones. Focus on relationships with existing clients and be creative in finding ways to keep them. Every client should be given a questionnaire to complete each year — something on the order of a report card — to measure your relationship with that client and his or her satisfaction with your service. Always ask for and encourage client input. If a client leaves, do as much research to find out why as you do to seek out new markets.

6. Project a big image.

It doesn't cost anything to aim high. Think of yourself as owning a "macro" not a "micro" business. Remember, most home-based businesses are relatively small operations — but the smart ones don't advertise it.

Look around you, listen to other business people, analyze business advertising — newspapers, magazines, newsletters, television, signs — and become aware of all the marketing techniques you are subject to as you go about your day. Most of this advertising has been produced by top professionals. Try to build on these ideas and apply them to your business in ways that fit what you are selling. There are no new ideas under the sun, just different ways to use them.

You may find creative marketing a challenge at first. Although being innovative isn't difficult, trying new ideas isn't easy either. Don't be discouraged. With a little practice, you'll soon get a feel for it.

MONEY-SAVING MARKETING IDEAS

If you are on a budget, as most of us were when starting our businesses, here are some very inexpensive ways to market your service.

1 . Develop a 30-second commercial

It is very important to market yourself at every opportunity. The best tool for this is a rehearsed 30-second commercial about yourself and your business. State your name, the name of your business, where it is located, what type of business it is, how long you have been in business and your specialties. End your commercial by handing that person your business card. If you catch someone's interest, you will have time to expand their understanding and may even gain a new client or a referral.

2. Become an expert

Television and radio programs, especially local shows, are always looking for programming. Many business organizations are looking for speakers for meetings. Become an expert who is available and agree to appear without charge. Become such an interesting, informative guest that word begins to spread about your speaking abilities and the great information you have to share. Schedule at least one appearance monthly. The medical transcription home-business industry is growing by leaps and bounds. Who better to be an expert than you?

3. Get your business mentioned in the media

Develop both a press kit containing interesting and pertinent information about you and your business and a media list (a list of all newspapers, radio and TV stations, and publications in your community) of those sources that communicate with and reflect the demographics of the group you believe will buy your services. Using a newsworthy "hook" (an interesting and attractive idea), write your own one page press release. Distribute the release to the media list you have developed. Within one week, contact every source on your list and sell them on running your story. The best part, it won't cost you a dime.

4. Advertise in newsletters

Many associations publish newsletters which are mailed directly to members at their cost. These newsletters may target individuals or groups that you really want to reach. Often they sell ads at minimal rates. Identify the newsletters you want to reach and send a press release, flier or advertisement to the membership. Also, think about advertising in your local medical association newsletter. Every county has a medical association and most will take advertising. These newsletters are sent to every doctor in your county who is a member.

5. Network, network, network

Networking is more than just going to special business events to specifically market your business. Networking is a way of life.

Every day, everywhere, every person you meet socially, professionally or athletically is a part of your network. You should always sell yourself and your business. Remain open to going to new places and meeting new people. You never know where that next contact will lead.

Contact the medical staff secretary at your local hospitals to see about possible referrals. These people are the first contacts that new doctors make when moving to a new community and setting up practice.

6. Have a positive, professional attitude

Treat people with respect. Be honest. Be consistent. Be credible. Be nice. Great service is never forgotten.

ESTABLISHING A BUSINESS PLAN

As stated earlier, numerous businesses fail within the first year because of poor planning. Ask any successful business owner, and he or she will tell you that the first step for assuring success is developing a business plan.

There are three main reasons for having a business plan.

- It helps you to visualize your business before it actually gets off the ground.

- It is required if you are seeking financial help from lenders or investors. They want to see that your business idea has been well researched and well thought out.

- You will be able to determine from the business plan if the business has a reasonable chance of succeeding.

Here are steps toward developing a business plan:

- Define your business mission and your business goals. What do you hope to accomplish? List your personal as well as your professional goals.

- Describe your anticipated market and client base. Indicate your fee structure and develop a marketing plan.

- Prepare revenue and expense projections on a monthly basis for two years. Determine how much profit you want from your business. Be realistic. Carefully evaluate whether your projected net income will satisfy your personal financial needs.

- Define your market and your competition. Demonstrate that you can generate enough work to produce your projected revenue.

- Indicate the legal form of your business. Is it going to be a sole proprietorship, a partnership or a corporation?

- Indicate how your home business will physically operate. Is your home or apartment large enough to accommodate living quarters and the business you are considering?

- List the assets required to operate your business and estimate their costs. Determine how much money will be needed to meet all start-up expenses, including your living expenses during the hungry, start-up phase. Refer to Budget Assumptions on the next page.

- Identify actual and potential funding sources for your business.

- Indicate if you will need additional personnel to get your business underway and as it grows. If so, identify potential personnel sources.

- Evaluate risks involved with the business and decide what measures you need to take to cope with these risks.

Using these steps, you should have a highly detailed statement as to why your business is being formed, what personal and monetary goals can be realistically achieved, and where and how it will operate.

If the plan looks good, then GET INTO ACTION. If it looks dismal, keep your full-time position and postpone your plans for a home-based medical transcription business for a year or two — or until the prospects for success can be improved.

It is very important to have a business plan. You should closely evaluate what type of income you are expecting to generate from your business and if you are being realistic in your income and expense expectations. In order to help you assess this, we have included a budget assumptions list for your use.

Estimate your monthly expenses by reviewing your actual expenses for the prior six months. After you have completed this form, you will have an excellent idea of how much money you will need to make every month in order to meet your obligations.

Since some of you are just starting your businesses and have not yet paid quarterly taxes, use the formula found in the finances section of this book to guesstimate what your taxes would be for the amount of income you expect to earn based on your plan.

BUDGET ASSUMPTIONS
FOR HOME-BASED BUSINESSES

CATEGORY	ASSUMPTION
Gross Income	_____
Advertising	_____
Automobile	_____
Bad Debts	_____
Business Gifts	_____

Business License   _____

Continuing Education   _____

Depreciation
- Office Space   _____
- Office Equipment   _____
- Car   _____

Insurance
- Health   _____
- Disability*   _____
- Life*   _____
- Liability   _____
- Equipment   _____

(*for corporations only)

Interest (business loans)   _____

Office Equipment   _____

Office Supplies   _____

Lease Payments   _____

Marketing Promotions
- Brochures   _____
- Mailing Lists, etc.   _____

Rent   _____

Repairs & Maintenance   _____

Payroll (employees)   _____

Subcontractors (Outsourcers)   _____

Subscription/Dues   _____

Taxes
- FICA   _____
- Federal Income   _____
- State Income   _____
- State Disability   _____
- Payroll Taxes   _____

Telephone   _____

Utilities   _____

In the appendix is an example of an effective budget worksheet from the book *Easy Financials for Your Home-based Business*, which can be photocopied for your use.

GETTING FACTS/ADEQUATE INFORMATION

- Total market and demand

- Competition

- Industry trends

- Your target market

Familiarize yourself with the resources in your area. If you have been established in an area for some time, this can be an advantage as you may already be familiar with the available market. On the other hand, if you are new to an area, there are various resources for obtaining market information.

YOUR TARGET MARKET

The medical transcription marketplace is broad. Determining **your** target market, zeroing in on the specific area for **you**, is important, and it isn't difficult to do.

Evaluating your background experience will help determine your target market. Are you a student of medical transcription who is considering self-employment upon completion of your education? An experienced, currently employed transcriptionist? Are you crossing over from a related profession or an unrelated profession? If so, you will discover that each of the above will have a different target market.

If you are new to the field of medical transcription, your target market will probably be limited. We recommend starting with one medical specialty, focusing on that specialty until you have developed a high level of skill and confidence. At that point, consider expanding your business.

```
┌─────────────────────────────────────────────┐
│                                             │
│                 WARNING                     │
│                                             │
│          Don't take on too much too soon.   │
│                                             │
└─────────────────────────────────────────────┘
```

Medical transcription is a challenge even for experienced professionals. If you are a novice transcriptionist, you will be wise to allow yourself time to develop additional skills, insights into your work style, and confidence. Spreading yourself too thin at the beginning of your career may result in unnecessary failure.

With adequate experience, your career future offers exciting opportunities and your business will grow. The more experience you have in medical transcription, the more diversified your service will become. Your service will be in demand by hospitals, medical clinics, physicians, and others within your market area.

Evaluate the overall transcription service need of the medical community in your area and then target a specific segment of that need. This is your target market.

You may decide to transcribe for hospitals and medical clinics, or limit your accounts to physicians' office records.

You may prefer to work as an independent, on-site/off-site, for a transcription service, home-based, or develop another option. There are various directions you can take, depending on your qualifications and experience.

Identifying the total market is the basic step. Make a list of what is available in your area.

DIRECTORIES

If you live in a large metropolitan area and decide to target hospital accounts, the best source for getting names and addresses of hospitals is *The Thomas Guide*, available in major book stores. In the back is a list of all hospitals within the county.

Another excellent tool is the yellow pages of your telephone directory. Not only are hospitals listed, but also physicians within the area you are targeting. Directory information includes addresses, phone numbers, and in larger institutions and clinics, departments. Physicians are listed alphabetically and by specialty. If you are marketing your service outside the area in which you live, review the telephone directories for every county and city on file at your local library.

Local medical societies also have directories. Call or write for a physician reference directory.

Classified "help wanted" ads provide additional information.

There is a directory called *The Little Blue Book*. This is a complete physician directory that includes pharmacies and related health professionals in 157 metropolitan areas. It lists physicians in alphabetical order, and includes their specialty, address and phone number. This publication, which costs $12.00, is a great marketing tool. To see if *The Little Blue Book* is available for your area, contact **InSight Media** at 1-800-345-6865.

PTD also offers advertising that is very inexpensive ($25 for a two-line listing).

As you network and become more familiar with your area, you will discover other directories that will be helpful in your marketing. Always be on the lookout for them.

ADVERTISING IN THE YELLOW PAGES

The Yellow Pages Publishers Association (YPPA) in Troy, Michigan reports that almost 60% of all adults use the Yellow Pages weekly. Eighty four percent read two or more ads, suggesting that users are not just looking up telephone numbers but are shoppers who can be influenced by the quality of the ad. For those of us on a budget, this is an excellent advertising alternative.

There are about 6000 Yellow Pages directories nationwide. Some areas are served only by one, but others have many. Los Angeles County has 28. Telephone companies publish the most widely used directories, but there are now many independent companies that publish directories, too. The cost of an ad in an independently published Yellow Pages directory is usually less expensive (often one-tenth as much!) as an ad in a phone company directory. However, an independent directory may not give you the exposure you are seeking.

A Yellow Pages sales rep will pressure you to place ads under several headings, i.e., Medical Secretarial Services, Medical Transcription Services, Secretarial Services, Word Processing. That may be a good investment, but be careful; many headings is usually a waste of money. The best way of finding the most productive heading is to look where the competition places its ads. If you see competitors under the same headings year after year, you should be there too. Remember, too, that these sales reps work on commission and may also pressure you to use color, have large ads or use other expensive options.

Consider using an outside agency or graphic artist. Yellow Pages advertising is different from conventional print, so if you decide to use someone other than a sales rep, use only a person with experience in this medium. You may even discover that you are the expert in designing your own ad.

Always track your ad responses or you will never know what works and what doesn't. Make sure you ask every caller how they learned about your service — from a friend, physician or hospital referral, one of your speaking engagements, an ad, etc. — and write down their responses. If they saw your ad, and if it is appearing in more than one directory, ask callers for the ad's page number, which will tell you what directory they are using. This way you will know exactly how many sales each directory or listing produces.

EVALUATE THE COMPETITION

It is important to research service demand in your area. Is there a need for additional transcription service or is the local market pretty well saturated?

For information regarding the industry, contact local employment agencies, employment development departments, personnel departments and other medical personnel service agencies, trade schools, and community colleges that offer courses in medical transcription.

Do not hesitate to make phone inquiries and check out the trends in your area. Review the yellow pages of the phone book for transcription services and talk to managers in clinic and hospital personnel departments to see if there is a need for medical transcriptionists.

When you have completed your investigation, carefully analyze the facts you have gathered and determine the potential market for your transcription services.

TRANSCRIPTIONIST NETWORKING

Communication and networking with other medical transcriptionists is beneficial in fact-gathering. Make a list of local transcription services and file information you obtain about self-employed transcriptionists in your area. If you are not already online, consider accessing the Internet. There are approximately 750-1000 MTs online networking via chat rooms or through newsgroups.

ORGANIZING A NETWORKING GROUP

If there is no medical transcription networking group in your area, consider organizing one. Kathryn Hunter-Dyer, CMT, in Orange County, California, organized Networking Entrepreneurs in Transcription (NET) and directs quarterly medical transcription networking meetings for service owners and independent contractors.

NET is an excellent forum for discussing and solving business problems, as well as for increasing communication and networking. The group is self-supporting. There are no dues but each participant is encouraged to make a donation to help cover the cost of printing and mailing business meeting fliers.

For further information about starting a similar group, contact **Kathryn Hunter-Dyer** at 714-965-3288.

COMPUTER ONLINE INTERACTIVE INFORMATION AND COMMUNICATION SERVICES

Networking is a key element in any successful business because the more people you connect with, the more business you will obtain through referrals. If you don't have access to a local networking group, consider joining one of the computer online services. To get started, all you need is a computer, a telephone line, a modem and a basic online service package. Many personal computers and modems are now being marketed with online services preinstalled. You can get a membership kit, which includes software for connecting to the service and often a usage credit, from the online service you have subscribed to. Kits cost about $30. Most of them have bulletin boards for every facet of business including medical transcription.

It's great fun talking with MTs all over the country. Heard a new word that you can't document or need a business question answered? No problem. Your question can be answered twenty-four hours a day on a bulletin board. Following is a list of bulletin boards currently available for a one-time subscription fee and monthly fees based on the amount of usage:

- **America Online Incorporated**
  8619 Westwood Center Drive
  Vienna, VA 22182-2285
  800-827-6364

- **CompuServe Information Service**
  5000 Arlington Centre Boulevard
  Columbus, OH 43220
  800-848-8199

- **GEnie**
  General Electric Information Services
  401 North Washington Street
  Rockville, MD 20850
  800-638-9636

- **Prodigy**
  Prodigy Services Company
  445 Hamilton Avenue
  White Plains, NY 10601
  800-PRODIGY

> *"Networking is a key element in any successful business because the more people you connect with, the more business you will obtain through referrals."*

GATHERING FACTS AT
THE CHAMBER OF COMMERCE

The local chamber of commerce is generally helpful in providing and recommending resources for businesses. Visit your chamber office to find out what is available.

Consider joining your local chamber of commerce, which offers many benefits to members: informative speakers; educational presentations; business tours; fact-filled seminars; fun-filled business open houses and parties; well-researched booklets, brochures, directories, and newsletters; information about state and national business trends; updates on relevant legal and tax issues; insurance programs; and other benefits specific to local chambers. Although some chamber programs and printed materials are available to the public, many are not, which gives chamber members an inside track in the race to business success.

Chamber of commerce membership dues vary from community to community so check with your local chamber office regarding its dues schedule. Most members find that business generated by referrals from the chamber office more than covers their annual chamber dues. In addition, dues are a tax-deductible business expense.

Chamber membership cannot substitute for your medical transcription association memberships, but it will build friendships beyond your medical transcription environment and broaden your knowledge of diverse businesses. To locate a chamber of commerce near you, contact your state's chamber of commerce office listed in the resources at the back of this book.

STAYING ABREAST OF MT NEWS
AND INDUSTRY TRENDS

If you are beginning your independent medical transcription career with little or no background information, spend some time researching the history of medical transcription, current trends, and what is forecast for the future.

If you are an active member of AAMT, you will receive the bimonthly *Journal of the American Association for Medical Transcription (JAAMT)*. Health Professions Institute publishes *Perspectives*. *MT Monthly*, a monthly newsletter by Computer Systems Management contains word lists, new medications, and a variety of articles pertaining to the medical transcription industry.

ROMANCING THE $$$

In the past few years, in order to reduce overhead, there has been an industry trend toward contract services. This is good news for independents because contracting offers increased opportunities for skilled transcriptionists working outside a hospital or medical office setting.

A few years ago large medical transcription services dominated the medical transcription industry. They made huge investments to be on the cutting edge of technology because they realized that health care facilities were finding it increasingly more difficult and less cost effective to maintain in-house transcription departments. With increasing volumes of dictation and lack of physical space to expand, many facilities were contracting part or all of their transcription work to outside services. In many cases, it was not a positive experience. Some services failed to meet commitments for turnaround and transcription quality was poor. In addition, they had their own staffing problems, legal difficulties and so on.

Now the industry is fragmenting, with frequently breaking news of mergers, acquisitions and takeovers. The home-based business movement is definitely changing the marketplace and the future of the medical transcription industry. As information and technology become more affordable to one-person businesses, we are providing the same services as the industry giants, often at a lower cost and with better quality.

Everyone is romancing the client and there is a niche in the marketplace for all. Independent contractors are not capable of servicing 2500 bed facilities, but they are more efficacious for smaller hospitals, physicians, clinics, and hospitals in rural settings. Large services are romancing their clients for total contracts — extended contracts to guarantee their investment in equipment and technology. Some are even offering to place the technology on-site.

Many hospitals are now shifting direction and, with the help of their financial departments, discovering that they can decrease costs while bringing work back "inside." As a result, many hospitals are not renewing contracts with larger services. "If a service can utilize home-based medical transcriptionists, why can't we?" they ask. The answer is, of course, they can! So they are placing their own employees at home or are using independent transcriptionists with excellent results.

Competition is fierce, but there is more than enough work and funding for all skilled transcriptionists. Health care regulators now allow the use of contract services to be included in health care providers' operating expenses. This is good news for independent medical transcriptionists because it means more work is coming our way!

DEFINING YOUR MARKET

Define your market. Do you want to work for hospitals, offices, multispecialty clinics, or a combination of all three? Will you mail, modem or personally transport transcription work? How far are you willing to travel to pick up and deliver work? Remember, depending on the priority of work types, hospital work turnaround times will vary from two-, four-, or six- to twenty-four hours. Offices and clinics are generally more flexible. Turnaround time will also vary, of course, depending on clients' needs. With technology now available through telecommuting, the trend is toward shorter turnaround times, so make sure that you evaluate this factor when defining your market.

YOUR CLIENT BASE

Another key factor in success is determining the number of clients needed to support your business. A good rule of thumb is to follow the old adage: *Do not put all your eggs in one basket.*

A hospital overload account is wonderful, but it can be a fickle market. For instance, the hospital census may decline or a new medical records director may decide to keep all work in-house or switch to a larger service. If you are dependent on that one hospital account, you may suddenly find yourself with no income.

A market mix is much better, perhaps one hospital and two or more small accounts comprised of doctors' offices or clinic transcription. In this way, if one account disappears or declines, you may still have a solid business base and adequate revenues.

ANCILLARY DEPARTMENTS

Another excellent market is hospital ancillary departments, which include specialties such as cardiology, gastroenterology, radiology, pathology, physical therapy, occupational therapy, and emergency rooms. In the past, these ancillary departments relied heavily on the hospital's main medical records department for transcription service, but that is changing.

Recently, there has been a trend toward separating ancillary department work from that of the medical records department, mainly because the primary hospital transcription pool is finding it increasingly difficult to keep up with inpatient work, let alone outpatient services.

MAILING LABELS

Another great marketing tool is mailing labels, which may be ordered from a wide variety of marketing consultant firms. One such firm is American Data Consultants, which sells 3000 mailing labels for approximately $200.

When ordering, specify market type and target area by zip codes. You will receive lists, on preprinted mailing labels, of hospitals and/or physicians, by specialty if you wish, for a particular area. Call for a free catalog.

- **American Data Consultants**
  800-634-2547

NEWSPAPERS

Local newspapers are another good resource. Hospitals, clinics, and physicians often advertise their services in space ads. Review classified "help wanted" ads for transcription positions, and don't overlook any opportunity. Even if the advertisement is for an in-house position, consider interviewing for it. You may convince the interviewer to work with you instead. Stress the advantages of an outside service over a full-time or part-time employee, including dollars saved on benefits packages, vacations, sick leave, and holidays. Tell the prospective client that studies have been done that show it costs an employer between 45-75 cents a line to hire an in-house employee. Hospitals, clinics and physicians almost always respond to new ways to cut operating expenses.

PERSONAL ADVERTISING

There are many ways to reach your market, including business brochures, cold calling, fliers, and letters. You can network in elevators, parking lots, hospitals, office buildings, emergency rooms, and by word of mouth (doctor to doctor). You can advertise in the Yellow Pages, local newspapers, trade newsletters and journals, as well as local county medical society newsletters for a very nominal fee. The Internet allows one great exposure. Many MTs are regularly tapping into resources by surfing the Net. Many MTs are even publishing their own Web pages.

THE BOTTOM LINE — OBTAINING CLIENTS

Medical transcription is a multibillion dollar industry and the competition, big or small, can be fierce. Read and learn EVERYTHING you can about marketing because if you are to succeed professionally, YOU MUST MARKET YOUR GOODS AND SERVICES. If you don't, your business will fail. Marketing should become second nature to you, and if it doesn't, seek help from someone skilled in marketing.

Be bold in promoting your transcription service. "Press the flesh" as often as you can. Tell everyone you ever knew or come into contact with that you are in business and would appreciate their business and/or referrals. Pass out your business cards and brochures as though your life depended on it ... and when they're gone, order more. Business cards do you no good unless someone sees them. Plaster your fliers on every bulletin board you can find.

Consider giving clients a packet containing information on charges, turnaround, delivery, stat work, availability of services beyond basic transcription, i.e., DTP, fax, phone-in or modem capabilities, samples of reports and references. The key word here is BENEFITS. Convince the client that the services you are providing are BENEFITS to them. The more BENEFITS you offer customers, the more work you're likely to get.

When approaching a potential client for the first time, present a personally addressed letter (not a form letter). Follow up with a phone call, and if there are no available openings, offer to fill in on an as-needed basis during employee vacations, holidays, or other absences.

When soliciting new business, some transcriptionists offer to transcribe a tape of dictation or a few reports at no charge to demonstrate the quality of their work. This can be effective because the client feels under no obligation to commit to using your service. HOWEVER, don't make the mistake one transcriptionist made. At the start of her career as an independent, she sent out a great little flier that offered *one week of free transcription*. She got takers — absolutely! They literally bombarded her with tapes of transcription. Unfortunately, she could not complete the work, and finally had to return some of the tapes. It was not a good beginning for her business.

Don't be overly generous to clients even though you are anxious to get your business started. Clients may take advantage of your free offer and then bid you farewell. A large transcription service once offered a month's free transcription to a large hospital, hoping to impress the medical facility with quality transcription produced in a 24-hour turnaround time, which would result in a substantial transcription contract. The hospital bombarded the service with work. The transcription service hired numerous IMTs to service the account, and everyone was happy because they were working. Well, when the thirty days ended, the hospital said thanks and good-by to the service, the service had no more work for the IMTs, and that was that.

This marketing tactic proved to be financially devastating for the service. It worked for 30 days free but still had to pay its IMTs and cover its overhead. The service could not pay its IMTs as agreed and everyone suffered from the trickle-down effect . . . except for the hospital, which came out smelling like a rose!

MARKETING YOUR SPECIALTY

If you have special knowledge in a certain area, that is the area you should promote. After all, that is where you "shine" and will "outshine" your competition.

BUSINESS CARDS

Do you have a business card? How effective is it? How do people react when you hand them your card? Do they just put your card in their pocket or do they give it a second glance? If the latter is true, you have probably made a positive impression according to Paul and Sarah Edwards, authors of "Your Card: A Marketing Tool," which appeared in *Home Office Computing Magazine*.

The Edwards, leading authorities on working from home, recommend reviewing the business cards in your Rolodex and selecting those that stand out. What attracts you to them? How does yours compare? An effective business card is far more than a piece of paper containing your name, address, and phone number. It is a marketing tool that can serve several purposes.

Think of your business card as a mini-billboard, a brochure, or an advertisement . . . even an order form.

- **Coordinate your business card, letterhead and stationery.**

  For continuity, use the same typeface and colors on all your print communications. The investment you make in designing a consistent visual image for your business will return to you in referrals.

  Select a readable typeface that is not complicated or ornate. A business card is small, so use no more than two typefaces. Create variety with sizing, boldface type, and spacing. Avoid printing with only capital letters, which makes your card less readable and detracts from a quality image. And don't crowd the card with type.

- **Make sure your card talks to your market.**

  What do potential clients expect from a business like yours? The creative and unusual? Quiet elegance and professionalism? Tried, true, and trusted? Design your card to meet the expectations of your target market.

  Avoid cartoon characters, cute creatures, and hearts and flowers. They're unlikely to convey your professional image.

- **Cover the basics.**

  Your business card should contain the name of your business, your name (if different from the business), title, and your phone number(s). Your business card will probably also display your address (optional) and logo. If you don't have a logo for your company, consider using the logo of your trade to enhance your credibility, i.e., a computer screen, dictating unit, or the medical caduceus.

NOTE

The logo for the American Association for Medical Transcription is the sole property of AAMT and therefore, cannot be used on stationery or business cards.

Make sure your phone number stands out prominently.

- **Be open to creative alternatives.**

  Instead of simply using a standard business card, consider a card that fits a Rolodex. Or use a double-size card folded in half. Double-size cards become mini-brochures. Standard business information appears on the front; additional benefits and information appear inside. On the down side, bear in mind that such cards may be difficult to carry.

- **Add color.**

  An additional color, which can make your card stand out, may add only $15 to $20 to your printing bill, depending on the color. If your budget simply won't allow two colors of ink, select a single color in addition to black, and use it creatively. Alternatively, choose a card stock other than white. Consider various textures to complement your image — high gloss, matte, and rag for example. Each creates a different impression.

- **Make the most of your business cards.**

  Don't let them sit in your office. Carry them with you at all times and give them to as many people as possible. Remember, as you distribute your business cards to new contacts, they will give you their business cards in return, resulting in excellent leads that you can follow up by phone or mail.

  If you want advice about your business card ideas or need help designing your business card, contact a professional. Local printers are generally more than happy to advise potential customers, and graphic artists are readily available for design work. To locate skilled professionals, check the yellow pages of your telephone directory or get a recommendation from an associate.

THE BUSINESS ADDRESS

A business address communicates respectability, substance, and permanence. If you are home-based, you may be hesitant to publicize your home address for safety and personal reasons. You are not required by law to show your address on your business cards; however, most states do require that you show a street address on your business stationery. If you are hesitant to advertise where you live, consider renting a post office box for business mail or better yet, use a mail-receiving service like MAIL BOXES ETC®, which in our opinion offers service that is superior to that of the U.S. postal system. And don't forget, rental of either a public or a private postal box is a tax-deductible business expense.

At the time of this writing under current California law, independent workers are required to list a physical address for their businesses. Noncompliance carries a $2500 fine and a maximum six-month jail sentence for those not disclosing their home address when using the word "suite" as their box return address. As with anything else, do your homework before taking any action, and find out what the laws are in your state.

THE COVER LETTER

Cover letters should accompany material you send or hand deliver to others. These letters should be brief and to the point, courteous, attractive, and accurate. The main purpose of a cover letter is to introduce you and provide basic information about you and your service. Include a description of any additonal material you are enclosing or attaching. Request some action on the part of the letter's recipient — review of material provided, acceptance of your planned telephone call, scheduling an interview with you.

THE RESUME

Prepare and maintain an updated resume of your work experience. It will be helpful in promoting your service, especially if the content is professionally done. You can hire a professional resume writer to work with you or prepare the resume yourself, using resume-writing reference books that are available at bookstores and public libraries. Attach the resume to your flier, enclose it in packets of materials, or carry it with you to present on interviews.

FLIERS

Paul and Sarah Edwards point out that a flier is one of the easiest and least expensive advertising methods. Make it clever, to immediately capture the reader's attention, but don't make it too flowery or cute. Bunnies, kittens, or bridal bouquets may get immediate attention but will probably create a less-than-professional impression of your business!

Desktop publishing firms, and some printers who offer desktop design services, can be great help in creating a professional looking flier. Fees will be approximately $25-$35 an hour for the setup, a worthwhile expenditure if you are not able to design your own flier.

In your flier, state your objectives, the services you offer, and your background in medical transcription. It is not necessary, at this point, to quote a price and we recommend against it. Pricing should be presented only after discussing the account with the client.

After you have created the flier, take it to a print shop (unless, of course, you are already working directly with a printer) and have it photocopied, preferably on colored paper. Colored paper costs a little more, but it generates more interest and creates a longer lasting impression. Select a color that coordinates with your business cards and, for a dynamic visual impact, add matching colored envelopes.

Be sure to paper clip or staple a business card to each flier before mailing. This will ensure that either one or the other is kept by the client for future reference. If your flier is really impressive, the client may keep one and pass the other on to a friend!

On the following page is a sample of a successful flier.

A-ONE TRANSCRIPTION SERVICE

1-800-DICTATE

WANTED

— A FEW GOOD PHYSICIANS —

QUALIFICATIONS: • Must demand high quality transcription at an affordable price.
• Must have a need for an expert in the field of medical transcription.
• Must require an expeditious turnaround time.
• Must possess a dictating system (standard or micro cassettes).
• Must possess a fairly good command of the English language.

If you meet the above qualifications, then I would be very interested in talking with you. I am a certified medical transcriptionist with 21 years experience, who is presently home based, having worked in a variety of settings for many years. I can offer you high quality transcription at a very affordable price with an extremely fast turnaround time. I own the latest computer equipment with a letter quality printer and can transcribe from either standard or micro cassettes. I possess excellent written and oral English skills as well as a highly developed ear for dialects.

I know what you are thinking. **I CANNOT AFFORD SUCH A SERVICE.** However, in our litigious society, you cannot afford not to have this service. For less than the price of half of a first class postage stamp, one piece of chewing gum or one-tenth of a gallon of gas, you can get a quality line of transcription.

For a no cost personal interview, please contact me at the above number.

BROCHURES

After your business is established, you may want to consider investing in a business brochure, which will promote your transcription service and enhance your professional image.

A well-designed brochure conveys the message that you and your transcription service are professionally successful — facts that are true and should be publicized. Don't be shy when it comes to business promotion. After all, you have worked long and hard to achieve your excellent professional reputation. Develop a great brochure that showcases your service, and you'll soon have new clients.

Use colored paper for extra panache, especially if you don't have a color printer. Many paper companies offer trifold paper with colorful borders and patterns especially designed for brochures. Note: If you plan to fax your brochure, stick with plain white paper.

Office and art supply stores stock a variety of paper types. In addition, specialty mail-order companies offer extensive variety and some real bargains. For a catalog call these suppliers:

- **Quill**
  800-789-5813

- **PaperDirect**
  800-272-7377

- **Queblo**
  800-523-9080

- **Idea Art**
  800-433-2278

It is not necessary to design a complicated brochure. It can be as simple as an 8½" x 11" folded sheet of paper. By folding it twice, as you would a letter, then turning it upright so it opens like a book, you have the beginnings of a brochure.

On the outside, write a headline that stands out and gets the attention of the client. Immediately inside, elaborate on the headline's promise or claim. Then elaborate further about the benefits of your services in the remaining brochure space.

The overall look of your brochure is the key to making a good impression. Here are some ideas to help:

- Have the descriptive copy typeset in a fairly large size.

- Break up the copy with subheads.

- Add something unexpected visually. Avoid broad or slapstick humor, which may give the impression you are not serious or professional.

- The back of the brochure is a good place for a business biography or testimonials from satisfied clients. Briefly describe how your business began, how it has succeeded, and its current status. Include your professional affiliations (i.e., AAMT, state/regional association or local chapter of AAMT), any offices held past and present, any special schooling that you have received, etc.

- Add substance to your brochure by printing it on heavier paper stock than you would normally use for a flier.

Enclose your business card with the brochure. One or the other will generally be filed for future reference.

Don't be disappointed if after sending out a flier or brochure, your telephone doesn't ring off the hook. You may receive immediate responses, but prospective clients may not call for a few days or weeks. It isn't uncommon to receive calls even two years later.

It is a good idea to send out fliers and brochures every four to six months to ensure a steady work flow. As mentioned earlier, accounts will come and go for various reasons, and it is important to keep your name and business fresh in the minds of prospective clients.

MARKETING THROUGH NETWORKING

Networking with other transcriptionists offers excellent opportunities to share information and services and increase professional exposure.

As a member of your local AAMT chapter, you will be able to promote your business and word-of-mouth referrals will be readily passed on. At chapter meetings, announcements are made about who and where transcriptionists are needed. Don't be shy about passing out your business cards at meetings, and do send thank-you notes for referrals. That personal touch is important.

We recommend donating door prizes in your business name at appropriate professional functions. The door prizes will cost you very little, association members will remember you positively, and you'll discover that it's personally rewarding.

ADVERTISING IN TRADE PUBLICATIONS

Local chapters of AAMT offer business-card-size advertising space in their newsletters for as little as $15-$20 an issue. This is a cost-effective way to promote your business while contributing to your local professional newsletter. Consider advertising in other local publications and trade newsletters in your area. Look into the possibility of advertising in your local medical society bulletin, newsletter or physician directory. Don't forget the Internet!

Remember, marketing is an ongoing process. Successful entrepreneurs never stop promoting their business.

MARKETING THROUGH THE CHAMBER OF COMMERCE

Membership in your local chamber of commerce is another excellent way to market services. Through chamber activities, and with chamber support, your business will increase.

You will enjoy networking with men and women in a wide variety of businesses. These business people are dedicated to maintaining a strong economic base in their community, and they actively promote local businesses.

Medical doctors, chiropractors, podiatrists, and many other health care professionals are active in chambers of commerce, offering you added opportunities for one-on-one contact, professional recognition, and word-of-mouth promotion.

As a participant in chamber activities, you and your business will receive publicity in local media, and you will also receive coverage in the chamber newsletter.

WORD-OF-MOUTH REFERRALS

Word-of-mouth referrals are an excellent source of new business. Doctors talk to one another in elevators, operating rooms, and at business functions. If they have been provided with your business card, they can refer you to fellow physicians.

COLD CALLING FOR THE SELF-CONFIDENT

For those of you who are self-assured and assertive, cold calling may generate new clients. Spontaneous or semi-spontaneous introductions, when managed with a professional demeanor in a courteous manner, can be very effective. If you are energetic and have a spirit of adventure, give it a try.

Before setting out, verify that there are no local restrictions on cold calling, which is prohibited in some cities. And even if cold calling is legally permitted in an area, it may not be allowed in specific buildings.

When cold calling and meeting prospective clients, be positive about yourself and the transcription service you offer. Point out the exceptional qualities of your service and your skills, from which the client will, of course, benefit.

However, let us interject a word of warning at this point. Do not promise the moon to prospective clients! A foot in the door and enthusiastic self-promotion can be a heady experience. You may be tempted to offer more or better service than you can realistically provide. Don't do it! Know yourself and know your limits! Both you and your clients will be better served when you are able to follow through on professional commitments.

ARMED WITH BUSINESS CARD AND FLIER

Brief visits to medical offices and one-on-one contact with front-desk receptionists is an effective way to market your service. Select an appropriate medical building and go from office to office armed with your business flier and business card. Some transcriptionists also leave note pads and/or pens imprinted with their business name, logo, and telephone number. Introduce yourself to the receptionist and leave the material for later review. You may experience some rejection, but nine times out of ten the material will be accepted with a smile.

MANAGING NO-THANK-YOUS

Your service may be excellent and your promotion superb, but some professional contacts will say, "Thanks, but no thanks." Don't take it personally or let it get you down. Rejection happens. It's part of the keyboard of life! We can assure you that clients will come your way if you are persistent. In fact, the very next person you call on may be a new customer.

FIRST IMPRESSIONS LINGER LONGEST

Long ago, humorist Will Rogers said, "You don't get a second chance to make a first impression." The statement is as true today as it was then. Your initial impact on business contacts will leave a lasting impression, so make your initial impact magnificent.

Before you open your mouth, the person standing before you will quickly review your appearance and demeanor, and make an instantaneous value judgment based on what he or she sees. You may be exceptionally competent, capable, intelligent, educated, and efficient, but if you don't look like a professional, your credibility will suffer.

When meeting a client for the first time, look as professional as possible. Basic squeaky-clean guidelines are a given, of course — face, hair, hands, nails, clothes, shoes. Leave the sweats and shorts at home. It isn't necessary to dress as though you are attending an afternoon tea at the Beverly Hills Hotel, but do dress for success. If you look professional and behave in a professional manner, you will generally be treated as a professional.

INFORMATIONAL PACKETS

Plan ahead. Well before a scheduled meeting, prepare and organize all appropriate materials in a neat packet . . . or several packets if you are scheduled for a number of interviews. The interviewer will be impressed with your organization and you won't be embarrassed by last minute fumbling . . . or missing information sheets.

> *"You don't get a second chance to make a first impression."*
> — Will Rogers

THE INTERVIEW

Be prepared for interviews. Have your resume up-to-date and readily available, as well as personal references attesting to your competence and skills. Some transcriptionists also provide a ready-to-sign contract, which demonstrates professional forethought and commitment.

Be ready to provide specific facts about your service to clients who ask for information regarding schedules, turnaround-time, and availability to clients who request this information. Give forethought to guarantees of service and confidentiality. Review your deadline procedures and backup systems for personal emergencies.

Be prepared to answer questions about your office and its location, type of equipment you use, your proposed method of operation, line counts, margin widths, type styles, quality assurance, and other facets of medical transcription.

When speaking, be as concise as possible, clearly explaining your service and how it will benefit the client. Point out areas of flexibility and offer to tailor your service whenever possible to meet the client's needs.

If the interview goes well and you negotiate a contract, state your terms succinctly and logically at the outset. Carefully explain your fees, billing dates, payment schedules, and other important business factors to avoid confusion later.

In an interview, **do not answer statements**. If a prospective client states that using an outside service is expensive, don't try to convince her otherwise. Smile pleasantly and allow her to express her opinion.

Do not criticize or belittle your competitors! If a prospect baits you by praising your competitor, do not respond with a laundry list of your competitor's flaws or snidely point out that if the competitor was actually so fantastic, the interviewer would already be using that service! Instead, respond with a relaxed smile and "Hmmm," "Very interesting," "Ah, yes," or another ambiguous comment.

If you are familiar with your competitor's service and are asked a specific question about it, respond as honestly and as directly as possible, but phrase your response so the final emphasis is on the excellence and benefits of **your** service. Emphasize **your** experience, training, background, continuing education, and awards you have received.

If a prospective client asks about your competitor's credentials or urges you to corroborate negative rumors, simply reply that you cannot speak for your competitor's credentials or personal life. And then get back to business.

Try to maintain control of the interview from opening formalities to final farewells, moving the meeting along with pleasant efficiency as you systematically explain your service program, answer questions, and conclude the meeting. Your professional position will be stronger if **you** bring the interview to an appropriate conclusion and avoid an unexpected or abrupt ending initiated by the interviewer.

When you have concluded your presentation, ask if there are any further questions. If not, thank the interviewer for meeting with you and indicate that you will look forward to hearing from her or him in the future, at which time you will be happy to answer any additional questions. That's it! End of interview!

DO NOT BEG FOR BUSINESS

Do not say, "Let's draw up a contract" or "Won't you please try my service on a short-term basis?" Do not beg for work or offer bargain prices. Hold your head high and exit.

You are a professional medical transcriptionist and professionals adhere to standards of excellence. Even if this is your first client prospect, it is important to maintain and communicate an aura of professionalism and independence. Although your service may not yet have reached the pinnacle of success, it will eventually. Believe it, work for it, and it will happen. Don't settle for anything less. Communicate your future success now!

ADVERTISING

There are different approaches to marketing, but the most efficient and economical are mailings and handouts. Utilizing the information you gathered from the yellow pages and various reference lists, mail your fliers, brochures or cover letter with your business card attached.

Focus on a few clinics each week, perhaps ten, and build a solid base from there. Don't be tempted to market more widely, to 50 or 100, even though you feel secure in your skills and are eager for accounts. Trying to manage too much too soon can result in overwhelming problems and possible business failure.

It's important to direct your mailings to medical record/transcription supervisors, office managers, or medical transcription supervisors in specific departments. Be sure you correctly identify the department and contact person on your dispatch or it may never reach the intended destination. It may end up in health care limbo!

After a week or so, follow up your mailing with a phone call. Introduce yourself, verify that you are not interrupting your contact's work (in which case you offer to call at a more convenient time), and ask if your announcement was received. If not, indicate that you will send another packet and call again soon. If the mailing was received, continue your conversation.

Request an appointment, at the supervisor's convenience, to discuss your services. If the facility currently has no need for your services, encourage the supervisor to keep your card on file for future reference.

Conveying a positive and professional demeanor on the telephone is not easy, especially when you are feeling rejected, but it's vitally important. Don't allow yourself to label the negative response as "a turndown," when in fact it is only "a turning aside." The supervisor didn't say, "No." She merely said, "Not now." Continue to radiate enthusiasm and energy, and you can be sure your business card will go in her file.

PUBLIC RELATIONS

Develop rapport with lead and other transcriptionists and office managers at medical facilities. Often, the in-house staff may initially feel intimidated by you or they may even feel jealous because of the income disparity between independents and in-house medical transcriptionists. Always maintain a positive and friendly attitude, even though at first it may seem that your friendliness is not being returned.

You may discover that because of their resentment toward you, in-house medical transcriptionists may be inclined to route sloppy work they don't want to do to you and other independent transcriptionists. Our recommendation is, do it! Once you do the "slop" you will become very valuable to those in-house people, and their attitudes will change because they know that they can depend on you. Yes, learn to do slop. Through it you'll "earn your stripes," increase and diversify your skills, and find all other transcription easier.

MAINTAINING A CLIENT BASE WITH CREATIVE FOLLOW-UP

In any service-oriented business, finding and keeping clients is an ongoing challenge. Having an established business doesn't mean that you can take a rest from pursuing and nurturing new accounts.

Maintaining a solid client base requires follow-up and communication. There are various ways to do this including thank you notes, dependable service, prompt delivery of completed work, phone calls, personal visits, and other courtesies tailored to individual clients.

Call and make sure customers are satisfied with your services. Encourage comments and suggestions for transcription improvement, then respond positively and actively.

The cumulative effect of everything you say and do affects your clients' perceptions of you and your business, ultimately determining whether or not they continue with your service and refer others to you.

Whenever there is client contact, there should be regular, ongoing follow-up. This demonstrates to the client that you are concerned about their business needs, not just the account income. Your excellent service and personalized care will make your client happy; and a happy client is usually a loyal client.

FOLLOW-UP CHECK LIST

- Budget time for follow-up and make it a regular habit.

- Keep a 3 x 5 card, or use a software program such as *ASK!* for each client, listing name, address, and telephone number and comments.

- Remember to send thank-you notes to clients after the first meeting. The simple courtesy will be long remembered.

- Contact new clients five days after beginning the service to ask if they have any questions or concerns. This establishes a strong communication link and helps resolve problems or potential problems.

- Always deliver your work as promised. If for some unforeseen reason the delivery schedule cannot be met, contact the client immediately, apologize, and explain the reasons for the delay. Specify the exact time the work will be delivered and make every effort to meet that goal.

- Always be honest. Clients respect a transcriptionist who has integrity. Don't give creative excuses for delays or other business problems. "Computer trouble," "stuck in traffic," "sick kids," and "brownout" work only so many times before the frustrated client stops calling for transcription and calls it quits instead.

- Communicate promptly. Some days will be disastrous to your work schedule, but don't keep your clients pacing back and forth waiting for work that should have been delivered hours earlier. Call your clients as soon as possible about any significant delay or change in schedule.

- Consider taking clients out to lunch or giving them gifts occasionally. These professional courtesies are tax deductible business expenses. Keep your receipts.

- Don't forget to follow up. Keep a tickler file, mark your calendar with colored pens, or use sticky notes to flag dates and people to contact.

A LIST OF PROSPECTIVE CLIENTS

Medical Doctors/Specialists	Orthopedists
Cardiologists	Court Reporters
Internists	Family Practitioners
Neurologists	Surgeons
Radiologists	OB/GYN
Ear, Nose and Throat	Correctional Facilities
Dental Clinics	Industrial Medicine
Walk-In Clinics	Ambulatory Care Clinics
Urgi-/Surgi-Centers	Pathology Laboratories
Word Processing Services	Other Transcription Services
Hospitals Extended Care	Hospitals Acute Care
Chemical Dependence Facilities	Physical Therapy Clinics
Urgent Care Clinics	Group Medical Clinics
Rehabilitation Centers	Clinical Laboratories

Prospective Clients (*continued*)

Military Installations
Imaging Facilities
Mental Health Facilities/State Hospitals
Cardiopulmonary Rehabilitation Centers
Clinical Psychologists/Counselors
Workers Compensation Clinic
Veterans Facilities
Pediatricians
Dentists
Osteopaths
Health Centers
Insurance Adjustors
Disability Offices
Podiatrists
Radiology/Medical Imaging Facilities
Workers Compensation Clinic
Ophthalmologists
Immunologists
Pathologists

Teaching Universities
Urologists
Oncologists
Neurosurgeons
Plastic Surgeons
Pulmonologists
Veterinary Clinics
Psychiatrists
Veterinarians
Oral Surgeons
Insurance Agencies
Legal Offices
Surgical Centers
Chiropractors
Private Investigators
Authors
Gastroenterologists

Business Ethics

"Character isn't inherited. One builds it daily
by the way one thinks and acts,
thought by thought, action by action."
—Helen Gahagan Douglas

An ethical person is one who lives by a set of principles of right conduct, that is, a system of moral values. These principles of right and wrong serve as guides and help the individual make decisions that will have positive impacts on his or her life and on the lives of others. In the same manner within professions, ethical rules or standards govern the conduct of each profession and its members.

MEDICAL RECORD CONFIDENTIALITY

Confidentiality of the medical record and protecting patient privacy has long been a major health care principle. In today's health care world, medical record confidentiality continues to be vitally important because of ethical, medical, social, and legal implications.

Medical transcriptionists must be responsible in transcribing accurate medical records and maintaining patient confidentiality regarding those records. What is input into today's record will become a permanent part of the patient's chart, and the code of medical ethics must be upheld. If this is not done, the patient's right to confidentiality has been violated.

A patient's trust in the physician, a factor that is important to the patient's physical and emotional well-being, is directly affected by all personnel involved in that patient's care. Medical transcriptionists, because of our relationship with patient records, are in a particularly sensitive position. In the course of our work, we learn myriad intimate details about patients — more details than some members of the hands-on health care team learn. It is our responsibility to respect and protect that knowledge because of its privileged nature and its importance to patients.

AAMT CODE OF ETHICS

The American Association for Medical Transcription has adopted a strict code of ethics and, like other health care professionals, medical transcriptionists conduct their business in accordance with this medical/legal code. Noncompliance with this code of ethics can result in loss of professional credibility, loss of clients, and litigation.

> "Protect the privacy and confidentiality of the individual medical record to avoid disclosure of personally identifiable medical and social information and professional medical judgments."
> - Point 9, Code of Ethics
> American Association for Medical Transcription

Hospital accounts may require that you sign a nondisclosure agreement, which in effect states that if the confidentiality of a report is violated, you or your service will be terminated immediately. See a generic copy of a nondisclosure statement at the end of this chapter.

By California law, all health care professionals are required to maintain confidentiality of patients' personal and medical records. Legally, discussion of medical record information is allowed only in "legally privileged" medical/legal situations. Casual conversation with family and/or friends about a patient's condition is not legal.

The patient is *". . . to be assured confidential treatment of personal and medical records . . ."*

-72527 Administrative Code, Section 9

To adequately ensure confidentiality of the patient record within the medical transcription office, purchase a paper shredder. There are inexpensive models ranging in price from a low of $99 to more expensive models costing $700. Nothing should be put into your wastebasket that contains any identifying information, i.e., patient name, age, address, etc. All documents should be shredded so patients' rights are protected and you are not at risk for a lawsuit.

Keep your lips sealed where patient information is concerned. Derogatory comments about the patient — or even idle conversation you consider harmless — could be interpreted as slanderous if it gets back to the patient. And if his attorney is convinced that your comments have indeed resulted in "defamation of character," you may be sued.

"Slander is a false and unprivileged publication, orally uttered . . ." which results in *"injuries"* to the patient *"in respect to his office, profession, trade or business . . ."* or *" . . . which, by natural consequence, causes actual damage."*

-46 Civil Code

Written communication regarding patient medical records, except for legally privileged situations, is also illegal if it results in harm to reputation or income. In this case, the injured patient may sue you for libel.

"Libel . . . exposes any person to hatred, contempt, ridicule, or obloquy, or which causes him to be shunned or avoided, or which has a tendency to injure him in his occupation . . ."

-44 Civil Code

UNETHICAL TRANSCRIPTIONISTS

There are no ethical shortcuts through the forest of professional medical transcription. Those who are lured along the path of unethical practices usually regret their action sooner or later. UTs (unethical transcriptionists), who do not adhere to generally accepted transcription profession standards, face a number of risks.

Unethical transcriptionists who fail to maintain confidentiality of the medical record or refuse to comply with other quality assurance guidelines that result in patient injury may face legal action. Even if they are not sued, they risk losing their professional reputation, the friendship of their work associates, and their livelihood. The ethical breach will be recognized by peers, who will not sanction the unethical behavior nor support this transcriptionist professionally.

Unethical behavior can have far-reaching effects. Some UTs attempt to build their businesses "the quick and easy way," by "stealing" accounts from other transcriptionists. Eventually, the truth catches up with them and they lose all professional credibility, along with all their purloined accounts. Unfortunately, innocent individuals may be hurt in the process. Patients, clients and other transcriptionists may be harmed, too.

Although most transcriptionists are ethical, public reports about even one unethical transcriptionist can damage the credibility of ethical transcriptionists, especially if they are self-employed.

A few years ago, a large medical transcription service launched an advertising campaign that portrayed a home-based transcriptionist talking on the telephone to a friend, relating a report she had just typed on a mutual acquaintance. The ad asked, "Is this the image we wish for ourselves?"

Be a professional. Honor the patient's right to privacy and the ethics of the American Association for Medical Transcription. You will never regret it.

NONDISCLOSURE AGREEMENT (SAMPLE)

By signing this Nondisclosure Agreement, I indicate my understanding that:

Patients, physicians and other health care providers furnish confidential information to obtain or carry out medical services, and medical service information and records are confidential.

Patients depend on the providers of medical services to keep patient information confidential. The provider's reputation depends on this confidentiality.

If medical information has been used or disclosed inappropriately, patients or providers who have suffered loss or injury may seek legal action to recover damages from the person who used or disclosed the information. Specific violations of patient confidentiality resulting in economic loss or personal injury to a patient may be punishable by law.

Any breach of confidentiality will be considered serious and subject to investigation and possible discipline, including immediate termination of services.

Therefore, as a contract service provider, I agree that I will not at any time:

1. Disclose services given or information about patients.

2. Allow anyone else to examine or copy any records or documents having to do with patients, physicians, or other health care providers and services.

_____   _____
Independent Contractor   Date

Business Operations

" . . . it either is or ought to be evident to everyone
that business has to prosper before anybody
can get any benefit from it."

—Theodore Roosevelt

You decided to become an independent medical transcriptionist and have completed your homework. You have spent a great deal of time and energy accumulating information that will prove invaluable not only now, but in the future.

Now you must organize your business and make that organized system work for you.

GETTING STARTED —
STUDYING THE FACTS AND ORGANIZING

You now have at your fingertips a base of information that will be the foundation of your business. You have files on medical facilities available for your marketing, who and where your competition is, what transcription methods are being used in your area and in the transcription profession at large, and you have determined your target market as you review the following information.

- Set up specific reference files for the clinic, hospital, and physician reference lists you have obtained.

- Provide space for any journals or publications you may subscribe to for quick and easy reference.

- Set up a file (or files) of information you may have on other services in your area.

- Set up a "people" file in which you gather names, addresses, and notes on people you meet and may wish to contact in the future.

All of the above files, and others you may need in the future, can easily be updated as your business progresses.

By this time you have determined your specific market. You are ready for the next step.

CHOOSING A BUSINESS NAME

It is perfectly all right to name the business after yourself, i.e., Ima Mazing Medical Transcription Service. For you more creative people, let your imagination take charge. A business name, however, should be selected with great care. Here are some key guidelines to follow:

- Choose a name that is pleasant and easy to pronounce. If your client regurgitates your name every time it is mentioned, it is not likely to be repeated and people will not hear about your business.

- Choose a name that will do a little advertising for you, telling people what you do, i.e., Medi-Scribe, Healthline.

- Choose a name that will not severely limit you, a name that will stand up to the passage of time.

> *"A business name should be selected with great care. It should stand up to the passage of time and do a little advertising for you along the way."*

BUILDING A BIG IMAGE

Most home-based businesses are relatively small operations — but the smart ones don't advertise it or think of themselves as small. If you think small you'll be perceived as small, and chances are your results will be small. A major factor in establishing your professional image is your business name. In general, names should sound professional and tell something about the company. Avoid using the word "enterprises" as this is a name that has become synonymous with an amateur.

LEGALIZING THE NAME

If you select a name for your business other than your own, you should file a fictitious name statement, called a DBA (Doing Business As).

There are several ways to handle this. The first and easiest is to go to your local newspaper and file a fictitious name statement with them. They will then record the information with the city or county clerk's office and publish the DBA in their newspaper for the period of time required by law. Shop around for the cheapest newspaper prices as some newspapers charge $50; others, $100 or more.

You may go to your city hall or county clerk's office and review the alphabetical list of registered fictitious names. If you live in a small city and have no plans to expand, you may not need to search further.

However, if you live in a large city and plan to expand, consider utilizing the services of companies that specialize in name searches. Using computer data banks, they will review the millions of registered fictitious names in the United States.

If you live in a large urban area, you may discover your first, second and perhaps even third business-name choices are already registered.

You may wish to contact the person who owns the business name and find out if the business is still in existence. If it isn't, and if the owner of the name consents, an Abandonment of Fictitious Name Statement can be filed, whereby the previous owner gives up all rights to the name. You can then simultaneously file a Fictitious Name Statement for the name.

The Abandonment of Fictitious Name Statement procedures are identical to the Fictitious Name Statement procedures, including the requirement to publish the statement in the newspaper. The former owner will probably ask you to pay the cost of filing the statement of abandonment and may even want you to pay a fee for abandonment.

Avoid choosing a business name that is already being used by an out-of-county or out-of-state business. Corporations are usually granted exclusive statewide use of a business name, assuming they were the first in the state to choose the name.

Your state's secretary of state maintains a list of business names claimed by in-state corporations and by out-of-state corporations licensed to do business in your state. Contact your state's secretary of state to determine if your proposed business name will conflict with one already in use.

An even greater potential problem involves federal trademarks of business names and products. Most large and even some very small businesses obtain trademarks from the U.S. Patent and Trademark Office. Trademark law basically states that a business with a federally registered trademark sometimes has exclusive use of that name throughout the United States.

Public libraries usually have a copy of the current *Federal Trademark Register*, in which you can look up your proposed business name. If you discover that it is the same as, or very similar to, a trademarked name, you may avoid future problems by not using that name.

What happens if you start your business and discover later that some other business has prior claim to your business name? You may receive a letter from an attorney telling you that you are in violation of the law and that you must cease using that business name or they will sue you.

If you receive such a letter and believe you were not in violation of the law, you must then decide whether or not to fight for your business name in court, which can be an incredibly expensive and time-consuming process.

Another way to avoid infringing on someone else's business trademark is to check your local telephone directories and review national trade directories for your type of business. Trademark or no trademark, avoid a business name already in use.

Once again, if you use your own personal name for your transcription service, you are not required to file a Fictitious Name Statement.

In summary, do your homework before selecting a business name to minimize any future liability. Be bold, brave, and daring when selecting a name, but don't be too cute. "Frenetic Fingertips" may be a delightfully creative name for a medical transcription service, but it does not promote a very professional image.

LICENSES AND PERMITS

Studies show that among self-employed individuals, 95% of those who succeed in business have obtained business licenses. Entrepreneurial consultants are not surprised by this pattern. They believe that obtaining a business license is a primary indicator of the commitment and planning necessary for career success.

In California, you will probably be required by town, county, or state to have a business license. However, some rural areas are excluded from this requirement. Required or not, a business license may be helpful to you. Many banks will not open a business account without verification of licensing, and in addition, operating a business without a required license can result in fines and business closure.

The first step in acquiring your business license is to investigate your city and county codes and zoning restrictions. If you are in a residential neighborhood there may be stricter policies than in commercial zones. Check on rules and regulations at the zoning department at your city hall or county administration office.

If you live in a small town, you may only need to go to the city hall, fill out a request to operate a home-based personal service and obtain a business license. This license must be renewed each year.

On the application, you will probably be asked whether or not your business operation will create additional pedestrian/auto traffic. If yours is a personal service in which you provide pick up and delivery with no clients coming in and out, your business should easily meet legal requirements. On the other hand, if your business will increase traffic, you may face restrictions. Standards vary so check with your city, county, or state on local zoning regulations before opening your doors to business.

When processing your business license, double check your assigned business classification and the fee rate. Most city clerks do not understand the work of a medical transcriptionist so they may classify you incorrectly and charge you an excessive license fee. We have found that business license fees generally average $50 to $75. If you are charged over that amount, don't hesitate to question the licensing clerk.

INCORPORATION

If you are considering incorporating your business, investigate the costs in your state or region. Attorneys' fees for incorporation vary, but many attorneys discount their legal fees in hopes it will generate future business.

The incorporation fees you are charged should include all filing fees, a corporation kit with a seal and a set of bylaws, and at least two hours of consultation time with your attorney, during which you can discuss your business and ask questions. You will receive a corporation tax ID number and in some cases, a DBA (Doing Business As) certificate if the corporation will be conducting business in a name other than its corporate name.

Some lawyers charge "a la carte" for their services, and some will tell you to buy your own kit and seal. Shop around, and ask what is and is not included in the fees you are quoted. The total cost of incorporation should be less than $500.

Some attorneys recommend against incorporation if they think your benefits from incorporating will be outweighed by the added expenses and time required to maintain and administer the corporation, which will include additional record keeping, tax returns, and corporate filings.

FINDING A MENTOR

Home-based medical transcriptionists experience an isolated career world, especially those who work for services that pick up and deliver work materials to the transcriptionist's home.

The transcriptionist is plugged into a machine all day, listening to others' voices, having little or no personal contact with anyone but the mail man and delivery person. In earlier chapters of this book, we explained why networking with other transcriptionists is essential to a successful transcription business. For those new to the field of medical transcription, it is also a good idea to seek a mentor.

MENTOR

A wise and trusted counselor.

—*Random House Dictionary*

How does one find a mentor? Probably the most efficient way is to network with other medical transcriptionists and determine who inspires you, shares your philosophy, and has qualities you wish to emulate.

This admirable professional is someone who, if willing and able, will advise you and nurture you as you establish your career. Your mentor will have in-depth knowledge and experience as a medical transcription business person and will help you with specific questions and provide you with a wealth of emotional support.

Be sure to thank your mentor. There are givers and takers in every profession, and medical transcription is certainly not an exception. Some of my dearest friends have acted as mentors for ten or more years and while 99% of the medical transcriptionists they have helped have been extremely grateful, there have been a few who have turned around and stolen accounts from them. Unethical? Yes! You don't have to give your mentor your first born child; a pretty bouquet of spring flowers, a nice leisurely lunch or just a pretty thank-you card will suffice. Remember, these people have taken time away from their lives and work to help you and have asked nothing in return. Let them know how much they are appreciated.

The authors of this book have served as mentors for many novice transcriptionists. It has been a pleasure helping them solve problems we have faced, nurturing their professional development, and seeing their businesses succeed. More often than not, mentors and those they nurture become close friends and confidants in their personal and professional lives.

THE WINNING ATTITUDE

The large majority of men and women who are successful set goals for themselves. Setting goals consciously moves them toward those goals and nurtures a positive attitude.

Set goals for yourself. Make them measurable goals so you can monitor your progress, make adjustments as needed, and reward success points.

Be enthusiastic and positive about your medical transcription service, and others will be enthusiastic, too. With excellent knowledge and skills, you should radiate the exhilaration you feel about the services you provide the medical industry and the patients it serves. When meeting a potential client, remember that the client has a need and your service will fill that need.

When results don't turn out as planned, a winning attitude helps you look ahead to the next opportunity. People only fail when they give up. Trying again means they have learned one way in which their goal cannot be achieved.

SETTING BOUNDARIES IN YOUR BUSINESS

For better or for worse, we are now living in a world without boundaries, in an era in which we are frequently dealing with issues that are no longer crisp black and white but hazy gray. Often it seems that no one is certain what rules to follow, and rules can change from one day to the next. Regrettably, in this fluctuating setting, instead of working together for the greater good, we frequently find ourselves working against one another.

For the most part, doctors are really fun to work with. Most of them are undemanding and are grateful to have their work completed in a timely fashion. When giving doctors excellent quality at a fair price, a transcriptionist will usually have them eating out of her hand. Unfortunately, dealing with office personnel is usually not as simple. Issuing a title to some people gives them delusions of grandeur.

It has been our experience that when contracting with a new client, the proposal is usually made to the office manager, not the physician. In fact, most physicians delegate all office decisions to the office manager, and sometimes, the office manager begins acting like the GREAT AND POWERFUL WIZARD OF OZ.

The GREAT AND POWERFUL WIZARD OF OZ (or G-WOZ) begins to make decisions about how we should conduct businesses and, feeling great and powerful, has no qualms about telling us how to run our businesses even though he or she may have no idea precisely what we do. The G-WOZ is condescending and demanding. Out of the blue we receive a phone call demanding 24-hour turnaround instead of the agreed-upon 48 hours. The contract provides for the original work only; now the G-WOZ demands two copies. And the format is all wrong. Instead of block style, she now wants indented style; instead of 10 pitch, 12 pitch is required. Next, morning pickup and delivery is changed to afternoon.

COMMUNICATION AND ASSERTIVENESS SKILLS

It is important to have solid, clearly defined personal boundaries when facing the likes of a G-WOZ. Every independent transcriptionist must believe and act upon the knowledge that no one can dictate to us how we should run our businesses. Only we, as highly trained medical transcription professionals, can judge what works best for us and what doesn't.

If you do not have a firm grasp on your strengths as well as your limitations and weaknesses, do some personal analysis and list your qualities in writing. This way you will be able to set healthy boundaries for yourself and make decisions based on your own knowledge about what you will or will not accept.

Fear is the biggest drawback to healthy communication and assertiveness when conducting business. Often, we devalue ourselves by acquiescing to another's demands even though deep down we know that decisions should not be made for us but by us. To overcome the fear of speaking up for yourself, develop a stronger, more rooted sense of who you are and what you believe in. That is why making a list is so important.

In every relationship, especially business relationships, give and take is essential. Any type of relationship that is one-sided will only lead to resentment, anger and cessation of all communication. The following are some keys to open the doors to communication and negotiation.

1. Be a good listener

The first and most important step is to learn to be a good listener. All of us *hear*, especially in our particular line of work, but few of us truly *listen*. Listening is a normal physiological process. Sound is transmitted to the ear and is transported to the brain for interpretation. However, listening is a more complex psychological process requiring us to interpret and understand what we just heard.

Skilled communicators know that they need to listen first to persuade or negotiate later. They do not make requests or plead their case until they have paid close attention to others. The single biggest mistake made by poor negotiators is their tendency to rush ahead of themselves and start talking before making an effort to understand their audience. If you want to assert yourself more forcefully in your business relationships, make a commitment never to speak unless and until you have prepared and listened first. Resist the temptation to interrupt, daydream, jump to a conclusion or change the topic abruptly.

2. Assess ideas and viewpoints

Do not dwell on whether you agree or disagree. Listening does not oblige you to pick a side. Keep your mind focused on the message itself, not on judgments of right-wrong or good-bad. Don't feel pressured to respond immediately to every comment made; it's better not to. Rather than talk back, assess the speaker's ideas and viewpoints in a clearheaded, unbiased frame of mind. Let the message hang out there, in beautiful silence, without the static that so often turns a conversation into a contest.

3. Set your boundaries

After listening to the speaker without any bias, then you and only you will have to decide what you will and will not accept (setting your boundaries).

4. Be persistent

To be effective in your assertiveness, you must be persistent. Continue repeating what you want again and again without getting angry, irritated or loud. More often than not, to communicate in a conflict situation, you have to be persistent and stick to your point. By practicing speaking as if you were a "broken record" you will learn to be persistent, keeping your focus on the point of the discussion and saying what you want to say while ignoring all side issues brought up by the person you are negotiating with. Continue in this manner in a calm, repetitive voice until the other person accedes to your request or agrees to a compromise.

5. Offer a workable compromise

You may find it practical to offer your prospective client a workable compromise. This should be done, of course, only after you have determined that the compromise will not have a detrimental impact on your business or negatively affect your sense of personal and professional self-respect. A successful compromise results in a win-win situation for both negotiating parties. It should also help you move closer to your material goals.

TAMING THE GREAT AND POWERFUL G-WOZ

For example, imagine you are negotiating with the GREAT AND POWERFUL WIZARD OF OZ, who suddenly demands 24-hour delivery after having accepted the conditions set by you for 48-hour delivery. After listening very carefully ask, "Is this being done at the physician's request?" If you determine that the physician knows nothing about this and that the new demands have been initiated by the G-WOZ, take some time to evaluate the situation. Calmly but firmly tell Oz you will return shortly with an answer.

If after having looked at your schedule you realize that 24-hour turnaround is impossible, call the G-WOZ and state that you cannot comply with that request because of time constraints. If the G-WOZ becomes angry, hostile and will not take no for an answer, keep repeating your message in a very matter-of-fact, firm voice, reiterating that you cannot possibly comply with that demand. Say it as many times as necessary until the G-WOZ accedes and accepts your answer.

What if the G-WOZ does not accede after your broken-record method? Try another tactic! If you feel you could comfortably return the work within a 36-hour time frame, offer that option as a workable compromise. Nine times out of ten, the situation can be remedied without you or the G-WOZ feeling manipulated. A potentially harmful situation has been averted and you have both maintained your self-respect. It's a win-win situation.

COMPLAINTS

No matter how hard you try, you will not be able to avoid a few complaints . . . even if you and your service are excellent.

Some complaints will be anticipated. Other complaints will appear unexpectedly, perhaps about something you never considered a potential problem.

How do you solve problems, keep clients happy, and maintain your personal integrity?

- When a complaint arises, allow the client to ventilate, expressing his or her feelings.

- Verify the problem. Listen carefully. When you feel you understand the problem, repeat it back to the client for verification.

- Suggest a resolution to the problem. In a calm, matter-of-fact, professional manner, explain what you can and cannot do. Suggest a solution to the problem or give the client a choice of solutions.

- Be willing to compromise. If initial suggestions don't solve the problem, consider alternatives.

- Accept the outcome and move ahead. Solutions that result positively for both transcriptionist and client are ideal, but occasionally a client cannot, or will not, be satisfied regardless of how hard the transcriptionist tries to accommodate. In these situations, don't berate yourself, acquiesce to guilt, or dissolve in feelings of failure. You've done your best, so get on with your work.

WHY CLIENTS WILL STOP DOING BUSINESS WITH YOU

- 9% die, move away or develop other friendships.

- 91% leave for competitive reasons.

- 14% are dissatisfied with the service provided.

- 68% quit because of the service owner's attitude of indifference toward the client.

Medical transcription is a service-oriented business. We must offer quality service without jeopardizing our integrity. Regularly talk with your accounts about their interpretation of the services you are offering. Remember, many accounts are lost due to indifference or a laissez-faire attitude on the part of the service.

Remember the days of old when you walked into a department store, a bank, grocery store, library, post office, restaurant or gas station and were greeted with a smile, a hello and "please let me know if I can be of assistance?" Remember the old adage, The customer is always right? Today, too many businesses have an attitude of disdain and sometimes even contempt toward a customer who asks for assistance. From time to time, each of us needs to look into the mirror and ask if we have developed the same posture.

One of the best ways to judge the quality of your service is to prepare a questionnaire asking clients to rate your services in a variety of areas including turnaround time, quality of work received, completeness of work received, as well as your working relationship with them. Ask for their input regarding how you might improve service and leave plenty of room for their answers. You might be shocked to learn that what you thought was an excellent relationship is only rated fair or good by the client. Just as we were given employee evaluations when we belonged to the 9-5 work world, we must take it upon ourselves as micro-businesses to make sure we are offering the best service possible. We alone are responsible for our mistakes, and we certainly can't remedy problems if we don't know they exist.

Remember, you are only in competition with yourself.

THE THEORY OF NEGATIVITY

There are times when we long for the not-so-long-ago days when people treated one another with respect and dignity, the office of the President of the United States was looked upon with awe and reverence, our lives were centered around families, friends and communities, the work day lasted from 9 a.m. to 5 p.m., job loyalty was a reality and not a myth, and life was more gentle, secure, peaceful and relaxed. In that atmosphere, our country grew by leaps and bounds, because individuals were nurtured, new ideas were encouraged, creativity was applauded and ingenuity was revered. People had hope, rose above fear, welcomed change, and pursued their dreams.

In contrast, as we near the close of this millennium, it sometimes seems as though we're living in a lost world. A whirlpool of negativity surrounds us. We see it in every facet of our lives — home, personal relationships, workplace, social scene, entertainment, and government. Many politicians no longer confront issues directly, and they use character assassination as a routine and acceptable political tactic. American corporations have grown greedy at the expense of the people who made them great — their employees; reorganizing, downsizing, outsourcing, and decreasing employee benefits to keep stockholders happy and the CEO assured of a job for the coming year.

People are frustrated, angry and, most of all, tired. There is never enough time, especially for our families and communities. Our children are no longer sustained by traditional values and are often overwhelmed with a sense of hopelessness, We blame one another for our misfortunes, and America appears to be at war with itself. Citizens are arming themselves to drive the freeways and hostile confrontations are increasing.

We find it easier to talk to one another through our computers than to spend personal time over a cup of coffee. Some of our professional associations are instilling fear in us by giving us no hope for the future. We are told that outsourcing medical transcription will replace us, especially work being done overseas, or that we are going to be replaced by voice recognition technology. We are being fed a daily diet of doom and gloom and now the ultimate insult . . . Negativity on the NET. The NET, a forum meant for exchange of new ideas, problem solving and promotion of our profession, has become infatuated with itself and thrives on the unhappiness it spreads through Negativity.

Being negative is a nonproductive waste of time, and it eats at our souls. In our negative world, it seems that people are no longer responsible for their words or actions. They blame bad childhoods, bad people, gender discrimination, racial discrimination, bad marriages, people they work for, addiction problems, and so on ad infinitum. The US versus THEM mentality results in blaming everything and everybody else for the sorry lot of one's life. If you doubt this, read any newspaper, magazine, or watch one of the regular daytime talk programs on TV. It's time we take charge of our lives and make healthy decisions about ourselves, putting the responsibility where it belongs . . . on our own shoulders!

Negativity feeds on itself like a cancer. It rears its ugly head with one comment or one diatribe and before you know it, we are all feeling sorry for ourselves. It is making us sicker and sicker in our thinking, and the sickness increases as negative people gravitate to one another, finding comfort and encouragement in their misery. How did this happen in our industry?

MEDICAL TRANSCRIPTION AGE OF INNOCENCE

When we began our careers as medical transcriptionists, collectively 55-plus years ago, there were no schools of medical transcription and no reference books, but there were people willing to mentor us and answer our sometimes silly and mundane questions.

During that era, some great and wonderful people in our profession had a vision: They would form an organization to introduce us to the world and to our peers, to provide us with education and instill pride in what we do. The dream became reality. The early years of that organization were wonderful. Members were encouraged to share in the vision, to network with one another and solve problems, to broaden our horizons and, as the U.S. Army's slogan says, "be all that you can be," and more.

There was a whirlwind of activity. Policies and bylaws were written, committees formed, conventions planned and leaders elected. The organization prided itself on its membership and began working for the betterment of all. People who had never belonged to an organization were invited to participate, to become members and leaders. Nurturing souls encouraged others to get out of their comfort zone and expand their horizons, to not be afraid, to take risks and to accept challenge. It was an exciting time for all involved. The members became a part of the dream and worked long, tedious hours without compensation and without complaint because they had hope for a brighter tomorrow.

The incredible minds — ours! — behind the machines were acknowledged. Suddenly there were reference books — tons of them — and abundant educational opportunities. Seminars and symposiums offered presentation by, and direct interaction with, the greater medical community, satisfying our never-ending thirst for knowledge. We began calling ourselves professionals and believed we deserved that title. A certification program was established that validated our knowledge and skills and instilled pride in our accomplishments. We were empowered because we were part of something greater than ourselves. We felt there were no boundaries, no barriers, and the sky was the limit for all who participated.

Then FEAR raised its ugly, foreboding head and before long, medical transcriptionists began feeling less confident. Lawyers sprang out of every crevice, talking authoritatively about "risks," "liabilities," and "lawsuits." We had to be careful, we were warned. If we said or did the wrong thing we could be sued . . . even by fellow members of our own professional organizations. We could be discredited; we could lose something called "face."

Faced with such dire warnings, transcriptionists grew overly cautious about expressing new ideas or discussing professional issues with peers. It seemed safer to say nothing at all and to warn others to say nothing, too. Fear began to replace the old joyous feelings of freedom and hope. Distrust and paranoia followed, preventing much meaningful communication, positive networking, mentoring, and professional growth.

Regrettably, fear has also crossed the borders of the Internet as transcriptionists talk endlessly about professional problems and negatively rehash old issues without working toward solutions. Instead, we should be brainstorming for workable solutions and make our feelings known through positive statements. If we are to take charge of our future, we must toss aside paralyzing fear and negativity, empower ourselves as a group and work together for the good of all.

The face we are presenting to the world on the Internet is sometimes ugly and unbecoming to our profession. Imagine physicians, hospital administrators, and even legislators coming on the Medical Transcription Bulletin Board at any given time. What must they think?

Let's quit dwelling on problems — perceived or real — and together welcome change and diversity, find and implement solutions, and pioneer new territories. Then and only then will fear and distrust disappear because they are cowards in an environment of positive thinking.

FACING OUR FEARS

Fear can be bold or subtle. It can come in millimeters or centimeters, inches or feet, years or decades. Fear instills insecurity, anger, self-loathing, and negativity. It tells us that we must be afraid of change, off-site transcription, large medical transcription services and independent medical transcriptionists, because they might take our jobs. It tells us to fear medical transcription teaching programs, which may produce too many MTs and dilute our job market. It tells us to fear independent thinkers who advocate change and visionaries who look with hope to the future. It tells us to fear even our thoughts, actions, and words — even when they are correct — because we might be sued.

Be clear about this: Fear is powerful. It keeps people in line, keeps them quiet, and keeps them inactive. Fearful people are not dynamic entrepreneurs, innovators, trend-setters or leaders. And, generally, fearful people are not happy.

• **Should we be afraid of overseas competition?** No. Like so many other businesses, we will soon be a part of the global economic scene. Think of the potential opportunities! Those wishing to travel and perhaps live in another part of the world may someday be able to do so as new businesses evolve or by working via the Internet, using new technology that offers worldwide phone lines for telecommunication and new software, which is now being developed, that will bypass the telephone companies.

• **Should we be afraid of large medical transcription companies?** Absolutely not. There will always be a need for experienced independent medical transcriptionists, especially for smaller hospitals, clinics and physician office accounts. If during the next few years standardized health care becomes a reality, and when 100% of this country's population will have free access to medical care, just think how much work will be available. We must learn to work together and not be divided.

• **Should we be afraid of medical transcription teaching programs?** Of course not. Most of the old guard medical transcriptionists are getting very tired, and some are even retiring. We need to encourage new people to enter the field to carry on our noble work. We must be willing to look at teaching programs, however, to see which are offering students the most for their money and time. We should praise the ones that are excellent and discourage students from taking classes that we know will only familiarize them with medical transcription equipment and a few medical terms. Many of you could start your own medical transcription schools to ensure quality education. Who better to teach medical transcription than an experienced MT?

Mentoring is another aspect of teaching. We must all be willing to mentor people new to the field and serve as their guides, not discouraging them with horror stories of impossibly hard medical transcription work. Remember, most of us were once mentored by experienced medical transcriptionists, to whom we owe a debt of gratitude. Experience the joy of helping another who is following a dream to be self-employed. It's a satisfying pleasure no one should miss.

Mentoring is needed for non-novice, transitioning professionals, too. These are the displaced, the wounded and the courageous, following their dreams to be self-supporting business owners. They come to our field with all the hopes and dreams many of our ancestors carried with them to the Promised Land. We might even learn from them as a majority of these people bring expertise from their previous work lives. Before choosing medical transcription as a career alternative, they were accountants, nurses, computer technobots, marketing professionals, business executives for large corporations, and others. They have much to teach us.

• **What purpose is served by fearing voice recognition technology?** None at all. Instead, let's analyze how we can use this technology to our benefit? We all know that physicians are not likely to spend weeks teaching their computers to speak for them. So why not form our own companies singularly or collectively to offer this technology to the medical community, edit reports and charge for our services as we do now? Can you imagine not having to keyboard 8 to 14 hours a day. Hallelujah and sing a joyful song!

We must not let the world of technology pass us by. In preparation for the future, we must continue to educate ourselves about new technology by taking computer courses, learning more about telecommunication, and maybe even taking coding classes to increase our marketable skills. Just as in any field going through transition, we must learn as much as we possibly can to stay current, because only the most knowledgeable and skilled will survive.

• **Should we fear our medical transcription peers?** No. Fear stifles professional communication and relationships which should nurture and sustain us. Fear also incites negative behavior as people who feel threatened lash out in defense of their territory or against someone they perceive as "different" or "wrong." No one is a winner in those situations.

Let's not hurt one another by being cruel and spiteful. Instead, let's treat others with the respect and dignity that we wish for ourselves. Helping strengthen our peers also strengthens us and our profession. Maligning another's character only drags us down. Diverse personalities — yours, mine and theirs — make this country great. We must learn to listen to others, welcoming all ideas with vigor and enthusiasm even if we don't always agree with them. In other words, agree to disagree, but do it with kind words and statements.

If we are going to survive as a profession and succeed as individuals business people, we must step out of our comfort zone, embolden each other to be the best at what we do, and encourage everyone to bring to the table their own special talents and expertise. Otherwise, we will become as extinct as T. Rex.

SHOW ME THE MONEY! TAKING CHARGE

Your attitude can affect how much you earn, too. Do you feel that you, a skilled independent medical transcriptionist, are not making as much money as you deserve? Well, adopt a positive attitude and tackle the problem. The solution is in your hands. If you haven't raised your fees for awhile, do so immediately. Charge for extra copies, faxed reports, and extra trips for picking up work if you aren't telecommuting. Factor in your expenses for the most modern equipment demanded by your clients, telephone charges, utilities, car expenses, retirement and health care benefits. Look for more lucrative accounts.

We know many IMTs who are extremely happy and satisfied with their businesses. They are making more money than they ever dreamed possible, and it has nothing to do with the part of the country in which they live. Their success is a direct result of having positive attitudes and being willing to learn all they can about themselves as well as the world around them.

TRIUMPH OVER NEGATIVITY — A PERSONAL STORY

For forty years, one of the authors went through life mired in negativity. Nothing was ever good enough. How pitiful! She was never good enough, smart enough, thin enough, pretty enough. And, she kept telling herself — and others who would listen — that life was a living hell. You work and then you die! was her philosophy. She wouldn't let herself see the beauty around her and experience joy. Nor did she have hope or find ready solutions to her life's dilemmas. She did not realize that things could get better if only she would move away from her negative way of thinking. In other words, she was afraid and insecure.

Ten years ago, she had had enough. Her negativity had created a big hole inside her that nothing and no one could fill. She could feel herself dying from within and when she was finally ready to listen and willing to change, teachers appeared everywhere. They told her she had to take responsibility for her life; and, for every negative feeling or observation she experienced, there was also a positive side. If she practiced every day, she was assured, she too would find those positives in her life. You must be kidding, she thought to herself; but deep down she knew they were right. They had been practicing this way of life for some time, and she could see that they were much happier, more grounded, filled with self-assurance, patient and understanding and doing great things with their lives. She took on the challenge of a lifetime.

It was hard not being miserable all the time, blaming other people and circumstances for her troubles. It was equally hard allowing herself the freedom to be happy, to look for and expect the best outcome in every life situation. But she did it, and soon she began seeing significant changes in her life. By being positive, she found herself surrounded by like-minded people; people who were trusting and caring; people who taught her how to take chances and risk disappointments, how to learn from her experiences — good or bad — and how to be willing to help others facing negativity in their lives. In other words, her new acquaintances became her cheerleaders. For every success in her life, she was given kudos and a multitude of "'atta girls." For every disappointment, she received a patient and understanding ear, someone who listened and did not judge her or her actions. When she stumbled, they picked her up, dusted her off and set her off in a different direction. In short, she was given hope.

Hope minimizes negativity, allowing us to walk through and beyond fear with the realization that nothing we do is a failure but rather a life lesson. And when we have overcome negativity and are filled with self-confidence and joy, we are eager to share what we have learned and foster this same inspiring hope in others. This is definitely a better way to live, and we recommend it for everyone.

HOME-BASED TEMPTATIONS

As an independent medical transcriptionist, you will face myriad temptations: sleeping late, daytime television, the urge to "kick back" in sweats, personal telephone chats, shopping sprees, and other nonproductive and nonprofessional enticements so subtle you'll scarcely be aware of them until your business suffers.

PLANNING FOR SUCCESS

If you plan to succeed, and we assume you will, structure your workday as if you were employed in a standard office setting. One successful independent explained her action plan this way:

"At the beginning of my home-based career, I set short-term career goals and gave myself one year's probation. I made up my mind that if I didn't reach my goals by the end of that year, I would have to get a 'real' job.

Since I really wanted to remain independent, I made sure I was at my desk promptly on schedule each morning. At year's end, I had exceeded my goals."

One of the authors of this book accomplishes optimum productivity with an unorthodox 2:00 a.m.-10:00 a.m. transcription schedule. After 10:00 a.m., business calls are returned and priority business items completed. The rest of the day is filled with personal activities, including horseback riding regularly.

Some professionals begin work at 9:00 p.m. or midnight or work early in the morning, break for the afternoon, and work again at night. You probably know your most productive hours and will schedule your workday in that time period. On the other hand, you may have to experiment until you find what works best. This flexibility is fantastic and one of the primary benefits of being an IMT.

COPING WITH DISTRACTIONS

Medical transcription requires great concentration. Little interruptions can create big problems. Take control of your home-based career at its beginning and don't allow distractions to erode your business.

People: Immediate family, knowing you are readily accessible, will seek your personal touch and attention in a wide variety of situations. Establish your home-based-career ground rules immediately and adhere to them.

Extended family and friends will undoubtedly be delighted to learn that you are home-based and may drop by unexpectedly for visits. "It's okay to interrupt," they reason. "Working at home isn't a **real** job."

Be gentle but firm as you explain schedules, deadlines, and entrepreneurial responsibilities. Make it clear that although you look forward to having coffee, lunch, or a visit with them, you must do it around your work schedule.

Generally speaking, people who are unemployed during the day don't intentionally wreak havoc with home-based career schedules. They simply do not understand your responsibilities.

Telephones: An answering machine is a must! During peak work hours, let the machine take your calls until you have met your deadlines, then call back. One home-based acquaintance, whose work routine is very specific, announces on her machine, " . . . Laurie isn't available right now, but she will be returning calls this afternoon at 3:30 . . . " If your schedule is very regular, you may find this system works well for you.

Doorbells: Salesmen, political activists, religious promoters, and youthful fundraisers are just a few of the uninvited people who will arrive at your front door during the work day. You are not obligated to answer their summons, rushing to the door and wasting time on their pitch and your response. Such unexpected interruptions are inconvenient and detrimental to your work. Besides, you can always review the handouts they leave and contact them later if you wish.

Some home-based professionals post a "No Solicitors" sign at the front door. Others install a two-way speaker system so they can easily determine who is at the door without leaving their desk.

Food: Your desk is not a deli counter or a snack bar so save snacking for breaks and meals. Nora Nibbler not only slows her productivity but gains weight, too.

Television: Game Show Gertie finds herself consistently lured by fun and laughter. Soap Opera Sally is drawn to tears and trauma. Too much of either will result in poor transcription career ratings.

Housework: If you are a Nelly Neatnik, you will be tempted by dozens of household projects. If you take time to do them on a daily basis, you will scuttle your transcription work schedule. Instead, set aside blocks of time for housework and gardening. Train yourself to ignore noncareer tasks during transcription hours.

MAINTAINING THE MOTIVATION

Successful home-based professionals are masters of self-motivation and utilize a variety of techniques to maintain their professional enthusiasm. We hope the following suggestions help motivate you professionally, but we encourage you to modify and add creative inspirations to meet your needs.

- Believe and be proud that you are a professional. As frequently as necessary, remind yourself that YOU ARE A PROFESSIONAL.

- Look on the light side. Post inspiring verses and humorous cartoons around your work station and on your calendar. Smile frequently.

- Remember praises. Keep an "ego file" of letters of commendation, positive press/newsletter coverage, thank-you notes for transcription work, brief notations about verbal praises, and any other item that lifts your spirit.

- Dress for success daily. Not only will the drop-by client be favorably impressed, but you will feel better about yourself.

- Take breaks. Take regular ten or fifteen minute breaks and lunch during your work day. Also schedule occasional leisure activities with acquaintances. All work and no play makes Trish a dull transcriptionist.

- Exercise. Make it a regular part of each day, even if it's only twenty minutes per workout. Get outside when possible, away from your desk.

- Network. Professional communication and interaction is stimulating.

- Surprise yourself. Keep a list of intriguing things you haven't tried — massage, museum tour, Indonesian food, hike around the lake, exotic clothing shop — and try one.

- Volunteer time and talents to your children's school, your professional organization, or a community activity. This is a real "perker-upper."

- Reward yourself. For work well-done, pamper yourself with favorite things — bubble bath, movie, new dress, facial, mini-vacation, or time with a favorite book.

THE WORKPLACE

In order to make a full professional commitment and provide optimum opportunity for success, you must establish a proper workplace or office. A suitable workplace provides essential professional elements: tools capable of producing quality medical transcription and an environment that nurtures physical, mental, and psychological health, with all elements designed to meet client and government agency criteria.

AVOIDING ISOLATION AT HOME — DON'T GO THERE!

When working for someone else, you spend most of your time in a reactive mode, responding to other people's requests for action. As an IMT or business owner/operator, you must switch that mode to proactive, meaning that nothing happens unless you take action. For many, it is difficult to change from a reactive to a proactive mind-set, but it is essential if you are to avoid the negative impacts of work-at-home isolation.

Dixie Darr publishes a newsletter called the *The Accidental Entrepreneur*, which is targeted for "corporate refugees." She offers several suggestions for scheduling interaction with others during both work and personal hours.

Some of these include scheduling lunches, taking classes relative to your business, attending conferences and trade shows, writing for publications, giving speeches and/or participating in seminars, and even pursuing a joint project with another MT or home-based business owner. There are other useful tips in this publication, and it is worth reviewing. An annual subscription (6 issues) is $24.

- *The Accidental Entrepreneur*
  A bimonthly newsletter for corporate refugees
  3421 Alcott Street, Denver, CO 80211
  303-433-0345

SELECTING HOME-BASED BUSINESS SPACE

It is extremely important for your office to be comfortable and located in an area where you will have the fewest distractions.

A work environment that is light and airy is physically and psychologically healthy, so try to locate in an area that is open and has windows. Use draperies or mini blinds to cut down on computer screen glare. If you have worked for services, hospitals, or clinics, you know that it is very depressing to work in the basement or in dark, dank rooms in which you develop hidrosis in the winter and frostbite in the summer. Don't re-create that scene.

Since you now have control over where you will spend the majority of your day, make it great — or near-great. Establish a work area where you will not be disturbed by children, husbands, wives, pets, and the incessant ringing/chatter of nonbusiness telephones.

Establishing a separate work area is important for another reason. Internal Revenue Service guidelines for home businesses stipulate that the home office be separate from the living quarters of the home and used only for business-related activities.

If you are planning to cordon off a section of the living room for a home office, it should be separated by a partition from the rest of the living space. This can be done very simply and inexpensively. Use your imagination.

PRICING YOUR TRANSCRIPTION SERVICES

> *"He is well paid that's well satisfied."*
> —William Shakespeare
> *The Merchant of Venice*

Transcriptionists who began self-employment careers during the early days of transcription's modern era found pricing very difficult. Because the large majority of us were female, novices in the field, and working without benefit of adequate peer communication, we often set prices too low and sold ourselves short.

For many years, there was no professional organization (AAMT) and no networking between transcriptionists. When transcriptionists did discuss "business," we talked about improving our output, workplace, or equipment — rarely, if ever, about dollars-and-cents issues.

Back then, women accepted many less-than-ideal conditions without question. We generally fulfilled society's expectation that we be "grateful" for income-producing opportunities, and we avoided discussing issues considered inappropriate for females. Unfortunately, that lack of significant professional communication became a breeding ground for paranoia. We transcriptionists, fearing others might take our business, avoided asking questions and sharing professional facts regarding pay rates and income. While our silence may have protected us from others, it also impeded significant professional progress.

Today, transcriptionists take a more realistic view of career communication, are more confident and assertive in the workplace, and are reaping the professional benefits.

PRICING RESEARCH

Pricing research helps decrease the frustration many transcriptionists experience as they struggle to establish initial transcription rates. If you are a newcomer to transcription, we recommend immediate networking with other home-based transcriptionists in your area to determine the "going rate" for transcription and whether the price is by the line or by the page.

As a professional, you should charge professional fees, setting rates that correspond fairly and competitively with those of other transcription professionals.

Don't ever hesitate to find out what your competition is charging. It's good for you and your business. By being aware of current transcription rates, you will be able to set your own rates appropriately in the beginning and in the future. Never, never ask anyone what they charge their clients. That really is none of your business, and most people are offended by that question. Instead, ask what is the range of rates charged in the area, e.g., 12 to 16 cents per line.

> *"A desk is a dangerous place*
> *from which to view the world."*
> —John LeCarre

John LeCarre said, "A desk is a dangerous place from which to view the world." He's right. It is impossible to keep track of the competition with your eyes fixed constantly on the computer screen. Look beyond your office, stay on top of fluctuations in the transcription marketplace, and adjust your rates accordingly.

Ask yourself two basic questions when deciding how to generate income from your professional services:

• What should my fee be?

• How will I command that fee?

Your fee should reflect your professional competence as a medical transcriptionist who has extensive training, experience, and successfully manages a bona fide business. YOU ARE AN EXPERT IN YOUR FIELD. Your fee should be commensurate with your expertise. Clients who value your quality service will not hesitate to pay an appropriate professional fee.

PREPARE FOR THE EFFECTS OF CAPITATION

Recently a new factor has come to the fore in the contracting of medical transcription services . . . CAPITATION. Capitation is beginning to have a tremendous impact on IMTs looking for a new client base. If you haven't heard about capitation yet, just wait . . . you will.

Today, Managed Care Organizations (MCOs) are responsible for establishing protocols to ensure that quality care is provided in a cost-efficient manner leading to positive medical outcomes. To achieve their goal, MCOs work through vehicles such as provider review, utilization review, case management, formularies, primary care gatekeepers, and concurrent review.

In order to provide necessary services to its members while remaining financially solvent, an MCO must enter into reduced-cost contracts with providers. A simple method of reducing costs is to establish a contract through which the MCO pays the provider at a discount from normally billed charges. Similarly, MCOs may contract with providers on a procedural fee schedule or on a Diagnostic Related Group (DRG) basis. Using this method, the provider and the MCO essentially share financial risk and cost.

Another method is full shifting of financial responsibility to the provider, which many MCOs perceive as the most cost-effective method of providing care. The most common vehicle used to shift financial risk from the MCO to the provider is through a capitation contract. Capitation represents a fixed negotiated amount that the MCO pays to the provider on a per member/per month basis. By receiving the capitation amount, the provider is obligated to deliver or arrange for the delivery of the service required by the MCO member as designated in the contract between the provider and the MCO.

How do we medical transcriptionists fit into this equation? Simple. Since the doctor is receiving a set amount of money to care for each patient during a specific month, the doctor's volume will unquestionably be affected. The key word here is "volume." Physicians will be receiving less for each patient but, because of the added volume of patients they will be seeing, their income may remain the same or even decrease. The medical transcriptionist's income is predicated upon the number of lines/pages/bytes transcribed and is variable from month to month, season to season, and solely dependent upon the physician. When physicians receive capitated fees, they are able to control the amount of time spent with each patient. The independent medical transcriptionist does not have that luxury. We are totally at the mercy of the dictator. If the physician's practice balloons because of participation in an MCO, it is reasonable to assume we might be transcribing more and receiving less!

Let me give you an example. While negotiating a new contract with your client, you must establish a monthly capitated or flat fee for transcription services. Using standard MT methods, you determine your monthly fee by averaging the total past year's income from that account. If the physician enrolls in an MCO and his or her volume doubles because of increased access to patients, you will find yourself transcribing double the volume and not benefitting monetarily from that increase. In fact, you will probably be losing money on that account.

If you have been approached by a client to enter into a relationship to provide services for a capitated fee, do your homework. There are several factors you must consider before agreeing to a flat fee for service:

- Number of physicians in the group

- Volume of dictation and patterns (including level of technical difficulty)

- Current turnaround time (TAT) and expected turnaround time (ETAT)

- Projected increase in patient volume

- Your level of expertise in handling the account

- Sufficient staffing to handle the volume

We know of one independent medical transcriptionist who contracted for a capitated rate with seven orthopedists. This was a new account and a fee was agreed upon, which initially seemed like a handsome sum to the transcriptionist. Unfortunately, there was lack of communication between the medical transcriptionist and the office staff and the physicians in the practice. In addition, the IMT had not considered all factors that might negatively impact her work for this client and did not negotiate her contract wisely.

While picking up work on the first day, the IMT was shocked to be presented with work not only from the previous day, but two weeks of backlog work, too! Do we hear a collective gasp?

Who is to blame, you ask? Obviously, the independent medical transcriptionist, who should have done her homework, asked more questions, and communicated more effectively with the client. Regrettably in this situation, all communication was controlled by the office staff, who, as the medical transcriptionst later discovered, were deeply opposed to the physicians' decision to contract work out.

Significant information was not communicated by the office staff to the physicians. They were not told about the two-week backlog of dictation, nor that additional time should have been allowed for formatting adjustments. The doctors simply expected to receive **all** transcribed reports within 24 hours.

This account turned out to be a nightmare for the IMT — Physicians calling demanding their transcription, office staff faxing back document "corrections" for which they had not provided correct formatting instructions or client information, and so on. After several days dealing with the "office staff from hell," the IMT determined that this account was not worth all the money in the world, and she fired the client.

Fortunately, this story has a happy ending. Although the account turned out to be a disaster, the transcriptionist was able to extricate herself with little effort. Although terms of the contract had been verbally discussed, the office manager had never gotten around to typing the contract and obtaining signatures from the parties involved. The transcriptionist thanked her lucky stars, and never again made the same mistakes when evaluating potential new clients.

CHARGING BY LINE, CHARACTER, OR PAGE

Most independent MTs prefer to be paid by the line or by the page. Others, however, prefer charging by the character, establishing a set fee for a fixed number of characters. Please note that when using a character count, the rates are generally 10-15% less than when using a gross line count. This is important when computing your fees.

Line counts are more widely used because of their simplicity. What constitutes a line? Most independent medical transcriptionists charge for each and every line, whether there is one word or several. There is no standard for what constitutes a line. It is what you negotiate with your client. For some accounts, a line may consist of sixty characters; for another, eighty characters.

Character counts are highly confusing to most clients, and most prefer the straight line count or page rate. In 1993, the American Association for Medical Transcription recommended that the unit of measure for transcription be the character count. The character count unit of measure includes headers, footers and macros.

What constitutes a page? Whatever standard you set for yourself is acceptable, as long as the fee is within the normal fee range for your area. It is not uncommon to charge half the fixed page rate for a page that is only a quarter- or half-page. However, charging the entire page rate for half pages is also an acceptable practice.

When interviewing a prospective client, ask for samples of past transcription so you can judge the size of the line. This will help determine your pricing for services. Certainly an 80 character line would be worth more price-wise than a 60 character line.

Whether you count every line or half-line is not really important. What is important is to be consistent with your client from the beginning in order to avoid later confusion. When negotiating your service contract, be clear and concise regarding how your lines will be counted, and stipulate your terms for line counting in your contract.

COUNTING CALCULATIONS

In addition to determining how you are going to price your services — by cost, demand, competition, or going rate — you must also consider your pricing strategy. Are you going to base your fees on the word, line, page, keystroke, byte or character?

Submitting bids to your clients for your transcription services is very important. You must convince clients that you are offering them a cost-effective rate, but also take into consideration that you must incorporate your costs into your fees. Clients, on the other hand, must determine which service is the most cost-effective, and they will solicit bids from several services to do this. They will take into consideration that bids are based on factors such as varying units of work measure.

WHAT IS A UNIT OF MEASURE?

Since August 1993 there has been much discussion within the medical transcription industry regarding medical transcription units of measure — byte, character, line, minutes of dictation, reports by page, etc. — and more specifically, how they should be defined. Currently, there are no inclusive unit-of-measure definitions that are recognized and accepted as standards within the industry. As a result, numerous definitions abound, which often lead to confusion, inefficiency, and an unprofessional image.

At the current time, there are too many variables in measurements to standardize them. For instance, standardizing charges by minutes of dictation is difficult, if not impossible, because dictation speeds vary from dictator to dictator and from region to region. A minute of dictation in slower-paced Georgia, even though it may contain the same number of words, is likely to be very different from dictation in fast-paced New York.

Currently within the medical transcription industry, as transcriptionists seek logical solutions to transcription measurement confusion, increasing numbers are accepting *character*, *word* and *line* as the standard units of work.

There are those in our industry who believe clearly defined and easily verifiable units of measure would improve communication between health-information professionals, service owners and transcriptionists, as well as support work measurement across the industry.

WHAT IS A STANDARD?

An established measure of weight, length, quality or the like, especially one serving as a model by which the accuracy of others may be determined; any type, example or model generally accepted as correct.

Suggested standard units of measure are the following:

- **Character:** Letters, numbers, symbols and function keys including but not limited to the space bar, carriage return, underscore and all characters contained within a macro, headers and footers.

- **Word-five characters:** Total character count can be converted to words by dividing the total character count by the specified number of characters in a word.

- **Line, 65 characters:** The total number of lines for reporting purposes is determined by dividing total characters by the specified number of characters in a line. Margins may vary resulting in gross lines of varying numbers of characters.

- **Keystroke:** Strike of a single key. Measures the input only, reducing a macro to entry strokes rather than meaningful output terms.

- **Gross line:** Any line of print with one or more printed characters.

- **Minute of dictation:** Measure of access time to a dictation unit or system.

- **Page:** One side of any sheet of paper with one or more printed characters on it.

As technology continues to change, so will the needs of the our industry and units of measurement. Even those that are standardized will require periodic review and updating.

In summary, in today's medical transcription industry there is no standard for what constitutes a line. It is still what you negotiate with your client. If you are currently successfully using a measurement other than those recommended by the authors, continue with it. There is no reason to change a system that's working for you and your client.

LINE- AND CHARACTER-COUNT SOFTWARE

There are several utility line-counting programs you can purchase that work with WordPerfect. One is *Sylcount-II* from Sylvan Software. It counts lines, words, pages and characters and keeps a log and is priced around $55. The second is *WPCount* by Productive Performance. For more information, see the product reference list in the back of this book.

- **Sylvan Software**
  800-235-9455

- **Productive Performance**
  206-788-8300

Many clients remain confused about the character count; they find it easier to understand charges by straight line count or page-rate methods.

If you are defining your unit of measure by the character, there are several software programs available on the market to help you. Some of these are described as line count utilities. They are designed to produce line and word counts for documents. The macros in these utilities allow the user to decide the character length of the line and character length of a word. In other words, you can revise the macros to change the count options.

For example, if you negotiate with your client a 55-character line and the macro is set at 65 character, you can revise the macro and set it at 55 characters per line. It can also be revised to skip spaces, skip or add hard returns, count merge codes, skip or count headers and footers, etc.

With these software programs, character counts are easily converted into words and lines. You can count a block of text, a document or directory file. You can generate line count reports by directory or by report, which can then be printed and incorporated in your client billing. If you are using a program like WordPerfect you can build a character count macro.

Whether you count every line or half-line is not really important. What is important is that you be consistent with your client. Be clear on how your documents will be counted and stipulate your terms for line counting in your contract, thereby avoiding confusion between the client and yourself.

SAMPLE LINE COUNT DOCUMENT

Document Name	Words	Lines	Date Counted
22.06	10	0	6-24-1998 00:11
Brooks.H 06	344	31	6-24-1998 00:11
Bruce.D 06	562	51	6-24-1998 00:11
Cann.O 06	524	47	6-24-1998 00:11
Cristoph.H 06	582	52	6-24-1998 00:11
Croswait.O 06	417	37	6-24-1998 00:11
Fausto.D 06	584	53	6-24-1998 00:11
Goozee.O 06	457	41	6-24-1998 00:11
Hall.O 06	422	38	6-24-1998 00:11
Hamilton,O 06	467	42	6-24-1998 00:11
Kinlock.O 06	752	68	6-24-1998 00:11
Lewis.H 06	660	60	6-24-1998 00:11
Macgrego.D 06	749	68	6-24-1998 00:11
Total words/lines	6530	588	

UNDERPRICING

When setting up a medical transcription business, it is sometimes tempting to attract clients by cutting your fees and underpricing competitors, but that strategy could very well backfire on you. If a client spreads the word that you do great work for seven cents a line while others in your area are charging twelve cents, you may acquire a reputation that is hard to shake. Granted, your strategy may result in great quantities of work as people clamor for your low-priced service, but you will have to work twice as hard to earn an adequate income. Wasn't the idea of becoming home-based to work smarter, not harder?

Professionals with valuable skills should be adequately compensated for their work.

DOING BUSINESS AT ANY PRICE

Anyone who has been a medical transcriptionist for more than a year has probably experienced the service that undercuts transcription prices charged by other local services. Whether you are a sole proprietor or a service owner, there is nothing more depressing than receiving a call from a long-established client telling you they have decided to do business with someone who has undercut your price. Undercutting is not unique to the field of medical transcription; in our free market society, it often occurs in service-related fields.

Based on our experience in the medical transcription industry, we believe the primary culprit for underpricing is ignorance. Very few people who enter the medical transcription field take time to do the necessary homework. Not realizing what it takes to run a financially sound business, they undervalue themselves by undercutting local competition with misguided hopes of getting into the game quickly and painlessly. They don't network with local medical transcriptionists to discuss going rates for transcription. Most important, they don't realize how greatly they hurt others as well as themselves by taking the edge off competition. Yes, they are swamped with work for a period of time, but because they have charged too little, they have to make it up in volume. Within a short time, they burn themselves out and move on to less exacting careers, leaving their transcription peers and clients feeling cheated, angry, and bitter.

Some naively believe they should charge less because they are home-based. Well, where is it written in stone that a sole proprietor must charge less than a large service? Independent transcriptionists offer the same high-quality services, only on a smaller scale, and our overhead and expenses are much the same. There is absolutely no reason to charge (or accept) less for our work.

Several years ago at an AAMT convention, I attended a lecture given by an attorney who had been employed by a large medical transcription service. His job was to conduct medical transcription studies and to talk with prospective clients regarding how much the service would be saving them. After much research, the attorney concluded that in most cases a full-time, in-house medical transcriptionist with a full benefit package cost the employer between 45-75 cents per line. Considering that the going rate for a line of transcription nationwide ranges from 10-16 cents, we should never apologize for our rates.

In a cost comparison presented with a transcription service proposal, the following was noted:

MEDICAL TRANSCRIPTION EMPLOYEE COST COMPARISON

Base salary level transcriptionist	$ 11.50
Benefit package provided by hospital 18%	2.07
$13.57 x 2080 hrs.	$ 28,226
Vacation/holiday replacement cost ($13.57 x 80 hrs., 1 week vacation, 5 holidays)	$ 1,086
Cost of transcription station space, equipment, service contracts, supervisory expense, personnel department expense	$ 2,000/yr.
Total cost of FTE	$ 31,312
Shift differential of 15%	$ 15.30/hr.
TOTAL COST OF FTE PER YEAR**	**$ 35,048**

**Transcription service output based on
1000 lines per day @ .12 = $120/day x 260 days
(52 x 5) per year = $31,200

The Association of Business Support Services International, Inc. (ABSSI) —formerly National Association for Secretarial Services (NASS)—serves member owners of business support services through a variety of benefits. A partial list includes its monthly 16-page *Industry Focus* magazine, unlimited free consultation, and 15 discounted industry-specific manuals. One of these manuals is a 120-page blueprint for starting a business support service; another provides industry production standards which, when combined with your own unique hourly rate, is a useful estimating and billing tool.

- **ABSSI**
  714-282-9398; 800-237-1462

If someone in your area is undercutting your service, don't be intimidated and think you have to lower your prices to match those of your competitor. Find out as much as you can about your competition, their background and the services they offer. You will probably discover positive aspects of your service that give you the edge over their lower-priced business. Do you have more experience? Are your skills specialized? Then your services are worth more because you are a specialist. Plastic surgeons with skills beyond those of the family practitioner, athletes whose track records are outstanding, and attorneys who consistently win court cases are adequately compensated for their training, skills and professional attributes. Then why not the professional medical language specialist?

HIGHER FEES SUCCEED

Professionals who charge fees in the upper market range are generally the most successful, according to Howard Shenson, author of *Contract and Fee-Setting Guide for Consultants and Professionals* ($39.95; John Wiley & Sons, 1990).

Shenson, who heads his own Woodland, California consulting firm and gives popular seminars and lectures on consulting and practice management, has also written the *Consulting Handbook and How to Strategically Negotiate the Consulting Contract*.

According to Shenson, you must ask yourself two basic questions when deciding how to generate income from your professional services:

• What should my fee be?

• How will I command that fee?

Your fee should reflect your professional competence. As a medical transcriptionist who has extensive training, experience, and successfully manages a bona fide business, you are an expert in your field. Your fee should be commensurate with your expertise. Clients who value your quality service will not hesitate to pay an appropriate professional fee.

LINE RATE FACTORS

To our knowledge there has never been a book, newsletter or journal published for medical transcriptionists in which specific fee ranges were discussed. As stated earlier, people new to the field of medical transcription have a tendency

133

to undercharge for their services because they are unaware of the fee range in their area. Recently some surveys have been conducted via the Internet to determine what transcriptionists are charging, how they count lines, equipment, etc. The surveys have been published on some Web pages and are available upon request. For more information on these rates/surveys, hop on the World Wide Web and subscribe to the news group *sci.med.transcription*. You will connect with some medical transcriptionists who are eager to discuss these and other issues with you.

Pricing ranges have been recorded according to regions by postmark on the survey. Range is based on **cents per line** as follows:

UNITED STATES REGION	LINE RATE RANGE LOW	HIGH
Northwest	10-12	17-19
West	8-11	12-17
Midwest	8-9.5	16-17
East	10	12-15
South	10-12	13-16

Within the United States, subcontractors' fees ranged from 6.5-9 cents in the East; 8-10 cents in the West; 7 cents in the South; and 8 cents in the Midwest. Fees for telecommuters working for services ranged from 8-10 cents. There were also respondents working for services who were paid a flat page rate.

Although these prices vary from city to city, we feel this survey is an accurate representation of fees being charged by independent medical transcriptionists. Consider these factors when setting your price:

- **Geographical differences.** Rates vary from area to area.

- **Availability and competition.** If there is little competition and large consumer demand, you can charge whatever the market will bear. It is a matter of supply and demand.

- **Current market prices.** Like all economic factors in our free market system, transcription prices fluctuate. Generally, these fluctuations are not great but should be monitored regularly because they do affect individual transcription fee schedules.

- **Your experience.** If you have specialized skills you may be justified in charging higher rates.

- **Special services.** If you are offering unique or specialized services such as rush turnaround, after 5:00 p.m., curriculum vitae forms for a physician undergoing board certification, or medical manuscripts, consider incremental charges for the additional services you provide.

- **Overhead expenses.** Be sure to include your overhead expenses when arriving at a price for your services. New business owners often forget to include many expenses of self-employment when setting prices. These expenses include your transcription equipment, telephone, gasoline, electricity, rent, transportation, advertising and many other items. You can obtain a list of write-off expenses from your tax accountant, or from one of the references provided in this book.

- **Management time.** Do not underestimate the hours you spend managing your business. It takes time to pick up and deliver, count lines, do quality checks, produce statements, set up formats, purchase supplies and update books, to name a few responsibilities. Be sure you have incorporated your administrative expansion into your fees.

COUNT CALCULATIONS

Before deciding how much to bill for your services you must know your transcription production capabilities — by the line, page and hour. Do not *underprice* your services, which will hurt not only you, but your competition and the transcription profession as a whole. And do not *overprice* your services, which will make it difficult for you to attract clients.

Be sure to accurately determine your production capabilities. In other words, are you fast enough and efficient enough to make a profit while charging the going rate?

Here are some simple formulas to calculate by lines or pages transcribed per hour:

- **Lines transcribed per hour.** Divide the total number of lines or pages transcribed by the total number of hours worked.

- **Entire job, total lines or pages.** Multiply the total number of lines or pages by your rate per line or page.

- **Dictation transcribed per hour.** Divide the total minutes of dictation by the total hours worked.

- **Hourly rate.** Divide the total amount charged for the job by the total hours worked.

NOTE

It is important to remember that hourly rates are looked at critically by the IRS and could jeopardize your independent contractor status. It is wise to set your fees based on production or job, not by the hour.

COMPUTER LITERATE PHYSICIANS AND PRICING SERVICES

Computers have been a part of the American scene long enough for many physicians, especially those who are younger, to become computer literate. They use computers and understand the basics of word processing, boiler-plating and templating. Sometimes this presents a problem for medical transcriptionists.

Some physicians are now calling home-based medical transcriptionists to ask about their services and to request or demand that boiler-plate and macro work not be charged at the same line rate as work that is typed word for word.

This has happened to me four times in the past two years. Recently a local dermatologist called seeking information about my service and my line rate.

She then stated that many of her reports could be standardized and put into macros and that she didn't feel it fair that I charge her the same line rate for that transcription because I wasn't physically entering the data.

I reminded the doctor that I had invested a significant amount in purchasing the equipment and had also invested considerable time learning the technology so I would have the capability to put that information into macros and store it. Then I presented a hypothetical scenario and asked her a question. Our conversation went something like this:

"Doctor, from typing your reports I know that you do quite a bit of laser surgery in your office. One procedure takes approximately thirty minutes for you to complete, and the patient is charged a set fee for your work. If you bought a new adaptor for your laser machine that would cut the surgery time in half, would you pass the savings on to your patients and only charge them half the previous charge?"

As you probably anticipated, the doctor responded with a resounding NO! I then asked her why she was asking me to do something that she herself would not consider doing. She had no answer and did not complain further about my billing rates.

I believe it is important that medical transcriptionists — not physicians — determine how we enter and price medical data. This is a personal, professional choice, and if we have the technology to store information in macros, then so be it. We should charge physicians no less than if that information were entered repetitively.

SPECIAL CHARGES

At times, clients will ask for services above and beyond the call of duty. As with any other business, it is appropriate to charge special fees for these specialized services.

- **Lost Reports.** Clients, especially hospitals, are notorious for losing transcribed reports. There is no fixed charge rate for reprints; some services charge the original line count; others, half that amount, while some charge a flat page rate.

- **Stat Work.** Work requested in a short turnaround time, which obliges you to reprioritize your work schedule to accommodate the rush job, should be charged a higher rate, i.e., two to three cents a line more.

- **Faxed Reports.** Most clients have fax machines and as a result, some may request that you fax copies of each and every report and deliver the original copy as well. Although you do not pay a direct fee to send a fax from your machine, it does take time from your busy schedule, and your time is a valuable commodity. It is not uncommon, nor is it inappropriate, for independent medical transcriptionists to charge a fee for each page faxed, i.e., one to two dollars per page.

- **Copies.** When setting rates, most clients request only one copy — the original. However, some clients want more than one copy and this should also be factored into your pricing. Your final price should cover the additional printing supplies and the additional time you spend duplicating the requested material.

- **Special Deliveries.** If you have to take time away from your transcription during a work day to hand-deliver a report, you should charge a fee for this special service. You can determine your fee by the amount of time it takes to deliver the report and what it cost you time-wise in transcribing, i.e., if the trip took you an hour and you consistently earn $20 an hour transcribing, then a $20 fee should be charged for special service.

NOTE

Regular pickup and delivery charges are usually factored into your line rate when negotiating with a new client and should not be charged separately from the contracted line/page/character rate. Unless your contract indicates otherwise, a delivery fee should be charged for special deliveries only.

QUESTIONS FOR PROSPECTIVE CLIENTS

When talking with prospective clients, and before quoting a price, there are some key questions you should ask. For instance, what length of line do they require — 60, 65, 70 characters — and what kind of turnaround time are they seeking? Also ask if they have written policies for quality. If they don't have quality standards, tell them about your quality standards and describe the various services you can provide.

Define what constitutes an error, and set standards for editing and reprinting. Find out if there are penalties for failing to meet deadlines.

Ask the medical records director or medical transcription supervisor (when you are talking to hospital or clinic accounts) to specify the in-house cost per line.

If charging by the page, you may want to charge a minimum page rate and/or establish a minimum number of lines (perhaps 20) for each page. Both are frequently used, acceptable practices among home-based medical transcriptionists.

RAISING RATES

For most transcriptionists, there comes a time when they must charge more for their services. There are several ways to manage this. Some transcriptionists charge a lower rate until they are well established and have a comfortable working relationship with clients — usually within six months to one year. At this point, a rate increase is generally not difficult. For your first as well as future clients, also consider negotiating a contract for a low rate for perhaps 90-120 days, after which the rate automatically increases.

When you become more established and take on new clients — again, usually within 6-12 months — you might decide to raise rates for new clients while maintaining lower rates for older clients. By this time you will have established credibility with existing clients and you should feel comfortable taking on and successfully managing more work.

For existing clients it is acceptable to raise rates every 12-18 months with a 30-day written notice. Make sure your rate increase policy is clearly defined in the client's contract when you negotiate. You could provide a 30-day notice at the time of submitting your monthly invoice, perhaps at the end of the year, by stating "As of January 31, 1995 there will be a rate increase to XXX per line."

139

RULES OF ENGAGEMENT

If you think "Rules of Engagement" refers only to warfare, think again. With any relationship, whether it's professional or personal, ground rules must be established at the outset for it to be a rewarding and satisfying experience for all parties. Nothing is more devastating to an old-timer or a neophyte in the independent medical transcription arena than to have a new or an established account do a 180-degree turn and become an unhappy client. What causes such a breakdown? Lack of communication.

It is extremely important when speaking to a client for the first time to clarify not only what the client expects of you, the IMT, but also what you expect of the client. Are you crazy? you say. I cannot be so audacious as to dictate my expectations to the client! Let us assure you, if you are to succeed professionally, you will do it.

Give some thought to the following: When hiring an attorney, you are given a page or two of his or her practice standards before signing a contract. When taking your VCR for repair, you are given a contract specifying what type work will be done and when the work will be completed. When having clothes altered, specifications are written down, and you are asked to sign a contract. Why should our medical transcription businesses be run differently?

Rule #1 — Communication

Communication is critically important to business success. The cumulative effect of everything you say and do affects your clients' perceptions of you and your business, ultimately determining whether or not they continue with your service and refer others to you.

Rule #2 — Proposal

Before meeting with a potential client, draw up a proposal. A proposal is your sales presentation, your effort to persuade a prospective client to award you the contract or use your service. The proposal should include a description of the specific attributes of your service and working terms.

> *"Smart transcriptionists make professional decisions based on sound business practices."*

Rule #3 — Presentation

When meeting with a prospective client, you present not only your proposal but yourself as well, and both should convey professionalism. Your dress should be tasteful; your demeanor, confident and warm. Your proposal should be thorough, concise and accurate.

The first meeting can be held with the office manager, but to avoid misunderstandings and potential future problems, subsequent meetings should include both the physician and the office manager.

This is the time to sell your services on a personal level. With enthusiasm and energy, but without monopolizing the meeting, describe what you offer the client: skills, quality service, experience, prompt turnaround, direct phone-in line and other benefits. Make yourself available for all questions and offer to provide a resume upon request.

Rule #4 — Put it in writing

Gone are the days when a verbal agreement and a handshake were acceptable contracting practices. Today when dealing with a new client, make sure to put everything in writing.

WRITING A SUCCESSFUL PROPOSAL

Your proposal is the written document you prepare for a potential client in which you describe specific attributes of your service and the proposed working terms between you and the client.

Following are methods we have found successful in developing effective proposals.

• Introduction

Begin with a brief statement of who you are, your general qualifications, and a brief abstract of your approach to providing service to the client (you can be more specific in later sections of the proposal).

- **Discussion**

Discuss the benefits of using your service, how it could provide an alternative for staffing, overload, and other problem areas. Make it clear that you are aware of and committed to quality transcription and maintaining confidentiality of transcribed records and reports.

- **Defining Specifics**

List specific services you will provide the client, and the terms. Describe your transcription equipment, staff availability, method of pickup and delivery (by modem, etc.), quality, confidentiality, schedules and prices. When preparing a proposal, discuss tailoring your services to meet the client's needs and include special services in the contract.

- **Putting It In Writing**

Misunderstandings about agreements can occur so don't depend on verbal agreements alone. **Put everything in writing.** If you and the client later agree to changes in the original agreement, write a letter to the client, confirming the changes and outlining the new terms, and file that letter with the original agreement.

CONTRACTS

A written agreement — a contract — should be negotiated with all new clients. In this agreement, the contracting parties commit to specific professional responsibilities. At the start of any professional relationship in which a contract is to be negotiated, it is important to discuss policies and procedures and to reach agreement on items to be included in the contract.

A contract clarifies how work is to be done. It should spell out what services the client is to receive, provide adequate information on processing reports, specify the price of transcription and for how long the rate is guaranteed. In general, rate increases occur every 12-18 months, with a 30-day notice given. The contract should also indicate when billing will be sent and when payment is due.

Specify in the contract when work will be delivered — 24, 48, or 72 hours — and stick to that schedule. One of the authors once contracted for a 48-hour turnaround, but during a prolonged lull in her work schedule, actually completed work within 24 hours. That was a major mistake! When business picked up again and the transcriptionist resumed the original 48-hour schedule, the client was displeased and demanded that the 24-hour schedule continue.

In general, deviations from contractual terms usually result in unpleasant complications. Prior to negotiating a contract, all factors relating to the business relationship should be considered carefully. When the agreement is finally set down in writing, it should be followed consistently.

Other important items to consider in contract negotiations include: Nondisclosure agreement (confidentiality policy). Information on required transcription material to be provided by the client. Method of access and delivery. Schedules. Quality procedures. Error definition. Pricing policy, which should include line or page lengths and rate. Editing and reprint policy. Missing deadline penalty. Termination date or renegotiation date and waivers of liability.

OPEN-ENDED CONTRACTS

An open-ended contract is one that does not specify a time frame for service. If an account does not want to use your service any longer, it simply provides no work for you. You might consider inserting a clause in your contract regarding the volume of work you will   receive (minimum/maximum) and a termination or renegotiation date. Many hospitals use open-ended contracts so they can utilize the services of independent transcriptionists on an as-needed basis.

VERBAL CONTRACTS

No contract business should be concluded on a handshake alone; it is always best to have your contract agreements printed out and approved with signatures from negotiating parties. However, it should be understood that although we do not recommend them, there are legal verbal contracts, and courts of law sometimes find them as binding as written contracts.

A verbal agreement may constitute an "implied contract." That is, if a client verbally agrees to pay you a certain rate per line, a contract is clearly implied. Should a legal dispute occur, a judge could conclude that an implied contract was in force.

Settling verbal contract disputes is usually problematic because it is difficult to establish exactly what the contract provided. It's one person's word against another's. Such problems are avoided with a written contract. In a well-written, detailed, signed contract, the parties are protected in the event of subsequent disagreements or misunderstandings.

If you have only verbal agreements with some of your clients, follow up with a letter to the client summarizing the terms of the verbal agreement and asking for acknowledgment. Send this registered mail with "return receipt requested" or just ask the client to sign a copy of the letter if he or she is in agreement and mail it back to you.

FINE-TUNING THE CONTRACT

If the contract is entered into in good faith with complete understanding and agreement by both parties, it is considered to be binding. If the contract lacks these qualifications, a court could declare it invalid. Contracts are often overturned because they are defective in some respect. Since contract laws are not always crystal clear and straightforward, caution in writing and signing contracts is always advisable.

To fine-tune your contract, avoid misunderstandings during contract negotiations, and to eliminate or mitigate future legal problems, you should always review contracts with your attorney. He or she will evaluate contract details, advise you on contractual requirements and procedures, answer any questions you may have, and recommend changes that should be made prior to contract negotiations.

If an attorney reviews and approves the contract for your first two or three clients, you probably won't need an attorney to review it each time you get a new client. Use the same contract unless there are major changes.

NOTE

It is important to remember that the Internal Revenue Service does not recognize a written agreement as verification of your status as an independent contractor. Contracts and agreements only provide details and terms of your services with the client. Even if your contract states that you are acting and operating as an independent contractor in providing your services to the client, this has no effect on IRS determining whether you are an independent contractor or an employee.

Important items to consider in contract negotiations include the following:

- Nondisclosure agreement (confidentiality policy)

- Information on required transcription material to be provided by the client

- Method of access and delivery

- Schedules

- Quality management guidelines

- Special services, policies and procedures

- Error definition

- Pricing policy, which will include line or page lengths and rate

- Billing policy

- Length-of-time guaranteed rates and rate increase policy

- Editing and reprint policy

- Missing deadline penalty

- Termination date or renegotiation date

- Waivers of liability

To review a sample contract, refer to appendix of this book.

BILLING FOR SERVICES

Semimonthly billing is more cost-effective than monthly billing, especially for larger accounts, and will improve cash flow throughout the month. Although you will spend somewhat more time on semimonthly billing, the accelerated cash inflow will decrease your stress level immeasurably. Ask your clients about their payment policies. Some large companies and institutions insist on paying invoices according to their policy. Therefore, understand their payment policy so you can decide if you want to accept the account.

Ask who is the contact person for billing inquiries. Generally if your client is a hospital or large clinic it will be someone in the accounts payable department.

Be sure to record your invoices in your software accounting systems or in your bookkeeping ledgers by invoice number, date and when submitted to the client. (You should submit your line count logs with your invoice. Most clients and services require that you do this). Then record when it is paid and record the check number. Once your invoice is submitted to the medical records director or transcription supervisor, it is authorized and forwarded to the accounts payable department. It is then out of the hands of the transcription department. It is keyed into their computer according to your business or vendor name and invoice number.

When designing your invoice, be sure to include the company name, your name and title, business address and phone number. Include the invoice number and invoice date; client's name and address; date and time frame of services delivered; total number of lines calculated at rate, e.g., 1520 lines @13 cents per line — 3360 lines @ 15 cents per line; total lines and total amount due. If appropriate, add any past due penalties or payment discount policies on your invoice. Finally, be sure to add a closing remark such as "Thank you." (See sample invoice on the following page.)

TIP

Clearly explain your billing policies and procedures and payment terms to your client, and also include them in your contract.

Invoice #0123
Date: 5/17/98

HEALTHWORDS
California
1600 Adams Street
St. Helena, CA 94574
707.555.5979

To: Client's name and address

Transcription services — Medical Record Dept.

Date	Lines
5/17/95	2611

Lines @ $.13	2611	$339.43

Total amount due	$339.43

Thank you.

TWELVE WAYS TO GUARANTEE PAYMENT

1. **Call it a bill.** Your form should carry the title BILL or INVOICE in large letters at the top of the page. Never call it a statement. Always number your invoices sequentially.

2. **Include your terms.** Make invoices payable on presentation or due on receipt.

3. **Submit bills quickly.** If you have a major account, bill it bimonthly (i.e., 1st and 15th). Never go more than two weeks without invoicing. Remember, the payment clock does not start ticking until your customer opens the envelope.

4. **Follow up firmly.** Most accounts will pay on time. However, there are always slackers, especially with new accounts. Don't be afraid to follow up with a phone call if you have not received payment within 35 days. If an account refuses to pay, don't hesitate to use collection agencies or small claims court to collect what is owed.

5. **Accommodate where you can.** Ask your clients when they would like to receive their monthly invoices. If they say never, you know you have a problem.

6. **Offer incentives.** Many business owners report they get paid faster by offering a 5-10% discount to clients who pay invoices immediately. Many companies respond to a "2%-10"discount, which means they can take a 2% discount if they pay the invoice within 10 days of the invoice date.

7. **Carry a big stick.** On the bottom of every invoice, post a monthly rebilling charge of $15 if payment is received after 30 days. You may not get paid immediately, but you can be assured you will receive payment shortly after sending the second bill with the $15 charge added.

8. **Consider color.** The Xerox Corporation, which has studied every aspect of document design, reports that when color is used to highlight the all-important "balance due" section, invoices are paid up to 30% more quickly than when boring old black-and-white bills are sent.

9. **Pick a format and stay with it.** It's most helpful if the last line of your invoice showing the amount owed is clearly identified with words or phrases such as PLEASE REMIT.

10. **Curtail details.** The more details you give, the more questions you get. Include date of service, the line count total, and amount due.

11. **Find software solutions.** Decide what works best for you, whether it is a macro with your present word processing program or a specialized billing and bookkeeping program.

12. **Keep good records.** Use a system that works for you. For example, an invoice record keeping system can be as simple as one file of unpaid copies of invoices you've mailed and another file of paid invoices with PAID scrawled across the top.

MAINTAINING CLIENTS

As an independent medical transcriptionist, you will face the challenge of deciding what you are willing to do to keep clients. This is not an easy task. For instance, a client may want to negotiate a flat fee for your services such as XXXX dollars for each billing period. This is called *capitation*. The offer may seem appealingly simple, but it's risky because you could be bombarded with dictation far beyond what you are prepared to process. We do not recommend this. Tell clients you prefer to be paid for what you do. If you do a lot in a month, you should be paid for it. If you do little, compensation should reflect that, too.

Occasionally, a client whose contract demands have not been accepted will take the account and go elsewhere. Stick to your guns, but don't burn any bridges. Three months later the client may call you again, admitting they need you because they can't find a skilled transcriptionist capable of completing their work on a regular and dependable basis.

CLIENTS WHO DEPART UNEXPECTEDLY

It is a painful fact of medical transcription life that few physicians let you know when they are leaving town temporarily, making a practice change, closing their practice, moving away, or have decided not to use your service any longer. They just DO IT — without informing you verbally or giving you written notice. Our advice is, be prepared for this. Once you are psychologically and physically prepared, you will find it easier to make necessary business adjustments and maintain a happy balance in your professional and personal life.

We have come to the conclusion that doctors probably erroneously compare your business to theirs. Their patients usually don't notify them when transferring health care to another doctor so why should your doctor notify you regarding his or her life changes? Perhaps doctors believe their account doesn't make any significant difference to you because they think you have numerous accounts and a long waiting list of potential clients.

Some transcriptionists take the initiative and meet with the physician or office staff to discuss future scheduling. You might consider inserting a clause in your contract regarding the volume of work you will be receive (minimum/maximum) and a termination or renegotiation date.

There are very few situations where the client actually informs the independent medical transcriptionist that he or she is having someone else do work for them. This problem is a frequent topic of conversation in transcription networking circles. Perhaps we need to change our thinking and avoid the employer/employee mode; that is, expecting to be told if we are going to be fired. No matter what, don't get discouraged. There will always be another client needing your services if you consistently increase your networking contacts and continually market your services.

GIFTS FOR CLIENTS

We all need to know we are appreciated, and clients are no exception. I have always given gifts to my clients during holidays and in past years have had especially positive feedback about gifts the entire office can enjoy, such as food items. If your clients are physicians, you probably have very little contact with them during the year. However, their staff is, and will continue to be, your lifeline in the office, and they should be acknowledged.

If you know that your client enjoys a hobby, consider a gift related to that hobby. Donations, dinner or theater tickets, also make great gifts. Donations are wonderful, especially if your client has a favorite charity or is on the board of a charity. A donation to a charity in the client's name is also beneficial from the standpoint of tax deductibility, because you can include it on your Schedule A along with other personal contributions which are fully tax deductible. If you decide to take a client to dinner or a show as a gift, you'll only be able to deduct 50% of the cost on your federal taxes.

Gourmet fruit baskets such as those from Harry and David are fun to receive and can be shared with the whole office. Gourmet coffee baskets which include teas, scones, hot chocolates, flavored coffees and specialty cookies also make terrific gifts. Since many people are now becoming vegetarians or have dietary restrictions, these are gifts that can be enjoyed by all.

Keep your receipts organized and itemized, and for tax references, it's a good idea to note the purpose of the purchase on the back of the receipt.

CHARGING INTEREST ON ACCOUNTS

Some businesses charge a 1.5% service charge if a bill is not paid within 15 days; others give a 1% or 2% discount for payments made within 10 days of the billing. Such policies must be explained to your accounts when discussing terms and must be clearly printed on each invoice.

GOVERNMENT CONTRACT PAYMENT

Government clients can offer lucrative contracts, but beware of the fine print. Many of these facilities will not send a vendor payment for 90-120 days. You must ask yourself if you are prepared to wait that long for payment. If not, then a government contract is not for you.

COLLECTING FROM POOR PAYING ACCOUNTS

If you are in business for any length of time, you will probably confront the unpleasant task of collecting payments from overdue accounts. This can be a problem not only with hospital accounts but with single physician accounts, too. As stated earlier, when discussing your contract with a new account, be sure to stipulate terms of payment with your client. Small vendors are among the last to be paid by some hospital accounts; at times, checks may be held for an unacceptable length of time.

> *"It has been said that debt enslaves, so I feel it is my duty to free as many slaves as possible by promptly collecting all money owed me."*
> — attributed to Isaac M. Tarcher

If you have a problem with a client not paying on time, there are several steps you can take:

- Call the client and discuss the matter.

- Agree on a payment date and payment plan (which you should have done at the beginning of the relationship).

- Follow up the phone conversation with a letter outlining the agreement and payment arrangement.

If you have a question about a past-due invoice, contact the accounts payable department, not the medical records department. Be sure to identify your business name, the invoice number and amount of billing. It is very important when submitting billing statements that you include an invoice number. Most of these are keyed in by computer and your billings are tracked by invoice number.

If payments continue to drag out, communicate your displeasure to the medical records director or transcription supervisor. If they think highly of you and your service, they will probably do everything in their power to expedite payment to you.

Several years ago at a transcription convention, this author sat with a group of home-based medical transcriptionists and their husbands who were discussing slow-paying accounts. One man told about a psychiatrist his wife had once worked for — a doctor who had a tremendously large volume of work and was consistently late in making payment. Although the psychiatrist insisted he was very satisfied with transcription produced, he always had some excuse for delaying payment.

One day the husband reached his limit of frustration. He marched into the psychiatrist's office, picked up the office copier, told the receptionist that he was taking the machine hostage and would return it when payment was made. Within two hours, the copier was back in the office and payment was made in full. Needless to say, from that point on, the psychiatrist made sure the medical transcriptionist was paid within five days of billing.

Most of us will not go to such extremes to force payment, but this story demonstrates potential frustration in attempting to collect overdue accounts.

I have never withheld work from an account that was slow in paying, but I have refused to pick up additional work until payment was made. This seems to work well with smaller physician accounts. Fortunately, since I let my first hospital account go due to slow pay, I have not had a problem collecting from my other hospital accounts. I work with a delightful transcription supervisor, who is very conscientious about payment. On the few occasions when checks have been delayed, she has marched directly into the hospital controller's office and made sure the check was promptly mailed.

Remember, you do have options in pursuing nonpaying accounts. You can engage the services of a collection agent. For a nominal filing fee, you can file a petition in small claims court where the dispute can be settled in front of a judge. Never hesitate to use these avenues if the need arises.

Some clients refuse to pay medical transcriptionists until they have received payments from their own accounts. If you have the cash reserve to see you through this period, which may be as long as three months, you can probably afford to work for them. This is a matter of personal choice. Working with services that pay every two weeks, regardless of when they are paid, is preferable.

If you are subcontracting for another service, you may run into a situation where there are no funds to pay you. As an independent, you have the choice of not taking any more work from them until you are paid or continuing to work not knowing when you will be paid.

It still amazes us that some transcription services demand that you turn their work around in 24 hours or less but feel they are only obligated to pay you when they get paid. We have also met transcriptionists who have not been paid for their services at all because the companies they worked for went bankrupt. Investigate services you are considering working with, and be on the lookout for fly-by-night companies soliciting your services.

If you have to hire a collection agency to collect an account, don't feel badly. It is part of being self-employed. In the real business world, professionals sometimes have to be aggressive to collect what is owed them. After all, you did do the work!

In summary, be patient and persistent. Use all appropriate means to collect payments, always remaining calm. If you find that an account is unreliable about payment, network with other medical transcriptionists in your area so they won't fall into the same trap. If the reputation of slow-pay gets around, the physician or hospital will have a problem finding qualified MTs to take their work. That can be very effective collection leverage.

DEALING WITH A CHRONIC COMPLAINER

Few things are worse than unjust verbal assaults from an unhappy office manager who has decided you are fair game for his or her fury. Often, the physician is totally unaware of staff game playing and one-upmanship. If you find yourself in this situation, immediately make an appointment to meet with the physician or medical record director. At that meeting express your concerns and ask if there is anything you can do to help turn this negative situation into a positive one for all concerned. If you have given this client the best service possible and they cannot or will not be satisfied, then rest contented knowing that you have done all you can. If the situation cannot be resolved positively and you continue to receive unjust criticism, then cut your losses and fire the account. Yes, we said fire the account. There is nothing to be gained by continuing in an abusive relationship.

Michael LeBouef, a management consultant and author of *How to Win Customers and Keep Them for Life* (BERKELY) says you have to be careful with an unsatisfied client. "When you get a client who is never satisfied, you need to go along with them initially. But if you find that it's a recurring problem, you have to remember that you're not in business to lose money." LeBouef says it is a good idea to remind the client in subtle ways that you are taking special care of him or her. You might try pointing out that you are providing a variety of services tailored to his needs, more extensive than those for the average account, and that while you are happy to do this for him, there is only so much you can do.

BOUNCED CHECKS

No matter how long you are in business, you will occasionally get a returned check marked in big, bold letters NSF (nonsufficient funds). Most retail businesses charge clients for returned checks, and it is appropriate for professional medical transcriptionists to charge for returned checks, too. You may charge only what your bank charges you or add an additional fee for your time and trouble.

FIRING AN ACCOUNT

Transcriptionists rarely fire accounts although they sometimes should. Instead, they needlessly endure poor tape quality, inefficiency, rude behavior, slow payment, and a host of other torments. Why?

Within recent years, this author has terminated two accounts and has suffered no regrets. The first account demanded, and received, 12-hour turnaround time but refused to pay until three months later. It took almost a year of increasing frustration and resentment to propel me into severing the relationship.

I terminated the second account because the rules kept changing. One week after agreeing upon transcription specifications which included copies of all reports and establishing what I believed was excellent rapport with the office manager, she announced that only some reports required copying. Two days later, she once again ordered copies of all reports. Two days after that, she demanded 24- instead of 48-hour turnaround. Two days after that, she decided afternoon delivery was preferable to morning delivery. The account's front office staff was disagreeable and inefficient; hours were wasted waiting for tapes and transmit logs. In an attempt to solve the problem I met with the manager. We discussed the issues; she praised my work and continued to change the rules. Finally, I ended the relationship.

Transcriptionists should never sacrifice their integrity. Loyalty to an ethical account is admirable, but not all accounts are ethical. If you find yourself in an unpleasant and unproductive work situation, take action. Acquire and nurture accounts that are professionally rewarding.

ENDING A CLIENT RELATIONSHIP

Always leave an account with professional dignity and decorum. If you are informed that your services will no longer be needed, it is appropriate to inquire why. It is important for you to know if the quality of your service has been unsatisfactory. Do not, however, withhold work or refuse to finish work in progress simply to be vindictive.

Being released from an account is not necessarily a negative reflection on you or your work, and the separation may be only temporary. In a few weeks or months, you may receive a call from the client who discharged you earlier, once again requesting your services. Always leave clients with a memory of your smile and professional demeanor. It may result in future business when you least expect it.

SCANNED WORK

"Scanned work" refers to taped dictation the client has listened to and about which he or she has documented certain facts. This is called "scanning." These facts are recorded on a transcript log sheet which serves as proof of what is actually on the tape. This should always accompany the untranscribed tapes and should include the following:

• Name of patient

• Date dictated

• Type of report

• Dictating physician

When the transcription is returned to the client, a copy of the transmit log sheet should accompany the work. Be sure to keep a copy in your files.

There may also be occasions when there will be dictation on scanned tapes that is not recorded on the log sheet submitted to you. If this happens, be sure to transcribe these reports and add the names of additional patients dictated on to the log sheet before returning it to your client, making a note that these were additional unscanned dictations that were found on the tape.

UNSCANNED WORK

We recommend never taking unscanned work because it frequently results in problems for the transcriptionist. Often, when a client is not sure what work is being sent out and material disappears, the outside transcription service is blamed for the loss. To avoid this situation, make sure you always have completed log sheets to refute any unfounded allegations regarding missing material.

If a client is not inclined to scan work, explain that you require it in order to maintain professional quality assurance standards established for patient medical records. Also emphasize that scanned tapes help prevent errors and delays that might impact the client's work schedule.

As a professional transcriptionist and a member of the health care team, your goal is to provide prompt and accurate transcription to enhance patient care. A transmit log sheet helps you reach this goal.

DETERMINING TURNAROUND TIME

In order to accurately estimate hours required to transcribe dictated tapes, you will need to know how much dictation is on the tapes. A tape containing 15 minutes of dictation may take 30 minutes to transcribe; a 60-minute tape may require 1½ hours to transcribe. Knowing dictation time will eliminate much frustration and improve work flow.

There are varying sizes and types of tapes. The most commonly used are tapes that hold 30 minutes, 60 minutes, 90 minutes and 120 minutes of dictation (this includes both sides). It is important when making a work commitment that you know how much dictation is on a tape and how many minutes the tape will hold. The average transcriptionist can do approximately 20 minutes of dictation per hour. This includes time spent spellchecking, proofing, transmitting and counting the documents.

If you are transcribing physician accounts, which is the case for 75% of independent medical transcriptionists, it is important to know specific facts about the tapes being used so that you can more accurately determine your potential work load.

It is easy for a transcription supervisor to assign minutes of dictation off a digital system. If you take 80 minutes of dictation, which is assigned to you in minutes and rerecorded on tapes, it will result in approximately four hours of transcription.

The worst nightmare for any home-based medical transcriptionist is to request a certain number of minutes, be assured by the client that the 25 tapes contain only one dictation per tape, and later discover that each dictation is 25-30 minutes long (750 minutes of dictation = 37.5 hours of transcription). Hope you didn't guarantee 24-hour turnaround because this job will probably take you a week!

PRIORITIZING TAPES

It is important to ask your accounts to prioritize work in order to maximize work flow. If they do not, handle all dictation with the same consideration.

"STAT" WORK

"Stat" is a marvelous, and sometimes confusing, word. Derived from the Latin *statim*, which means *immediately*, stat is used frequently in medical settings to indicate activities requiring immediate follow up. In medical transcription, deadlines on stat work vary.

In a recent hospital survey of over 150 physicians, the following definitions of "STAT" and "ASAP" were given:

STAT

- Unstable patient or serious change in the patient's condition. Results affect therapy for the patient and results are required quickly. Critical findings are expected.

- Systems in the diagnostic service will be interrupted to work quickly on the stat order.

- Stat orders must be verbally communicated to the nurse and written in the MD's orders.

- Turnaround: 30 minutes, during regular hours; one hour, after regular hours.

ASAP (AS SOON AS POSSIBLE)

- Unstable patient or serious change in the patient's condition. Results affect therapy for the patient and results are required soon. Critical findings are **not** expected.

- Systems in the diagnostic service will **not** be interrupted. At the next possible break in sequence, the report will be done.

- ASAP orders must be verbally communicated to the nurse and written in the MD orders.

- Turnaround: 1½ hours for completed report.

As you can see from the above study results, the definition of "stat" varies remarkably. When stat work is requested, communicate with your clients to determine precisely what they mean by "stat" and when the work is **really** needed. For many hospitals, stat means one- to two-hour turnaround. On the other hand, a medical office may expect completion of stat work in 24 hours.

FORMATS

A format is a blueprint or arrangement of, in this case, the medical document. Each health care facility will have its own type of preferred format, so it is important that you consult with the client to assure proper format use.

HOSPITAL FORMAT

There are many types of medical documents that may be entered in the hospital record, but the most basic reports, which are included for **every** patient, are the following:

- History and Physical Examination (H&P)
- Consultation Report
- Operative Report
- Pathology Report
- Medical Imaging Report
- Discharge Summary

These reports generally have specific subheadings, and it is important for the transcriptionist to be able to identify these sections as the dictating physician does not always break down a report into the correct sections.

MEDICAL OFFICE FORMATS

Office and clinic formats can be quite different from hospital formats. Medical offices generally use a chart-note format, and a format for consultation and referral letters. As 75% of independent transcriptionists do medical office transcription, it is important to be familiar with these formats.

Chart notes can be transcribed in paragraph form with the patient's name and date seen on the top of the entry. The most common chart-note format is the SOAP format:

S: Subjective — chief complaint
O: Objective — physician or clinician's findings
A: Assessment — diagnosis
P: Plan — goals and direction of treatment

Another common format is HPIP:

H: History
P: Physical exam
I: Impression
P: Plan

Often, physicians will combine both the above formats by dictating: Subject, History, Impression, Plan, etc. In any case, they will have standard styles they prefer, some of which may be their own designs.

Letter formats vary from full-block to a modified-block style. Some physicians have no preference and will allow transcriptionists to develop their own style.

Sample H&P format, operative format, and discharge summary format are included in this reference. The consultation format may be similar to the history and physical examination format, but in some cases subheading will not be included and often the physical examination portion of the format is requested in paragraph form.

An excellent reference that provides medical basics and format guidelines for 27 medical specialties is *Manual of Medical Transcription*, published by W. B. Saunders.

DISCHARGE SUMMARY (SAMPLE)

Date of Admit: **Date of Discharge:**

ADMISSION DIAGNOSIS:
1.
2.

DISCHARGE DIAGNOSIS:
1.
2.
3.

HISTORY OF PRESENT ILLNESS:

HOSPITAL COURSE:

DIAGNOSTIC STUDIES:

DISCHARGE INSTRUCTIONS:
Diet:
Activity:
Medications:
Follow up:

CONDITIONS ON DISCHARGE:

_____

ANY TOWN HOSPITAL
Any Town U.S.A
DISCHARGE SUMMARY

HISTORY & PHYSICAL EXAMINATION (SAMPLE)

Attending Physician: Date of Admission:

CHIEF COMPLAINT:
HISTORY OF PRESENT ILLNESS:
PAST MEDICAL HISTORY:
Illnesses:
Surgery:
Injuries:
Allergies:
Medications:
Habits:

SOCIAL HISTORY:
FAMILY HISTORY:
REVIEW OF SYSTEMS:
HEENT:
Cardiopulmonary:
Gastrointestinal:
Genitourinary:
Neurological:
Muscuioskeletal:

PHYSICAL EXAMINATION:
HEENT:
Neck:
Chest:
Heart:
Breasts:

IMPRESSION (or ADMISSION DIAGNOSIS):
1.
2.
3.

/
d
t

> NOTE: Each dictating physician or clinician will have a specific style. In many cases you will be asked to follow not only institutional formats, but individual physician formats as well.

ANY TOWN HOSPITAL
Any Town U.S.A
HISTORY AND PHYSICAL EXAMINATION

PATIENT NAME:

MEDICAL RECORD #:

OPERATION RECORD (SAMPLE)

Date:
Surgeons:
Anesthesia:

PREOPERATIVE DIAGNOSIS:

POSTOPERATIVE DIAGNOSIS:

OPERATION PERFORMED:

NOTE: All operative reports must indicate the preoperative diagnosis, postoperative diagnosis and name of operation as well as anesthesia and operating surgeons. Some facilities prefer the surgeon and the assistant surgeons be listed separately; others prefer anesthesiologist and anesthesia be listed separately, and they will also request the operation start and stop times. In any case, the basic headings above must be on every operative report.

ANY TOWN HOSPITAL
Any Town U.S.A
OPERATION RECORD

DIGITAL DICTATION

Home-based transcriptionists who utilize a digital transcription unit and transcribe directly off a digital dictation system will find their turnaround time greatly decreased because they are eliminating pickup time entirely.

This transcriptionist's clients are long distance — anywhere from 75 miles to the other side of the United States. Transcribing from a digital dictation system can be done directly real-time or done by downloading off a digital system and rerecording onto cassette tapes. Technology is ever changing and continuously upgrading, offering better and faster methods for completing transcription work. It's an exciting time to be a transcriptionist!

Transcribing directly off the transcribe unit is like working right in the client's office. You do not handle tapes at all. Patient demographics and ID information are shown on an LCD screen on the digital dictation unit in front of you, which includes the medical record (MR) number, physician, date, length and time of dictation and other statistics. When transcription is completed, the transcriptionist signs off the job with the push of a button and another report comes onto the system.

After spellchecking and proofing documents, they are printed out and downloaded onto a disk for delivery to the client; or they are sent via modem back to your client. Digital dictation systems save transcriptionists vast amounts of time.

PIRACY OVER THE AIRWAYS

Digital dictating and transcribing equipment is wonderful! Imagine having a desk telephone that includes a simple headset and foot pedal; and with one stroke of your finger, the telephone will patch itself directly into the transcription pool of any hospital, allowing you to work at any time of the day or night.

Five years ago I attended a workshop on the **new** digital technology and swore under my breath "they will never be able to do the impossible." Little did I know that four years later, I would have that *impossible* technology installed in my office.

As with all new technology, digital wizardry requires safeguards to foil unscrupulous services or unscrupulous MTs. I had such an experience with airwave piracy not long ago. The hospital with which I contract bought a digital system and everything seemed to be working just fine. Then one Sunday around 9:30 p.m. I received a phone call from the hospital's transcription department. I was asked when I was going to finish transcribing, and the caller commented that I had been on the system since 8:00 a.m. Well, I had just stepped out of the shower, and I hadn't worked in my office all day so I knew something was terribly wrong!

I explained my situation to the hospital representative, but she insisted **my number** was showing up on their board. Short of having her send the transcription police to make sure my machine wasn't on, I didn't know what else to do. She simply refused to believe me. The next evening I was again asked if I was on the digital line. At that particular time I was, and had been since mid-morning. Again I was asked about the work I had supposedly completed the day before. I assured her that if I had worked 14 hours the day before, I would have made sure the 5000+ lines of dictation were delivered on time so I would be paid!

The next day I was informed that a service that had been contracted to work weekends only had used my number — as well as those of every other medical transcriptionist using the system — and had drained all work from the system over the weekend. Needless to say, I was extremely angry as the service had **stolen** my work. I realized then why there had never been work on the system early Monday mornings for the previous four months. This unscrupulous service had found a way to break the code and had taken work from everybody. The hospital fired the service and is now implementing passwords to gain access to the transcription pool.

If you are using a digital system and your client has not begun to use some kind of password system, please inform them that in order to protect themselves and you, they should implement one ASAP. The password system is simple and consists of either a four letter word or a set of four numbers. Each medical transcriptionist, whether an employee or an outside contractor, is assigned a different password that only they can use.

SETTING UP YOUR HOME-BASED OFFICE

Thoroughly research office equipment before establishing your business. It does not take professional marketing research to obtain the information you need. You can easily do this research on your own through a variety of methods including phone surveys, mailing questionnaires, and facts obtained from published materials.

You can work anywhere that is private, comfortable, has good lighting and minimal distractions. To avoid distractions, separate your work space as much as possible from your other living space. To separate work space from living space, you must use partitions if walls are not present. If your work space is clearly separated from your living space, either by walls or partitions, the work space can be written off as a tax deductible business expense. Check with your accountant.

You must establish a true office if you are serious about being self-employed. Create a working atmosphere — a room furnished with a desk, a good ergonomic chair, telephone, typewriter, file cabinet, computer, printer, phone, transcribing equipment, and answering machine. Adequate lighting and ventilation are also essential.

Don't settle for a part-time office on the kitchen table or for temporarily borrowed space elsewhere in your home. An established office space is very important. Creating your work environment will help you learn to take your work more seriously. If your office is home-based, you must create a separate environment from your residence, despite being located physically within it. You must feel as if you are truly "at work."

Your home-based office must be in legal compliance with local laws. Most municipalities restrict certain types of home-based businesses so check on local zoning laws. Businesses that generate heavy traffic are often prohibited from operating within certain areas. Generally speaking, one-person transcription businesses located in private homes face no restrictions.

For specific information, contact your town or county clerk and request pamphlets or other materials on ordinances related to home occupations.

Also check with your homeowners association and examine your house deed for possible restrictions. Zoning is probably the only legal barrier to starting your home business.

Your home-based office must be in legal compliance with local laws.

THE MEDICAL TRANSCRIPTION OFFICE OF THE '90s — EQUIPMENT

COMPUTER

- 486 or pentium, IBM Compatible.

- EGA or VGA color monitor and interface card — be sure it has a .28 dot pitch or lower and is non-interlaced.

- A hard disk with a gigabyte or more of memory.

- At least 16 megabytes of RAM. Get more if you plan to work with graphics, multimedia or lots of big Windows programs. Additional RAM is inexpensive, so don't let your computer's RAM level slow you down.

PRINTER

- **Dot Matrix:** Cheap, zero-maintenance, does fonts and graphics, color easy and can do multipart forms (get tractor-feed attachment if you need this capability). On the minus side, slow and noisy. Get one with a 24-character pin head for letter-quality printing.

- **Inkjet:** Medium speed, very quiet, laserlike output, color available, low maintenance and lots of fonts available. On the minus side, can clot easily, is sometimes messy and will not accept multipart forms.

- **Laser:** Great output, easily does hundreds of fonts, low maintenance, very quiet. On the minus side, this machine cannot print multi-forms, color, and it is a little pricey.

EXTERNAL MODEM

- Get Hayes Compatible, preferably 33.6K bps or faster but not less than 9.6K bps.

FAX MACHINE

- Plain paper fax machines use cheaper paper but are more costly than thermal fax machines.

- An automatic paper cutter will help you avoid wasting paper.

- An anti-curl feature keeps paper flat, especially helpful when filing.

- Fax-Tel switch call routes for fax or voice communication are helpful.

- A fax that can also be used as a copier does double duty.

FAX MODEM

- On the plus side, they are cheaper and let you send faxes directly from your computer. Saves paper, and the quality is better because the document doesn't have to be scanned.

- On the minus side, cannot be used to send printed documents such as newspaper clippings.

CD-ROM DRIVE

- Ranges are from 8X to 24X. The faster the better.

SOFTWARE

- WordPerfect 5.1 or 6.0 to 8.0 for Windows

- DOS 6.0 (probably comes with the computer)

- Norton Utilities or equivalent

- PRD + — Medical abbreviation program, around $400

- Smarttype — Abbreviation program, costs less than PRD+

- ProComm Plus — Enables you to telecommute

- Quicken — Bookkeeping software

- Line Count Programs — Sylcount II by Sylvan Software, WP Count by Productive Performance

- Medical Dictionaries — Dorland's and Stedman's
  (Book and computer disk/CD-ROM formats are available)

- Spellcheckers — Stedman's Plus

- Backup Systems

REFERENCE BOOKS

- *DOS For Dummies* — IDG

- *Windows For Dummies* — IDG

- *ABCs of WordPerfect* — Sybex

- *Word for Windows* — Microsoft

- *WordPerfect 5.1 Instant Reference* — Sybex

- *WordPerfect 6 Made Easy* — Osborne

- *Modems Made Easy* — Osborne

PLACES TO LOOK FOR COMPUTERS

- CompUSA

- Price Club

- Computer City

- Best Buy

When buying a computer, make certain you will get the technical support you need should your equipment malfunction. Most computers come with a 90-day warranty, but companies such as Dell offer a one-year, at-your-home-or-office warranty, which can be extended an additional two years. If they cannot tell you how to solve the problem over the phone, they will send a technician out the next business day. All this is included in the purchase price. So shop, compare and shop some more.

If you use your American Express card to purchase equipment, AMEX automatically doubles the manufacturer's warranty on the product, i.e., a computer bought with a one-year warranty will be extended to two years.

THE DESK

After selecting a work space, you will be ready to furnish your office. Your desk will probably be your first purchase.

When selecting a desk, make sure it is the right height for you. One that is too high could result in physical difficulties such as carpal tunnel syndrome or back and neck problems.

It is not necessary to purchase an expensive desk. Some very fine computer desks with shelves and drawers can be purchased for as little as $50, if you are willing to expend the time and energy to assemble them yourself. Watch the newspaper for businesses that are liquidating their furniture. You can save a tremendous amount of money this way.

THE CHAIR

Carefully select the proper chair. Every fiber of your body will thank you.

Most experienced transcriptionists have worked in offices where they endured THE CHAIR FROM HELL, which is a modern-day torture device with two square wheels and a back that flips you into abduction and external rotation every time you lean back too far. Avoid buying such a chair. If you do buy the chair from hell, we guarantee you a future of prolonged discomfort and many physical complaints.

If you live in or near a metropolitan area, go to a furniture manufacturing company and test-sit as many different chairs as possible until you find the one that is right for you. If you don't have access to furniture manufacturers, do your research in stores that sell office equipment.

The most important factor in selecting a good chair is adjustability. When seated, you should be able to plant your feet firmly on the floor. The height of the seat back should correspond to your lower back, where you need support for your spine. Arm rests should not interfere with free movement. Your typewriter or computer keyboard should be low enough so that you can hold your wrists straight without tiring your arms.

State-of-the-art chairs have 10-15 adjustment settings. The most convenient chair has pneumatic adjustments, allowing the user to pump the chair up and down without getting up. Pneumatic chairs can be expensive but many transcriptionists believe this investment is money well spent.

COMPUTER TECHNOLOGY

It has been predicted that during the 1990s, smaller companies will be the most significant driving force in our national economy. In such a setting, opportunities for independents will abound. To take advantage of those opportunities, you need a powerful computer.

Not too many years ago, correcting selectric typewriters were state-of-the-art for self-employed transcriptionists. There are some people who still manage their business without a computer, but their numbers are few and dwindling. Today's smart transcriptionists use state-of-the-art computers.

Since the first personal computers appeared in the late 1970s, our economy and lifestyle have undergone dramatic transitions. In the blink of an eye an "information highway" has appeared, redefining our personal and professional lives, the workplace, and the way we work. It has also been a catalyst for the independent medical transcriptionist movement. Home computers, sophisticated software, modems, and digital dictation systems have opened many new doors for independent transcriptionists, allowing them to operate small businesses as efficiently as large services. Many are operating the "paperless office" and servicing clients entirely through telecommunication. And the future promises more exciting innovations in the realms of voice recognition and optical imaging.

We can't imagine running a home-based business in the '90s without the aid of a computer. If you use a PC, you know what we mean. The computer IS the tool of the '90s. To remain professionally competitive, you must have a computer.

CHOOSING A COMPUTER

You may be surprised to discover that you can afford a powerful computer. Computer prices have dropped within the last few years, to the point where some computers are now less expensive than typewriters.

If you feel hesitant to use a computer, you are not alone. Most people who have never used a computer are initially fearful, but it doesn't take long to feel comfortable with this great technology, and once you do, you'll wonder how you lived without it. And if you think computers have too many capabilities that you'll never use, think again. You will soon be using most or all of them and looking forward to more.

Although there are many types of computer hardware available, the following is a list recommended for the PC. Remember, more is better — the more memory your system has, the more software you can run.

Frequently, computer salespersons don't understand the type of work medical transcriptionists do nor comprehend how much capacity we need in our computers for document storage. When shopping, be prepared to inform them of the facts and don't settle for less than a computer system with a storage capacity that will meet your needs.

Consider at least 16 megs of RAM and even 32 megs or more if financially feasible. This makes the system more expensive, but it is worth it in the long run if you run Windows. Many applications (programs) will not even run on systems with less than 6-8 megs of RAM. Not long ago a large application took about 3-6 megs of hard drive space, but today the average application is 10-15 megs, and large means somewhere in the range of 30-60 megs. RAM is the temporary storage in the system, just like your hard and floppy drives are used for permanent storage. Make sure your hard drive is at least 340 megs and that there are expansion capabilities and floppy drives, 5¼" and 3½", preferably high-density. Make sure your computer comes with adequate expansion slots in case you want to add a fax/modem board later.

Computer consultants recommend that you have a Windows environment loaded. You can still run WordPerfect from DOS (or Windows) but with a windowed machine, you will also have multi-tasking or background processing capabilities. This will give additional flexibility, allowing you to work in several different environments at one time.

Effectively, this means that you can send or receive files or faxes while processing documents, spreadsheets or other items at the same time. Even if you aren't interested in windows and think you won't run WordPerfect in it, we recommend getting it anyway with the thought of learning it when you have the opportunity. Indications are that future software developments will utilize the Windows environment, and it does offer exciting possibilities.

MONITORS

A color graphics monitor will be easier on your eyes. Monochrome is much cheaper, you can get them for around $99; however, a good VGA color monitor is the most effective in running programs.

LEARNING ABOUT COMPUTER EQUIPMENT

If you have had little or no experience with computers, it is important to do some networking. Ask fellow transcriptionists in your area where they bought their computers and about the quality of any follow-up service they are receiving.

Visit a local college that offers computer courses. Talk with the instructors, especially those who teach word processing, and ask for advice concerning the type of computer they recommend for your work application.

Attend computer swap meets and small business shows. Review the many excellent computer magazines such as *P.C. Computing* and *Home Office Computing*, which can be purchased through newsstands and book stores. After you have completed your fact finding, it is time to visit the dreaded "C.S." — the computer store. We **do** recommend purchasing from a computer store or dealer — especially for first-time buyers — rather than from discount or department stores.

Computer dealers are specialists and generally provide more prompt and skilled service when you need help. They are invaluable for initial training, ongoing guidance, and computer repairs. Remember, if your machine is down, so is your business.

Small, independent computer manufacturing companies can also be helpful in initial computer purchases. They are usually eager to work with you and their prices may be lower than those of some larger computer franchises. It has been our experience that small, independent stores usually provide excellent in-house service, which shortens a transcriptionist's downtime. In addition, many of these small firms loan backup units while machines are being repaired.

Computer downtime is not common, but when it happens, it may take five to ten working days to get the required service performed. As a professional, you probably won't be able to delay work for that long. Therefore, when computer shopping, find out about the system's guaranty or warranty, whether repairs will be done in-house or sent out, and about the company's policy regarding computer "loaners."

BUYING A USED COMPUTER

Consider buying a used computer. There are many computer "teckies," also known as computer "nerds," who frequently upgrade their computer systems. They then sell the older computer model, which is generally in excellent condition, throwing in software, disks and accessories at no extra charge.

However, if the seller gives you used software, make sure that he gives you all the original diskettes and manuals and agrees to help you get the software license transferred into your name.

COMPUTER SERIAL NUMBER

Do not buy a used computer that lacks the manufacturer's serial number. Serial numbers are printed on adhesive labels, which are peeled off when the equipment changes hands illegally. If you can't find a serial number on the equipment, it may be stolen property, which could cause you problems. Remember, if there is no serial number, beware!

Look for computer bargains in your local newspaper's classified ads or on the bulletin board at computer stores.

An important feature to look for in a computer is how much available software the machine will accept. Don't limit yourself in your software capabilities. Your software is your computer's real power. Be sure you buy a machine that can be upgraded as your business expands.

KEYBOARDS

There are two major keyboards available for personal computers — the standard keyboard and the enhanced keyboard. We recommend the enhanced keyboard because it has more keys than the standard model, and it is the preferred model sold with most personal computers (PCs) today.

In addition to the keys found on standard typewiters, all PC keyboards include a few keys not found on typewriters. These are keys that move the characters around the screen — error and cursor control keys, keys that let you page through entire screens in a single keystroke, page up and page down keys, home keys, end keys, and function keys that will perform special actions and help access the systems in many programs.

Personal computer keyboards also have caps lock keys that shift keyboards into capital letters, number lock keys, and more. There are also insert keys, delete keys, and keys that let you print screen contents. Most keyboards for desktop computers have both standard numbers and separate number keys in ten-key-format for quick entry. Finally, all keyboards have **Esc**, **Ctrl** and **Alt** keys, which, when pressed with other keys, access special program operations.

Most newer keyboards have function keys at the top of the keyboard, and some special keyboards have function keys at both the side and top. There are also *kinetic* or contour fit keyboards of various types. These are designed to prevent repetitive strain injuries such as carpal tunnel syndrome. Some are quite unusual so try them out before you make a final selection.

Selecting your keyboard will be one of your most important decisions, because when your hands feel comfortable and the keys feel "right," your productivity will soar. Keyboards all have a different fit and feel. You may try out dozens before you find one that feels good to your touch. Also evaluate a "nonclick" keyboard, which eliminates that constant, potentially annoying, keyboard clicking. If you prefer a quiet office setting, you'll probably find the nonclick keyboard more efficacious for you. It is for me!

THE KINESIS ERGONOMIC KEYBOARD

Unlike the traditional flat computer keyboard, the kinesis key system is contoured to fit the shape and movements of the human body and integral palm supports. The design puts less stress and strain on muscles, reduces the user's risk for fatigue in hands, wrists and arms as well as identified risk factors for developing or compounding painful injuries such as carpal tunnel syndrome, tendinitis or other cumulative trauma disorders (CTDs).

Results from a pilot study have demonstrated that keyboard users adapted quickly to the kinesis ergonomic keyboards. Participants in the study acclimated quickly to its unique contours and most equalled or exceeded their speed and accuracy as measured on the traditional computer keyboard after only eight hours of use on the kinesis keyboard.

The kinesis keyboard is available directly from Kinesis Corporation at a suggested retail price of $390. It has a 30-day money back guarantee and a three-year warranty. To order the keyboard or for additional information, contact Kinesis.

- **Kinesis Corporation**
  800-454-6374 (orders)
  206-455-9220 (office)
  fax 206-455-9223

COMPUTER PRINTERS

The computer printer is an important purchase. Clients demand professional looking documents, and many transcription services suffer because they lack quality printers.

Some clients require that their reports be printed on a laser printer while others don't have a preference. By networking with other transcriptionists, you will discover which printers are most reliable.

When you begin your search for a computer printer, look for one that will best meet your professional needs and perform the functions your transcription work demands. The most efficient approach is to use seven major criteria to evaluate your options:

- Price

- Print quality

- Speed

- Flexibility of paper handling

- Software compatibility

- Durability

- Cost of operation

If you buy a dot matrix printer, which you will need for clients who have tractor-fed paper for chart notes or if you use roll stick-back paper, make sure it is a letter quality printer. It should have a 24-pin dot matrix with near letter quality and various font options. Dot matrix printers with two paper paths will save you considerable time.

NOTE

Do not buy a used or rebuilt dot matrix printer, which may not function dependably and result in major problems.

If your work requires a laser printer, Hewlett-Packard's are some of the most well-built and require very little maintenance. However, there are several other brands on the market that are also very good and cost 20% to 40% less than the Hewlett-Packard brand.

Purchasing a used or rebuilt laser printer may be a viable option for you depending upon how much you will be using the printer. If you need it only for your personal use and a few business items, a used model might be satisfactory. If, however, you are planning to print reams of reports, you will probably be better served by a new printer. Laser printer prices have decreased considerably in the last few years and there are now some very affordable models on the market — at prices we were paying for dot matrix printers not long ago!

Another major consideration in purchasing a laser printer is your day-to-day operating costs, which can run four to five times higher than a dot matrix printer. Replacing the toner/developer cartridge usually costs around $75 and must be repeated every 5000 to 6000 pages. Laser printer image drums cost from $100-$125 each and with heavy use, may have to be replaced two or three times a year. These figures will vary between printer types and models, so check details at your computer store.

Another aspect that makes laser printers somewhat less attractive than dot-matrix printers is their paper-handling limitations. The most popular laser models have a single paper tray that holds about 100-200 sheets of paper. If you want to print letterhead and second sheets, you will have to feed one paper type manually or look for a more expensive model with dual paper trays.

When print quality is your major concern, a laser printer usually is the way to go. Laser printers are wonderful and quality is unequaled, but if your major clients are going to be hospitals or large clinics, a laser printer probably won't be necessary. These facilities generally use impact printers or request that transcriptionists modem to their in-house printer. Impact printers use tractor fed NCR paper, which has an original and two or three copies.

Inkjet printers represent the smallest market segment of the three technologies, but for some, they are an adequate alternative to laser printers. Inkjet printers spray tightly controlled streams of ink onto paper to produce text and graphics, and print quality is only slightly less than a laser printer's high-quality output.

The primary difference between ink-jet and laser printers is price. If you need print quality and are on a budget, ink-jet is worth investigating. The trade-off, however, is operating speed. What you save in dollars you will make up for in waiting time. A single ink-jet page takes about a minute to print, which is extremely slow compared to laser printer output.

Two other important printer features are 1) tractor feed and 2) automatic single sheet feed. Some accounts use continuous paper and others use single sheets, so it's best to be prepared for both.

Ribbons are another consideration. Ask your computer dealer for information about ribbon types, features, and costs. A printer may look desirable because of its cost, but the cost to replace ribbons may be excessive.

If the printer you are considering is not a name-brand, ask the dealer to recommend other ribbons that are compatible with it. You can then shop for ribbons under that compatible name-brand and may get a better price.

If you plan to print graphics — designing your own fliers, brochures and letterhead — we recommend purchasing a Post-Script™ compatible laser printer or one with Post-Script upgradability.

Purchasing additional printer memory at the time of the initial purchase is more economical than adding it later. Check with your computer dealer for more information regarding this and other upgrades.

You will save money in the long run if you buy a quality printer in the beginning. And, ALWAYS plug your printer into a surge protector.

DICTATION AND TRANSCRIBE UNITS

A dictation unit is a small machine with a built-in microphone that a person dictates into for recording purposes. As a transcriptionist, you will not need a dictation unit; your clients will use these. You will soon discover that the better the dictation unit, the better the clarity and ease of transcribing.

As an MT who learns as much as possible about the medical transcription industry, you will find it useful to have a basic understanding of dictation units. Spend some time with sales representative and learn about the various types of dictation equipment currently available. This information will help you speak more informatively with clients about their dictation units and their needs. Also, a new client may ask you to recommend a dictation unit he or she should purchase, and given such a golden opportunity, you will want to recommend the best unit available.

A transcriber is a machine with a headset and foot pedal attached, so that it plays a dictation tape back for listening and typing purposes. You must have a transcriber to do your job as a transcriptionist. There are four types of transcribe units: standard, micro, mini and digital.

At the present time, standard and micro transcriber units are used most often in the medical transcription industry. However, digital dictation units are rapidly growing in popularity. *(See page 183 for more information on digital dictation units.)* Occasionally you will run across an account still using a mini cassette, or God forbid! an old Grundig Stenorette (a reel-to-reel unit as old as Methuselah).

No matter what system your clients use, you must be prepared to accommodate them. If a client uses micro dictation, you must have a micro transcriber available or purchase one. Some transcriptionists purchase a standard transcriber with micro and mini adapters. In today's market, these adapters are not as readily available as they were ten years ago. Product representatives rarely, if ever, offer them. They prefer you buy a separate unit for standard, mini, and micro transcriber (which they have in ample supply and which provide them greater profits). If you are interested in acquiring adapters, ask about their availability for mini or micro tapes when purchasing your standard unit. Remember, however, if you purchase a Lanier transcriber, **only** a Lanier adapter will work. Mismatched brands won't work together.

Although transcribers sold in office supply stores sometimes appear to be considerably less expensive than those sold by authorized dealers of dictation and transcribe equipment, they may cost you more in the long run. Equipment purchased from non-authorized dealers is sometimes lower quality and may break down more easily. Also, you may not have local service available when you need it. The non-authorized store may have to send your machine to the manufacturer to get it repaired.

Quality is the key here. Dictation and transcribe equipment sold in office supply stores are generally not commercial quality but rather consumer grade equipment; therefore, stores set prices so it is more economical and easier to replace broken equipment than to repair it. We recommend splurging a little and buying commercial-quality equipment from an authorized dealer.

To save money, consider buying a used, rebuilt, or reconditioned unit from a dealer. These usually carry a 90-day warranty on parts and labor, and a maintenance agreement for future repairs can be obtained at the time of the purchase or any time thereafter.

> ### WARNING
>
> If you decide to buy a used transcriber, be sure you don't get an obsolete machine for which obtaining replacement parts will be difficult, if not impossible.

Besides equipment quality, the most important factor to consider when shopping for transcription equipment is future personal service. Will you be able to get immediate service and loaner equipment when needed? If you don't get an affirmative answer to this question, buy your equipment elsewhere. Don't hesitate to ask what type maintenance service is available and find out how quickly the store responds to breakdowns. Service should be provided on the same day you make the call for assistance. Eliminating downtime is crucial to your work.

Whether you buy, rent or lease equipment, you can test reliability by using equipment for a short period of time on a free trial basis. Equipment should also come with a 30- to 90-day warranty, and you should have the option of returning any item that does not meet your professional needs. Among other things, watch out for dirty or faulty equipment, which can keep you from hearing dictation clearly. Be sure to test transcribers and dictation units sold at office supply stores; you will be amazed at the differences in the quality of transcribe machines. Again, **always** plug your transcriber into a surge protector.

Plan on spending more for a transcribe unit from an authorized dealer such as Lanier, Dictaphone, Sony, Phillips, or VDI than from a local office supply store. Exactly how much more depends on whether the unit is new or used and how great a negotiator you are. Yes . . . dealers **will** negotiate. Whether purchasing, leasing or renting, start by looking at what each vendor has to offer to meet your needs. Get quotes. It's better not to buy the machine on your first visit. Take time to research and shop around before you make your final decision.

When working with an authorized sales representative, it is usually possible to negotiate an equipment price reduction — sometimes as much as 30%-45% off the list price. Therefore, take 30%-45% off the lowest list price and consider this amount the price you will accept. Tell the sales rep that this amount is the maximum your budget will allow. He or she may not meet your price but may make a counter offer. And, it never hurts to let salespeople know you plan to purchase additional equipment and supplies from them in the future.

After writing down the sales representative's lowest offer for the equipment, call other vendors and repeat the scenario. Once you have all the quotes, take the lowest quote, call the higher priced vendors and tell them that XXX company will do business at XX price, and ask if they can beat the price. Continue your negotiations until you believe you have the lowest quote. At this point, make your actual purchasing decision based on the best quoted price **and** services offered **and** attributes of the sales representative.

When evaluating equipment or other products with a sales representative, most transcriptionists logically and intuitively know whether or not they would enjoy working with this person and the company they represent. In addition to personal rapport, you should determine the company's average response time to service calls, their loaner policy in case your equipment breaks down, warranty and maintenance agreements, number of free cassettes you will receive, other freebies or benefits they may offer, and the price.

If you are considering purchasing a digital dictation system, be prepared to pay considerably more than you would for a regular transcribe unit. This is because digital dictation systems **cost** more to produce as a result of sophisticated technology used in their manufacture. As a transcriptionist, you benefit from this technology, which allows you to directly access dictation without downloading onto cassettes, handling tapes, pickup, etc.

There are several companies that offer digital dictation systems. If you are considering this investment, be certain it is compatible with your clients' transcription system. Lanier will not work with Dictaphone, and vice versa.

DIAL-AND-DICTATE TRANSCRIPTION

Another option for the home-based transcriptionist is the call-in dictation system. This is also known as a "dial-and-dictate" system, which allows your clients to dial in and dictate on your unit. There are also new products that can be installed in your PC that allow clients to phone in and dictate. You can transcribe dictation as they are dictating. Some of these systems cost over $1000 so you may want to forego this added expense, especially in the early stages of your business.

Phone-in dictation systems cost $3000-$5000, which is admittedly pricey but may be well worth the investment because this system eliminates pickup of tapes, which cuts delivery time in half instantly. Transcribed documents can then be sent electronically to the client, be hand-delivered, or sent by express mail. If you transmit electronically, you save almost 100% of normal delivery time, which greatly facilitates turnaround commitments.

Phone-in dictation systems are very effective for physician office clients. Doctors are often reluctant to invest in expensive dictation and transcription equipment. They like the option of calling right into the transcriptionist's dictation system. These are available in digital and tape systems that hold several cassette tapes.

DIGITAL DICTATION

Over the past ten to fifteen years, computerization has touched all facets of our personal and professional lives. Home computerization has changed everything from alarm clocks to video cassette recorders. In the workplace, computers have revolutionized the way medical documents are transcribed through the use of word processing systems. Just as we have become proficient with word processing systems, the computer has changed the way physicians and transcriptionists dictate and transcribe reports.

WHAT DOES "DIGITAL" MEAN?

Digital means conversion of analog voice wave forms into a series of numbers (usually 0s and 1s) that can be understood by a computer. Within the computer, the numbers go through a digital-to-analog conversion, and a very high-quality replica of the original dictation voice is audible.

HOW DOES DIGITAL DICTATION WORK?

Physicians dictate into telephone or specialized dictation stations. The procedure is much the same as it would be with an analog tape system except that the dictator must enter certain identifying information — author ID#, work type ID, or patient ID — through a telephone key pad or bar code scanner. Physicians benefit from a number of special control options unique to digital systems. They can mark the spot where they start dictating the impression, jump instantly to the beginning or end of their dictation, and take advantage of numerous other exciting options.

All dictation stations or telephones are connected to a central computer by direct wire or standard phone line. Both the ID codes and dictator's voice are received by the port board, which digitizes the voice and transfers it to the systems disk to be stored along the code, thereby providing instant selective access by any user who needs to listen to the report — just like data with text retrieval on a more traditional computer system.

Currently, reports can be dictated, digitized and listened to, but they still have to be typed. It is difficult to predict how long it will be before speech recognition technology is sufficiently advanced to be truly user friendly and unambiguous, but we think it is safe to say that most medical reports will require human transcription for at least several more years.

Digital dictation systems facilitate the transcriptionist's work by eliminating cassettes and providing instant selective access to any dictation. These jobs can be routed by supervisors, who assign a number of jobs to each transcriptionist through a management terminal. For self-selection, jobs can be accessed through the digital keypad controlling the type of report to be transcribed. Selection is by author, work type, and patient ID. Standard earphones and foot pedals are complemented by special controls on the transcription station. There are systems which offer undistorted speed control. These have LCD screens that display report type, length, patient ID, author ID, and other necessary information.

Prices of digital dictation units vary widely so comparison shop and find the best system for your needs. Attend transcription conventions and seminars to evaluate and test products and systems that vendors exhibit.

Digital dictation equipment maximizes productivity by providing the transcriptionist with many timesaving features including instantaneous playback, digital audio voice quality and easy location of dictated reports. Digital sound quality is unparalleled, and there are no tapes to lose or damage. A digital dictation system will provide a crystal-clear recording without static.

The digital dictation system is a computer with very few moving parts and therefore it is very reliable. Problems such as tape breakage, battery failure and poor sound quality no longer occur. Digital systems can be accessed remotely from literally any location that has access to a telephone line, including cellular phone lines. Dictated reports are transcribed through telephone lines by use of a telephone transcribe station.

Once you have accessed a digital dictation system through a telephone line, reports can be transcribed online or actually rerecorded to a desktop cassette unit for transcription at a later time. This latter method is very cost effective for long-distance clients because you avoid transcribing "online" long distance, which can be very expensive. Work can be downloaded via virtually any touch-tone telephone with an inexpensive telephone coupler and a basic cassette recorder, either standard or micro.

The cost of a telephone record coupler is approximately $75. The cost of a desktop recorder ranges from $50-$600. In addition, if you are purchasing a digital dictation system — a specific unit such as Lanier or Dictaphone — the cost for your digital transcribe unit will range from $800-$1750.

THE VIRTUAL REALITY OF VOICE RECOGNITION TECHNOLOGY

Nine years ago, I attended a workshop on voice recognition technology that left me feeling very unimpressed. The dictator spoke in a very slow, monotonous tone (which we all know is not the real world of transcription) and spent much time editing and correcting text. We medical transcriptionists were told that within five years our jobs would be in jeopardy as a result of voice recognition technology, but after seeing the demonstration, none of us felt the least bit threatened.

Every transcriptionist in that room knew that few doctors would be willing to spend the time and the money (at that time the system cost $50,000) to train a system to accept their dictation. Doctors are busy people and most would not have the patience to speak at a rate of 30-50 words per minute, let alone clearly and succinctly. Doctors love to dictate on the run, especially while eating breakfast, lunch and dinner, enjoying quality time with the children and assorted pets at night, calling from their car phones on the way to an emergency or dictating late at night when narcolepsy overtakes them. Sometimes while dictating, they also chomp on snacks, drink, belch, yawn, snore or follow ambulances with lights and sirens running.

Some doctors have a phobia about dictating and even though they may be the most articulate member on staff, when faced with a microphone their natural speaking skills disappear. I once worked for a physician who was the worst dictator I had ever heard, which surprised me because he was normally a very engaging and happy man. When he dictated, however, he stuttered, slurred his words and spoke as if having a panic attack.

One day this doctor told me his story. As a young intern, he had worked in a large metropolitan hospital. He'd been there about seven months when one morning the chief resident grabbed him in the hallway and took him to the medical records department. The chief resident stood the baffled intern in front of a mountain of medical charts and asked why he had not dictated his reports. Try as he might, the intern couldn't recall ever having been told that this was his responsibility. That, he said, was his initiation into dictating and from that day forward, every time he picked up a microphone to dictate, he broke out in a cold sweat and envisioned that endless stack of charts.

WHAT IS VOICE RECOGNITION TECHNOLOGY?

Voice recognition technology was developed to recognize the spoken word, which activates computer input on the screen. This ability to interact with a computer system in the same fashion that we communicate with one another is almost universally appealing, and during the last 15-20 years, the technology has been researched extensively by many firms.

The earliest voice recognition systems depended on the user to chop their utterances into distinct words, which is an unnatural, robotic way to speak. Even then, reliability of spoken-word recognition was poor. The 95% accuracy rate sounds impressive until one realizes that 5% inaccuracy means the system missed one word out of 20. Most people would find it frustrating to speak to someone who misunderstood 5% of their speech. We think they would reach their boiling point even sooner if they were talking to something as impersonal as a computer.

Eventually speech recognition will be a standard feature of new PCs. It will be the ultimate in user-friendliness. In the not too distant future, this technology will allow us to use voice commands to operate our front door locks, turn lights on and off and operate televisions and stereo systems.

The exciting future promised by voice recognition technology is not here yet, however. Although brochures from various companies promote their technology as offering continuous speech, that simply is not true. Why? Because micro-processors are too slow at this time. Continuous speech at a normal speaking rate is between 125-200 words per minute, 200-250 for the majority of doctors, and current technology is limited to 30-70 words per minute.

Until a 686 computer is built, continuous speech will not exist. With systems available today, current technology can only process speech in discrete utterance, requiring a pause between every two to three words. However, it can be modified by building voice macros and single word commands that represent larger groups of words or keystrokes, thus speeding up the process. Such modifications are similar to our methods in using PRD+ and other abbreviation programs.

In any speech recognition system, speed and accuracy of the system is affected by vocabulary size and the number of users recognized. At this time, many highly skilled MTs are keyboarding in a continuous speech mode, using faster computers, ergonomic keyboards and abbreviation programs. There are four major voice recognition programs currently available:

- Kurzweil Voice for Windows

- IBM Personal Dictation System

- Dragon Dictate

- Phillips Speech Processor 6000 or SP6000

Kurzweil Voice for Windows contains a 60,000 word vocabulary and claims a 95% accuracy rate. It works in either WordPerfect or Microsoft Word but only in the Windows format. Kurzweil designed the Voice Medical System which is being used primarily by emergency room, pathology and radiology departments as well as by orthopedic and primary care physicians.

Kuzweil's technology uses predefined templates and words. For instance, if a doctor dictated, "Thirty-two, WF, twisting injury, left ankle, September 25th," the system would type, "This is a 32-year-old white female who sustained a twisting injury to her left ankle on September 25, 1997." For more information contact Kurzweil.

- **Kurzweil**
  800-390-1234

The **IBM Personal Dictation System** is designed to be used in the OS/2, DOS or Windows configuration and can be used with either Microsoft for Windows,

WordPerfect or Lotus Notes. It provides a 20,000-word standard vocabulary that includes a 30,000-word journalism vocabulary, 16,000-word emergency medicine vocabulary and 19,000 word radiology vocabulary. The system transfers text to an application by cut-and-paste or by keyboard emulation. Instead of continuous mode, it works in a discrete speech recognition program, requiring a short break before and after each word. Accuracy is rated at 90%. Contact IBM for more information.

- **IBM**
  800-426-2968

Dragon Dictate works with DOS or Windows and includes a 110,000 word backup dictionary as well as a vocabulary optimizer. Unlike other systems, it is phonetically based and requires a pause between words. A unique feature of the software is that it "learns" as you dictate by moving the most frequently used terms into a priority scale. Call Dragon Dictate for more information.

- **Dragon Dictate**
  800-825-5897

The **Phillips SP6000** is a digital dictating system that is currently limited to radiology reporting. A 45-minute to two-hour setup period is required per author. The system offers continuous speech recognition and can be used with WordPerfect for Windows or Microsoft Word.

To whom are these systems being marketed? Mainly to the keyboard illiterate, the disabled, doctors, nurses, reporters, loan officers, lawyers, auditors, insurance personnel and researchers. The Kurzweil system is being primarily used in emergency rooms, radiology and pathology departments. The IBM Personal Dictation System is being marketed to physicians, lawyers, and word processors while the Dragon Dictate is being marketed to anyone who uses a computer.

How well do these systems work? Well, I was given a private demonstration of the Dragon Dictate system by an attorney who had been using it for 1-1/2 years, and I was not very impressed. This lawyer was very articulate but even so, in the one paragraph he dictated the system made four glaring mistakes.

I was more impressed with Barbara Grow, a medical transcriptionist from York, Pennsylvania, who has been using Dragon Dictate since October 1993 and is a true believer in the system. Through a series of unfortunate mishaps and a multitude of surgeries including bilateral carpal tunnel releases, two cervical fusions, a laminectomy, biceps tendinitis, adhesive neuritis in her neck and entrapped ulnar nerves, she found it impossible even to hold a hair brush.

Barbara's chances for employment were slim to none. She was rated permanently and totally disabled as an MT. The thought of sitting home and collecting SSI was not appealing so, with the help of her vocational rehabilitation program, she looked into retraining for another career path. Vocational Rehab thought she should be able to operate a computer with a stick taped to her forehead, until she reminded them about the wires in her neck from the fusion and expressed her concern that they might break. She also explained to the rehab counselors that by typing this way, she would probably earn no more than $19.00 a day, not even enough to pay for her electricity and telephone charges.

One day someone mentioned the Dragon Dictate System and Barbara set out on her own to find out about this technology. After gathering information and convincing the Voc Rehab people that she could work full-time with such a system, they agreed to pay for it. Barbara spent three weeks full-time mastering and training her program before accepting any work and another three months getting up to speed. Her biggest adaptation was synchronizing her voice with the physicians' voice for system input. Currently, Barbara is "typing" between 1800-2000 lines a day and working full-time as an IMT. These days instead of contending with "typos," Barbara must deal with "mouthos." With modest pride, she reports she has never had work returned because of mistakes.

Using voice recognition technology, Barbara Grow is now able to work faster and with much less physical stress. Instead of carpal tunnel, her only work hazard is hoarseness. She's tackling new projects, too. Recently, in addition to her daily transcription, she also worked with Dragon Dictate to develop an updated medical dictionary for their systems. Barbara Grow is a remarkable person who has shown us not to be afraid of new technology but to use it to our advantage.

TAKING ADVANTAGE OF TECHNOLOGICAL TRANSITIONS

Who will survive technology's many transitions? Those with excellent skills. Excellent computer skills. Excellent medical transcription listening skills — for accents, in multi-specialties, etc. Excellent grammar, punctuation and editing skills. In the future, all will be in great demand.

It is predicted that within the next two decades, the number of acute care hospitals, both rural and urban, will be reduced by at least 20%. Hospitals, especially smaller ones with fewer than 200 beds, will increasingly outsource a wide variety of services in an effort to reduce operating expenses in favor of a more "variable cost" management philosophy. Outside contractors will provide services now covered by ancillary departments and specialty care units, including their costly high-tech equipment.

Physicians will continue to consolidate their practices and hospital corporations will continue to form alliances with one another. Hospitals that survive beyond the year 2010 will be run without the current departmental system, with less management and more technology. The future will favor managers who can manage resources, particularly human resources.

The future will also favor those who are flexible and stay alert for new opportunities. Each of us must take charge of our life, beginning today to prepare for the future. In large part, future employment opportunities will be determined by how we prepare ourselves right now, during the next decade and beyond. The era of the dedicated word processing system has come to an end. These systems can no longer meet the needs of the changing and evolving health care environment.

Since longer than most of us can remember, other professionals (and the general public, as well) have viewed medical transcriptionists as merely typists. Fortunately, thanks in large part to today's excellent communication and networking systems, that attitude is changing. People are learning about our specialized education and skills. We have no doubt that once consistent emphasis is placed on our true skills instead of just keyboarding, transcriptionists will become highly respected health care professionals, and we will be in greater demand. Imagine our future opportunities and benefits. The demand for our advanced skills will open doors not accessible to those with only limited medical language training. New and exciting medical language careers unheard of today will evolve. And, we will be able to work faster with less physical strain.

We can empower ourselves by working with, not against, new technology. Perhaps we will provide voice recognition technology to our clients. Perhaps we will work with companies developing voice recognition and other technology, not only for MDs but for MTs. Perhaps we'll develop our own new technology. In the future, medical transcriptionists will no longer be the invisible profession, but a very visible and a vocal one.

OTHER EXCELLENT COMPUTER SOFTWARE

A few years ago, **WordPerfect Corporation** and **Williams & Wilkins Electronic Media**, a division of Waverly, a leading independent publisher of medical reference books and electronic media, teamed up to produce the most comprehensive electronic medical/pharmaceutical spellchecker. The latest version is *Stedman's Plus 5.0* and *Stedman's Electronic Medical Dictionary 3.0*, a complete pop-up electronic medical dictionary.

Stedman's Plus 5.0 spellchecker contains more than 350,000 medical, pharmaceutical, surgical/surgical equipment, and biotechnology terms. It is compatible with all versions of WordPerfect 5.1 and up, MS Word, AmiPro, Word Pro, and MacIntosh and is available on diskette and CD-ROM on DOS, Windows and MacIntosh platforms.

Stedman's Electronic Medical Dictionary contains more than 100,000 medical and pharmaceutical words and is available on diskette and CD-ROM on DOS, Windows and MacIntosh platforms. It works seamlessly with WordPerfect, AmiPro, MS Word, WordPro, and Mac.

OTHER COMPUTER HARDWARE AND SOFTWARE

Other office necessities include computer cables, additional surge protectors (surge protectors do go bad), diskettes and diskette filing cases, antistatic computer cleaning cloths, chair mats, pads, monitor screen to reduce glare, foot rests, computer paper, additional toner cartridges, extra ribbons for dot matrix printers, printer paper, plastic covers for all components, and a switch/box if you are using more than one printer or computer. All of the above can be purchased at your local computer store.

SOFTWARE BY THE TRUCKLOADS

Today, there are countless software programs available, but the most popular by use and demand are the following:

• Microsoft DOS (MS DOS) — try to purchase the most recent version.

- WordPerfect (WP) for DOS is one of the most popular, but Word for Windows is being aggressively promoted. It is difficult convincing a die-hard DOS user to switch to a windows environment, but this appears to be what the future holds for our industry as well as many others. It's not as bad as it seems. Having worked in both environments, and as a former die-hard DOSsie, I have become spoiled by many windows enhancements. WordPerfect for Windows is also being utilized.

- Utilities Program: *Norton Utilities*, *PC Tools*, and *Central Pointe* provide shell and data recovery utilities, hard disk backup and restore, disk compression and desk top organizers.

- Bookkeeping Software: *Quicken* or *Quick Books* by Intuit, *Peachtree Accounting*, and *ACCPack*. The latter two are more sophisticated and expensive accounting software programs.

- *Quicken*, which seems to be most popular, costs about $49 and will save you countless bookkeeping hours. It is very easy to learn and will make completing your tax return a breeze.

- Legal Software: *It's Legal* is a program that produces boiler plate legal agreements and contracts, which are useful in writing client agreements.

WORDPERFECT 5.1 VERSUS WINDOWS

The fastest word processor on the market is still Wordperfect 5.1+ (for DOS) running on anything 386 or higher. The second fastest word processor on the market is WordPerfect 6.0 or 6.1 for DOS running in text (not graphics) mode on a 486 or higher CPU. These are also the most economical versions available and have proven to be among the most tried and true, bulletproof and bug-free programs available. Another reason that MTs and services are reluctant to change from this environment is because DOS is such a stable platform.

If you are working with Win95 and Word, the faster processors such as a Pentium will make large programs such as this run faster. WIN95 can run acceptably fast on a 486 if you run only one major application and you have lots of memory, at least 32 MB. If you really want to upgrade you might consider a 200 MHz Pentium processor with MMX technology.

REGISTER SOFTWARE

Fill out all registration and warranty cards that come with new equipment and software. As a registered software user (WordPerfect, Quicken, etc.) you will readily obtain online help and service. You will also be notified by the company when software upgrades are released, allowing you to upgrade your system at bargain prices.

You can spend a small fortune on computer software so shop wisely, networking with other transcriptionists and people in the business community to see what works well for them and their home computers. Read *Home Office Computing*, which lists best selling software in each issue, and research some of the other computer and software publications for updates on products.

NEVER, NEVER, NEVER!
BORROW SOMEONE ELSE'S SOFTWARE

Only buy new, unused software. It is against the law to copy software, because it is copyrighted. Some software is copy-protected, which makes it impossible or extremely difficult to copy. Additionally, according to the National Computer Security Association (NCSA), "borrowed" software sometimes contains a virus, which is put there by the manufacturer to deter copying. If a virus gets into your computer you will certainly have serious software problems. Use *Norton Utilities, DOS or PC Tools* to check for a virus.

COMPUTER AIDED TRANSCRIPTION (CAT) TECHNOLOGY — OR HOW YOU, TOO, CAN TYPE 225 WORDS A MINUTE

225 WORDS A MINUTE! This sounds like a sales pitch, doesn't it? Are you wondering how this is possible and thinking about how much you could earn if you could type this fast?

It's not a gimmick, and it is being done every day by court reporters all around the world. Now it is possible for medical transcriptionists to achieve the same typing speed by using machine shorthand and Computer Aided Transcription (CAT) technology.

Shorthand, of course, has been around for centuries. The mechanical device that is used to write shorthand is called the stenotype machine. It allows the simultaneous depression of multiple keys, and entire words can be written with one stroke. In machine shorthand theory, single letters and abbreviations are used to represent words; and students are taught to write words phonetically. For example, "Judge" is written J-U-J.

The keyboard of the stenotype machine has 23 keys. Since vowels come in the middle of words, the vowel keys are in the middle of the keyboard, and consonants are on either end. Letter combinations represent long and short vowels, and letters of the alphabet. Not all alphabet keys are present. There is no letter "C", for example. A "K" is used for the sound of the "C" in *car*; and an "S" for the soft "S" sound in *cease*.

Machine shorthand, as you probably surmise, is another language. The shorthand writer hears an English word, mentally and physically converts that word to shorthand, and presses the appropriate keys. When desired, the writer can read the shorthand, translate it, and either read or write it in English.

Computer Aided Translation software (CAT) does the same thing. After an electronic copy of the machine shorthand stroke is transferred to the computer, by modem connection or disk, the computer looks up each word in a shorthand-to-English dictionary and translates the words into English. The dictionary is created, a word at a time, by deliberately making dictionary entries from a list of words, or after the translation process, and untranslated words are translated and entered into the dictionary by the computer operator. As the dictionary grows, more and more complete translations are possible.

Some specialized CAT programs allow functions normally performed on a computer keyboard (block, move, delete, underline, etc.) to be performed on the stenotype keyboard, and most CAT programs also allow spellchecking with external medical/legal dictionaries. Generically described as "rapid text entry" programs, they are essentially high speed word-processing programs that use a stenotype keyboard instead of a computer keyboard. Medical transcriptionists will probably favor the program that uses WordPerfect for word processing.

Advantages of CAT technology: increased words-per-minute speeds; reduction in misspellings because the dictionary can convert "slop" shorthand strokes to correctly spelled English words; fewer repetitive motions because entire words can be written in one stroke; ergonomically satisfactory keyboard position because the shorthand machine sits on an adjustable tripod that can be positioned many ways.

Disadvantages of CAT technology: length of time required to become proficient at writing machine shorthand at high speeds; and equipment costs. CAT software prices average $3000-$5000; computerized shorthand machines average $2500 (although one CAT firm makes a $200 add-on device for the noncomputerized steno machine that would suffice for medical transcriptionists.

Most modern CAT systems will produce an ASCII transcript that can be imported into WordPerfect. The proficient WP user can then convert the document into the desired format. The most modern versions allow real-time translation, which can be used for captioning for the hearing impaired. This same capability allows for immediate onscreen correction or translation of the word just written.

CAT technology is made specifically to capture the spoken word, which is what court reporters and medical transcriptionists work with. Mispronunciations, inaudibles, bad grammar, and all other difficulties of transcribing the spoken word will still plague CAT users.

CAT technology is probably best suited to the many students of machine shorthand who are unable to achieve the 225 wpm speed required for court reporting jobs. (The dropout rate averages 95%). These students could use the skills and speeds they have acquired by using CAT technology for word processing and/or medical transcribing. (Of course, they would have to learn medical terminology and English skills as well.) Indeed, some court reporting schools are now teaching medical transcription using CAT technology. Call or write for more information on CAT technology.

- **Stenoware, Inc.** (makers of IntelliCat software)
  12337 Jones Road, Suite 200
  Houston, Texas 77070
  800-328-8220

TELEPHONE ANSWERING MACHINES

A telephone answering machine is vital to every home-based medical transcription business. It saves you time and money, because it is not time- or cost-effective for you to answer the telephone every time it rings. By having a telephone answering machine, you can monitor calls, immediately responding to those that are urgent or those from clients or potential clients. Non-urgent calls can be returned later.

There are a variety of answering machines on the market and brand-name should not be your main consideration. The key features to look for in answering machines are the following:

- A voice-activated, unlimited incoming message
  (This machine can also be used for stat dictation)

- Remote message retrieval capability

- Capability to change the outgoing message from a remote phone

- Recording of time, date, and number of calls

Low-end units cost as little as $50-$75 but lack voice activation, remote access, and some other features. Machines in the $75-$100 range usually include the extra features.

TELEPHONE COMPANY VOICE-MAIL SERVICE

Most local telephone companies now offer sophisticated voice mail that gives a small or home-based business the appearance of being a larger, more professional entity. The voice response sounds very professional, unlike some tinny-sounding tape-based answering units, and with this service, you also guarantee callers won't receive a busy signal. BellSouth's MemoryCall service handles up to six calls simultaneously even though you have only one phone number and one voice mailbox.

Some telephone companies charge a flat rate with unlimited usage for voice-mail service; others charge per minute beyond a fixed amount and for multiple mailboxes. For example, Bell Atlantic charges $8.50 per minute for a single mailbox with 45 minutes of storage and $10.50 per month for one mailbox that you can divide into eight submailboxes. This is an excellent alternative as the calling party never gets a busy signal and you don't have to interrupt one call to accept another as you do with call waiting.

If you already use local phone company voice mail, look into having the voice mailbox automatically notify your pager when a call comes in. For $10-20 per month you will be able to get back to your clients quickly. Your callers will appreciate being able to leave messages knowing you will pick them up and respond promptly.

If you only have one phone line, how can you tell if an incoming call is business or personal? With a distinctive ringing service, which you can purchase. Bell Atlantic offers *IdentaRing,* a system that allows you to add two additional dependent numbers to an existing phone line. Each phone number has a distinctive ring pattern — one long for the primary number, and a short-long-short or two shorts for the dependent numbers. With this system, it's easy to determine which number was dialed.

With the addition of a call-routing device, a switch that automatically identifies each ring pattern and directs the call to the appropriate telephone device, you can have a phone, answering machine, fax machine, or fax/data modem for a particular number. Call-routing devices are easy to install and cost from $50-$100. Contact your local phone company for information on this type service. The wonderful voice mail and fax-on-demand systems available today can make your home office sound like the corporate headquarters of YOU, INCORPORATED.

DIGITAL TELEPHONE ANSWERING SYSTEMS

Digital telephone answering systems are now available that give small businesses the same professional communications enjoyed by Fortune 500 companies. These digital systems answer your phone and route calls to one of four personal mailboxes, three announcement mailboxes or fax PC. One such product is called *FRIDAY, Advance Digital Answering System* by Bogen Communications. Contact Bogen for more information.

- **Bogen Communications, Inc**.
  800-456-5513

MODEMS

Consider purchasing a modem, either an internal modem or an external modem. Investigate the pros and cons of both to determine which you prefer. Both types connect to your computer via the telephone line and allow you to communicate with other computers and online data bases.

SAFETY THROUGH SURGE PROTECTORS

Electrical surges can destroy valuable data, so take extra precautions to protect your computer system by installing surge protectors, a cost-effective step that will prevent damage to computer hardware and software.

When one of the authors of this book bought her first computer, she learned about surge protectors the hard way. One day during a lightning storm, the lights flickered for just a moment, but in that brief power surge an entire half-day's work — about thirty pages — was lost. It was a devastating and needless loss.

Surge protectors/surge suppressors protect your computer and peripherals from sudden variations in electrical current. Underwriters Laboratory has established an objective rating guide for surge protectors. Look for the UL 1449 sticker on any surge protector you plan to purchase.

Surge protectors are not totally fail-safe, however. Experts caution against relying on any surge protector during a thunderstorm, since "lightning can arc across open contacts and do extensive damage to your computer."

Surge protectors (or surge suppressors) protect your equipment from power shortages and outages (not enough power) and power surges (too much power). We recommend that you purchase the best surge protector you can afford, with a built-in AC filter, and we cannot overemphasize the importance of plugging all computer and office equipment into surge protectors.

If you have a modem, it is suggested that you disconnect either the incoming telephone line or cable during a thunder storm. A lightning strike to the telephone line will zap your computer.

When setting up your home office, consider having an electric circuit dedicated to your computer and other electrical office equipment. It is hard on electronics to suffer power ebbs when a dishwasher, oven or other appliance kicks on. It's best to have computers on a circuit used only for low power consumers such as lights.

COMPUTER BACKUP

Every home-based medical transcriptionist should have a backup in case of a breakdown. It isn't necessary to buy a new piece of equipment for this purpose. If you have upgraded your existing computer to a faster, higher-powered machine, save that older computer for your backup. Although it may be somewhat slower, you'll be able to continue working. Believe us, there is nothing worse than an office full of work and no equipment with which to transcribe it!

TIP

Make backup copies of new software and store original diskettes in your safe, in a fireproof file cabinet or in your safe-deposit box at the bank.

BACKUP SYSTEMS

It is simply good business sense to protect your files by copying or transferring them regularly to removable tape cartridges or zip disks that can be stored in a separate location outside the office or in a locked fireproof safe.

While most computers have a backup system on the hard drive, if the entire system crashes, you'll lose that too. Floppy disks provide some backup protection, but their storage capacity is limited.

The newest tape backup systems compress data so you can transfer an entire database onto a single cartridge. For under $200 you can buy a basic backup system to create a taped library of all your files. More sophisticated, higher-priced version let you make selective backups or schedule unattended backups automatically, perhaps while you are out of the office or at night.

A tape backup drive operates much like a tape recorder, reading your files and copying them onto a tape. A special cassette tape, which must be pre-formatted, is inserted into the drive's slot; onscreen programs offer several options to choose from, including automated daily backup, backing up only selected files, scheduling after-hours backup and backing up files in the background while you work on other applications.

Several easy-to-use, easy-to-install tape backup devices are available for small business budgets. The internal models are sold with mounting hardware to fit into one of the existing 3.5.-inch or 5.25-inch floppy disk bays in your computer. External, stand-alone models are about the size of a hardcover book and plug into either a printer port or a Small Computer System Interface (SCSI) port at the back of the computer.

Most external backup drives have extra ports so printers can be connected to them; this feature, called a "printer-pass-through," reduces extra cables and ports needed. External drives are also a good solution if you want to backup multiple PCs with a single drive or for laptop computer backup and file transfer.

If you have a PC, your backup drive will connect to a floppy bay disk or your parallel port. Tape backup systems come with Windows or DOS software that is easy to install.

The advantages of a tape backup drive are that you can archive data, leaving more space on your computer's hard drive or use the backup system as an extra hard drive. Files can be transferred easily from one computer to another, enabling you to share removable tapes or take them on the road to use with your laptop. Most backup systems not only record files, but can also hold software programs, so rebuilding after a computer crash needn't mean refeeding dozens of separate disks.

When shopping for a tape backup system make sure the drive and the tapes you purchase are fully compatible with your computer. If you are short on ports, get a system with a printer pass-through. If you have hundreds of documents, look for a device with a cataloguing feature which allows you to create a directory of files for easy reference. Make sure the system has a "compare" feature so you can check the data on your tape against the data you have just copied. Be sure storage capacity and speed are sufficient for your present and future needs. Most manufacturers offer several models with different storage and speed capacities.

INTERACTIVE TECHNICAL SUPPORT

Technology is great, but it is definitely more beneficial and user-friendly when it is backed up by that "human touch," which in this case translates to "technical support." There are a multitude of high-tech ways to find answers to technical questions, but, unfortunately, they are not always reliable. Often, techs don't understand the medical transcriptionist's needs. And sometimes trying to get a live technician on the phone can take more time than building your own computer from scratch! Calls to technical support lines often result in hours spent on hold or worse, nothing but busy signals. Still, for desperate occasions, interfacing with a computer technician can be a lifesaver.

Most major computer and software companies offer technical support — often for a fee — and provide toll-free numbers for customer calls. Check your computer or software users manual or call your computer/software distributor for tech support numbers for IBM, Compaq, Hewlett-Packard, ACER, Dell, Gateway 2000, Packard Bell and others.

FAX MACHINES

Almost all home-based medical transcription businesses have purchased or are in the process of purchasing fax machines. This terrific technology is now reasonably priced and has become a standard office feature. There are many advantages to investing in a fax machine for your office.

A fax machine increases efficiency and profitability by providing 24-hour access to your business. It saves time and money over express mail, postal services or courier while improving your response time. It allows you to transmit documents across the street or across the world, and it reduces miscommunication by immediately transmitting hard copies of important documents.

A fax machine also enhances your professional business image. Today, business and nonbusiness contacts alike expect professionals to have fax machines. When business associates have something to send to you, more often than not they'll want to send it immediately via fax machine.

To further enhance your professional image and prevent great frustration for others, get a fax that responds automatically to incoming fax signals. Other professionals do not enjoy making one phone call to ask you to turn on your fax machine and another phone call to send the fax. And, if you aren't home when the first call comes in, additional calls are required. Telephone tag is especially irritating when someone urgently needs to send a fax. We know some business people who, after experiencing much frustration with this type of system, simply stop sending faxes. That can hurt business!

If you don't own a fax machine, you should have ready access to one, perhaps through a local copy center or drug store. Sending and receiving documents at a public location usually costs $1-$2 per page and is an expense the transcriptionist must bear. However, copy-center faxing is not ideal, and we recommend investing in a fax machine. It will save you much time and many dollars.

To get the most out of your fax machine, include your fax number on your business cards, letterhead, stationery, purchase orders, invoices, print and advertising. Use your fax for sending and receiving documents after hours, and encourage those who do business with you to fax rather than mail documents. For instance, you could have patient IDs, log sheets or tape logs faxed to you on a daily basis, which is especially helpful if your clients are long distance.

The fax has nothing to do with your computer, although it can be installed as a fax board in your computer or purchased as a stand-alone fax unit. There is now fax software that works on a dedicated PC with one fax board/one phone line and several network connections. Today's fax software allows you to convert and receive documents into files.

The issue of internal vs. external fax modems parallels the advantages and disadvantages cited for internal and external data modems. In brief, an internal modem requires less space since it is placed in the computer. Due to its internal location it does not require a separate power supply. However, there are no visible indicator lights like those on an external modem, and for some transcriptionists, indicator lights provide a comfort zone they need. Teckies even claim ability to *interpret* the indicator lights.

An external modem does require some desk top space and a power cord, but on the plus side, it is easy to install, is highly portable, and can be used with more than one computer. Ultimately, the internal versus the external issue is largely a matter of individual preference.

NOTE

Some computer consultants do not encourage installing a fax board in your computer but recommend getting a stand-alone fax because earlier modems have been known to damage PC hard drives.

Once you get a FAX machine, you'll wonder how you ever did without it.

ADVANTAGES OF OWNING A FAX MACHINE

• It can increase efficiency and profitability by providing 24-hour access.

• It saves time and money over express mail, postal service and courier while improving response time.

• It allows you to transmit documents across the street or across the world.

• It reduces miscommunications by having agreements/terms and other material in writing.

• It enhances the professional image of your business.

To get the most out of your fax machine:

• Include your fax number on your business cards, letterhead, stationery, purchase orders, invoices, print advertising, etc.

• Use your fax in place of first class or express mail.

• Use your fax for taking or sending documents after hours.

• Encourage those who do business with you to fax rather than mail documents.

MISCELLANEOUS SUPPLIES

Aside from your printed materials, equipment, computer hardware, software and furniture, you will need a calculator, adding machine, copy paper, printer paper, postage scale, tape, sticky notes, file folders, labels, binders, telephone message pads, pens, pencils, paper clip, stapler, etc. You may be tempted to buy everything in the office supply store but remember, office supplies add up fast so don't overbuy.

CALENDARS

Scheduling and short-range planning are key elements of successful home-based businesses. Every transcriptionist needs an efficient calendar to organize her life. Month-at-a-glance or three-to-four month wall-mounted calendars are very effective time-management tools.

There are some great computer programs, such as *WordPerfect Office Timeslips*, that offer calendars and appointment setups.

Whatever type calendar you choose, review it frequently. Scan not only the day ahead, but the upcoming week as well. This will remind you of regular monthly meetings, appointments, holidays and vacation schedules (for those hiring outsourcers), as well as scheduled time off, business lunches, etc. With a chart of future activities, you are less likely to overcommit yourself or make promises you can't keep.

RESERVE CAPITAL

At the start-up of your business, you can anticipate that no money will come in for at least six weeks. We recommend having reserve capital for unexpected expenses during this time and shortly thereafter. Be prepared to cover payments for rent, gas, electricity and telephone, as well as money for supplies, for at least four months. Under-capitalization is one of the main reasons new businesses fail within the first year. If you do not have enough reserve capital, perhaps you should consider getting a business loan.

When you are the business owner and have financial obligations, everyone else gets paid first — the phone company, the landlord, subcontractors, and employees. If you are like most independents, there will be times when you won't even be able to take a salary. Work volumes will probably fluctuate and your business may go through slow periods. Monitor your situation regularly. If you are not making enough money during the "good times" to make ends meet, you are probably not charging enough.

THE COST OF RUNNING A PERSONAL COMPUTER

A recent study measuring the energy used by different systems under test conditions found the wattage listed on the nameplate of each component is conservative. Actual electricity use is much lower. Costs range from ½ to 3½ cents per hour, depending upon what kind of components you have and how hard they're working.

Of the personal computers with monitors studied, use ranged from 30-210 watts. In a standby mode, dot-matrix, daisy wheel, and ink-jet printers used 3-45 watts, while typical laser printers use 40-130 watts. The study also showed that printers may use two to three times this much when printing.

ESCAPING DATA DISASTER

Insurers may cover the restoration of lost files if disaster strikes, but they still haven't come up with a way to replace lost business while you're re-creating those files.

Although there is no way to completely protect yourself from catastrophes, here are some strategies to safeguard valuable information.

* **Secure a second copy.** Backing up isn't hard to do, so make it part of your daily routine. Besides your database, creative works and billing records, other items that need duplication include investment documents, contracts, supplier lists and receipts.

* **Create an inventory list.** Most office components have visible serial numbers. Record them with such programs as Proof 2.0 (Fusion Software, 800-856-8566; Win; $9.95), print out two copies and store each in separate locations off-premises. For extra protection, videotape your office equipment.

* **Find a safe haven.** Stash your inventory lists and backup disks and videotapes in such places as a safe deposit box or your parents' home. However, avoid the basement to avoid possible flooding.

BACKING UP INPUT

Be sure to back up disks, copying material from your hard disk onto a floppy disk. One of your authors remembers an unfortunate early computer experience when an entire day's work was lost because she hit the wrong command. No one had told her about backing up input. Whether you operate from a floppy disk or a hard drive, back up your system every two or three reports.

Frequent backup of computer-generated data onto floppy disks, tape, or other media is insurance against hardware or software malfunction. Inexpensive backup software programs are fast and simple to use. Backup data is essential when you need to retrieve previous transcription.

Computer files are easily saved by patient name, medical record number, date of transcription, or any other system that works well for you. Once your files are on backup disks, you can easily retrieve the information. No matter how far in the future clients may ask for records they cannot locate, you will be able to quickly review your computer-generated list of files and print out the old transcription.

A tape backup system is optional since you can purchase backup software such as PC Tools or DOS. You should have either hardware backup capabilities or software backup capabilities to prevent losing data in the event of a hard drive crash.

If you are going to invest in a tape backup system, consider programming it to update your data backup every evening or during the time when you are not active on your computer. The system can be set to automatically back up your data to the point of the last backup. Ideally, data backup should be done on a daily basis.

DISKETTE CARE AND MAINTENANCE

Handle backup diskettes, the duplicate copies of your programs and records, gently. Computer disks are very delicate and should always be used and stored carefully.

- Make backup disks of your software and replace disks after 50-100 hours of use.

- Protect disks from dust, dirt, fingerprints, and old age, which can make disks unreadable.

- Store disks upright, away from excessive heat, cold, and moisture.

- Store disks away from magnetic interferences such as transcribers, computer monitors, television and VCR, magnetic paper clip holders, bulk tape erasers, and other similar technology.

COMPUTER CARE AND MAINTENANCE

Despite their hearty constitutions, personal computers need care and attention if they are to have a long life of reliable performance. Dust and dirt are always hazardous to a computer's well-being and home-based computers are at even greater risk.

When you work at home, your computer is subject to a variety of household pollutants that can interfere with its performance. Computer threats include dust, cooking grease, pet hairs, aerosol sprays, soft drinks, food crumbs, smoke, erasure particles, and numerous miscellaneous specks that float around our homes.

Just as there seems to be no way to avoid exposure to the common cold, there is no way to totally protect your computer from exposure to hazards. There are, however, several steps you can take to reduce harmful effects on your computer.

• Cover computer components when not in use.

• Periodically vacuum air intake vents. (Invest in a computer cleaning kit.)

• Vacuum and dust the computer area once a week, including printer and keyboard.

• Keep disk drives closed when not in use.

• Keep the computer area free from smoke and food.

• Print copies of important files.

• Replace filters regularly on forced-air heating and cooling systems.

• Keep the area around your computer clean, including floors, baseboards, bookcases and books, lamps, decorative objects, furniture, and windowsills. Clean the computer itself gently. Do not use detergent or chemical solvents to clean computer casings. Use a soft, damp (but not wet) cloth for dusting, or buy a commercial computer cleaning kit. You can also buy a disk-drive cleaning kit. In addition to cleaning, don't let stray paper clips or staples pile up around your equipment.

COMPUTER "HOUSECLEANING"

To lower the odds of a hard disk crash, do some basic computer file housecleaning on a monthly basis. Files get shuffled around from one sector to another when added or deleted frequently.

It's easy to tell when your hard disk needs maintenance: Its speed will decrease during basic functions. Keep your hard disk uncluttered and organized by regularly compressing, moving, or deleting files. This greatly decreases the chances of your disk crashing. Compress your disk whenever your computer's speed begins to decrease. Use PC Tools or Norton Utilities to compress your hard disk.

TIP

During thunder storms, disconnect your phone lines, cables and plugs, and make sure your computer is turned off. Never unplug your keyboard from your computer when the computer is on. This could "kill" your keyboard permanently and also do serious damage to the hardware.

FILE COMPRESSION PROGRAMS

Many of us are so busy with day-to-day activities of our business, most of which is keyboarding, that we have little free time to investigate alternatives that would make our tasks easier. When we discover timesaving products, it's very exciting. One great compression program called *PKZIP* is a real time saver. This wondrous little tool allows you to take a file or directory, or groups of files or directories, and compress them into a single file that is much smaller than the original.

Soon after I started using PKZIP, I discovered I was saving more than the cost of floppy disks because I used the "ZIP" to compress my old files. I can get 5 to 10 times more on my floppy disks than I could with just the old move/copy.

It you are online on a BBS or other service, you can save time and money uploading and downloading files. By zipping the file/directory first, you save 50%-90% in time and charges when sending and receiving files via modem. PKZIP is a shareware, and the newest version is 2.04G. With shareware, you are free to check it out before you buy it, but if you continue to use it, you must register (buy) it. The registration cost is $47 and it is worth every penny!

COMPUTER CONSULTANTS

Every medical transcriptionist, especially one new to the computer world, needs a computer consultant or "teckie." These are extremely warm and caring people, but they do have one flaw: They love computers more than life itself.

They eat, sleep, and breathe computers. They can be found in computer stores, or in the computer section of book stores, perusing the wonderful world of computers and the latest technology.

Computer consultants can take a computer apart and put it back together faster than the speed of light. Nothing excites them more than spending 24 hours (or more!) working nonstop on a computer glitch. If you don't have a computer consultant at home, shop around for one.

Join a computer club. Every area has at least one club, and they are loaded with computer teckies. There are even computer clubs for singles. In fact, we have a friend who met and married a wonderful teckie she found on a computer club's bulletin board.

Some clubs are for people who live in a geographic area, some are for people who have one specific type of computer or computer operating system, and some are for people who use a particular type of software. Whichever you choose, you might be bringing your very own computer teckie to the next transcription convention.

Computer publications are also good resources for information on computers and specialists available to help you solve computer problems.

UTILIZING VIDEO LIBRARIES AND AUDIOCASSETTES

Have you visited your public library's videotape section lately? If you haven't, you probably should. Public libraries have numerous computer applications videotapes that you can view at home simply by checking them out with your library card. For instance, if you use WordPerfect, you can begin with the basic WordPerfect video and move on to intermediate, advanced, windows, etc. These videos are wonderful references and you will gain an abundance of computer savvy from them.

There are also specialized videotapes on the market. These are a great resource for new WordPerfect users and others interested in learning WP tips and customized applications.

To get the most out of these videos, try to view them while actually sitting at your keyboard so you can practice the various techniques in the video demonstrations. If you do not understand something immediately, you can rewind the video and play it again. Through these various applications you will learn tips that will aid in cutting production time, improving transcription quality, and increasing profits.

You can easily bring yourself up to speed with self-paced audiocassettes. Put a tape in a Walkman™ or new transcribing machine, or slip a disk in your computer, and an instructor talks you through the program while you work directly on your computer. Two references for these self-paced audiocassettes are the following:

- **Personal Training Systems of San Jose**
  800-832-2499

- **Individual Software**
  800-822-3522

RECORDING YOUR COMPUTER AND SOFTWARE INFORMATION

It's a good idea to set up a file for detailed records of office equipment and computer hardware/software. It will be a valuable quick reference in case you experience office equipment problems. The file should include the following:

- Equipment model numbers

- Program names, dates of purchase, versions, serial and registration numbers

- Vendor names, telephone numbers

- Customer support phone numbers, software help line phone numbers

- Warranty information and expiration dates

BEWARE THE VIRUS

Software is subject to computer viruses that can contaminate data files and programs. To help prevent virus contamination, it is wise to invest in what the industry refers to as "virgin software programs" — software programs that are new and unused.

Invest in a virus check, too, even if you have purchased new software. Norton Disk Doctor, PC Tools and similar products are fine for this purpose. This is especially important if you plan on using a modem. It is truly sickening to see a software program self-destruct as a result of a virus.

As stated earlier, never borrow software because, according to the National Computer Security Association (NCSA), "borrowed" software could contain a virus that is put there by the manufacturer to deter copying. Viruses can also be introduced through other sources.

INCREASING TYPING SPEED WITH ABBREVIATION/EXPANSION SOFTWARE

I had seen demonstrations of abbreviation programs but was not enthusiastic about "retraining" in shorthand techniques . . . until I agreed to try PRD+ at the encouragement of a colleague. I was amazed at how quickly I adapted to it and soon found myself creating my own entries one after the other. Years later, I still feel that abbreviation software is the best invention since the agitating washing machine!

Even though abbreviation software can enhance efficient text production, it is not a substitute for in-depth knowledge of medical terminology and grammatical and transcription skills. Learning to spell and learning to type are two different things. One cannot be proficient in language skills without first having knowledge and understanding of the full word or combination of words that each character represents. Also, not all job settings will have abbreviation software available, nor will all those in charge understand and appreciate how they work.

A WORD OF CAUTION: Some home-based and classroom medical transcription training courses include instruction on abbreviation and word-expansion software programs, other time- and labor-saving devices, and information on how they can be obtained. However, we discourage taking courses that offer training in "shortcut" typing *in place of* learning the full meaning and spelling of the words and phrases being transcribed. Nothing can replace in-depth knowledge of medical language words.

KEYSTROKE/ABBREVIATION SOFTWARE

A keystroke/abbreviation software program can be a useful medical transcription tool, but it is most effective when used by a competent MT.

PROS

- **Reduces keystrokes** ... by compressing frequently repeated words, sentences and paragraphs into tailored abbreviations as short as two letters.

- **No stretching** ... to reach **ALT** or **CTRL** keys. With the stroke of a space bar or any "hot key," the abbreviation is expanded.

- **The savings** ... are in time and stress. Some transcriptionists report these programs save two or three hours in a 12-hour day.

- **Compatibility** ... with most word processing packages. You can easily customize your own abbreviations, phrases and formats.

I save approximately 45-60 minutes of keyboarding time in an eight-hour day with the WordPerfect macros and standard boiler plate documents I incorporated into my programs.

CONS

- Abbreviations can be mistakenly activated, so transcriptionists must edit documents with extreme care.

- Large abbreviations may sometimes be the same or similar (ASHD — arteriosclerotic heart disease and AHHD—atherosclerotic heart disease). Transcriptionists must be cautious when creating abbreviation menus. There is a toggle "on-off" switch that can be activated if you do not want phrase expansion, which would be helpful if you are typing a letter where a name like PAT might otherwise expand to a complex medical term.

PERSONALIZING AN ABBREVIATION SOFTWARE PROGRAM

Here are some of my favorite personalized abbreviation features:

- I enjoy the ease with which I can take the periods out of abbreviations like b.i.d. With abbreviation software, I type "bid" and it automatically expands to b.i.d. and includes the periods.

- Hyphenated terms are a snap because I've shortened words like "cul-de-sac." Now I just type "cds" and hit the space bar — the word appears as cul-de-sac.

- I use shortened forms for words my brain has difficulty transmitting correctly to my fingertips — words like "epididymis" and "sternocleidomastoid." Now I just type "epd" and "scm."

- Other words I've included are those I tend to transpose — such as and (adn), with (wiht) and the (teh). Even if a word has been transposed when I type it, at the tap of the space bar it is automatically corrected.

Prices for these software programs range from as low as a few dollars for shareware to over $400. One program we like very much and recommend you learn more about is the following:

- **PRD+ MedEasy** — around $400
  (Productivity Software International, New York)
  212-818-1144, or
  fax 212-818-1197

> *"I save approximately 45-60 minutes of keyboarding time in an eight-hour day with the WordPerfect macros and standard boiler plate documents I incorporated into my programs."*

213

- **ShortCut** (Healthcare Technologies, Inc.)
  610 Village Trace
  Bldg. 22
  Marietta, GA 30067
  Tel. 404-850-9300
  Fax 404-955-7555

Other abbreviation software programs include Smarttype, Instant Text and Explode-It!

WHAT TO DO WITH THAT OLD COMPUTER

Well, suppose you have been in business for a few years, and during the past year you have made an excellent income. So, you decide to take the plunge and exchange your 386 for a 486 or pentium super turbo charged computer. What do you do with that old computer? Don't let it stand in a corner collecting dust; give it a new lease on life.

- **Pass it on.** Do you know a child or, better yet, have a child of your own, who would love to have their very own computer?

- **Sell it** . . . and brace yourself for rock-bottom pricing. If you thought your car depreciated fast, you're in for a real shock. Old computers depreciate faster! Don't ask a high price and expect to have people banging at your door. Be realistic. If you don't want to haggle with anyone, contact the United Computer Exchange, 800-755-3033, which has a database of buyers and sellers of used equipment.

- **Donate it.** Many schools, churches and charitable organizations desperately need computers. You might even be able to count your computer contribution as a tax deduction unless you have already written it off as a business tax deduction.

- **Dedicate it to a specific task.** Save memory on your primary computer by installing your database on the old one. You can even turn your old standby system into a useful telecommunications tool by installing a voice/fax/modem board.

MACROS

Macros are subprograms that assign a complete sentence, paragraph, page or document to simple keystrokes. For example, if a doctor dictates that a pelvic examination is negative, the typist, with a single keystroke, can initiate a macro that prints out the doctor's standard description of a negative pelvic exam.

If you have not yet learned to create macros, I suggest you take the time to do so. The keystrokes saved will result in valuable time saved.

If you use WordPerfect, you'll find several easy macros already built into the program, and each upgrade you receive will give you even greater flexibility. Try attending a WordPerfect workshop and learn even more about macros and other great techniques.

COMPUTER REFERENCES AND RESOURCES

Generally speaking, there are two types of computer users: 1) users who want to know how their computer works, and 2) users who simply want the computer to work. When it comes to computer operating functions, I am no "teckie." I have learned about my computer through trial and error, and the more I learn, the more fascinated I become.

Through the years I have discovered a number of excellent computer references that have worked well for me. As many of you know, trying to decipher computer manuals that come with hardware and software can be like trying to learn a foreign language. Well, the light bulb finally went on and some enlightened soul came to the conclusion that all users aren't teckies. Here are some very readable computer references.

- *DOS for Dummies*. This is a lighthearted reference that takes you through the operating system, provides the essentials and leaves out the heavy technical stuff you don't need to deal with. Helpful little hints and warnings are sprinkled throughout the text — a feature I especially enjoy. You will become computer literate after reading this, and the best part is, you will realize you are not a dummy after all!

215

There are many *"Dummies"* books including the following:

- *DOS for Dummies*
- *Dummies 101: Word for Windows 95; WordPerfect 6.1 for Windows*
- *Dummies 101: The Internet*
- *WP for Dummies: Windows 3.1*
- *PCs for Dummies*
- *AmiPro for Dummies*
- *UNIX for Dummies*
- *Word for Dummies*
- *QuickBooks for Dummies*
- *Quicken 5 for Windows for Dummies*
- *1- 2- 3 for Dummies* … and more.

- *OOPS! What To Do When Things Go Wrong*, Que.
  This reference offers computer basics for the technically timid. It lists the ten most common computer problems and offers advice on trouble shooting and problem solving. This is a very readable, fun, and easy-to-follow book.

- *Modems Made Easy*, McGraw-Hill.
  This is a great reference for telecommuters. It defines all basic aspects of communication, what is needed to set up, how it integrates with your other computer systems, different types of data and modem software, etc.

- *Voodoo Windows, Tips and Tricks with an Attitude*, Ventana Press.
  This is a well written, creative reference for learning Windows. The book is very understandable and eliminates much of the fear involved in working with windows. Technical details are simplified, which creates a comfortable atmosphere for learning.

RX FOR PC HEALTH

> ### WARNING
>
> Using a PC may be hazardous to your health.

Prolonged sitting at a PC can result in physical disorders. Herb Brody, writing in "The Body In Question," which appeared in *PC Computing Magazine* (March 1989) points out that, ironically, PCs produce discomfort, in large part, because the machines are just too good. Never before has it been possible to accomplish so much while using so few muscles.

The PC has given new meaning to the word "sedentary." Unlike typewriters, which force us to use some muscle mass loading and unloading paper, computers allow us to sit for hours in front of our machines, absolutely immobile, with eyes fixed on the screen.

Serious computer users are reporting a bevy of symptoms such as headaches, dizziness and blurred vision that are known collectively as repetitive strain injuries or RSIs. RSIs result from the constrained posture or repetitive motion involved in most computer work.

MOVE IT OR LOSE IT

There is no getting around the fact that you must exercise in order to keep your muscles functioning properly. The next time you sit at your computer for six hours without a break, evaluate how you feel. Not great, right? It's important to get out of your chair regularly and take breaks. If you do, you'll feel better and your productivity will increase.

You can work out with old exercise programs or try something more modern. A software program, *ComputerHealth Break,* is designed to help you exercise at the computer screen. Compatible with IBM PCs and DOS 2.1 or higher, the program pops up on your screen at scientifically defined intervals based on your workload. Exercises are different from day to day, so boredom is never a problem. Remember, the more work you do, the more exercise you need. Studies show frequent but short exercise breaks are very effective in preventing computer related injuries. Your total exercise time need be only 10-15 minutes a day — the equivalent of one coffee break.

Most of us who use computers have a love/hate relationship with them. When they are working, they are marvelous inventions. When they are down, we feel like throwing them out the window. Nevertheless, transcription life is better with them than without, and this new technology has resulted in some exciting additional comfort benefits.

ERGONOMICS

We have worked as medical transcriptionists for over twenty years. Until the advent of the computer, medical transcriptionists had to suffer with the Chair from Hell (referred to in an earlier chapter), desks that were too high, bad lighting, and noise pollution from the constant drone of typewriters. Computer technology added a new word to the English language, *Ergonomics*.

Ergonomics! Almost overnight we were introduced to adjustable chairs that wrapped lovingly around our bodies, desks of varying heights, appropriate office lighting, quieter equipment, and reams of health and fitness information relevant to computer users.

We would like to think that all this innovative office comfort came about because someone was overcome with guilt about our Neanderthal-like office working conditions and was subsequently moved to improve our lot in business life. In reality, however, innovation probably occurred because individual and organizational office workers became a more significant market segment or because these improvements would result in fewer medical bills, physical and mental disability claims, and lawsuits. Whatever, we're delighted about the innovations.

We recommend that you take care of your body and maybe you won't end up in a retirement home for medical transcriptionists, sitting on a porch with your right leg locked into an extended position, suffering from severe kyphoscoliosis, and wearing double hearing aids that get tangled in your cervical collar!

THE EYES HAVE IT

Did you know that PC users blink less than normal people? We become so transfixed by the screen that we forget to blink, causing dry, itching eyes.

Blinking lubricates the surface of the eye and normally occurs about every five seconds. Medical transcriptionists sometimes work for an entire minute without blinking. Contact lens wearers are at even greater peril since their lenses require additional eye fluids.

Don't get smug, you bifocal wearers. You are particularly vulnerable to VDT-induced eyestrain. The near-focus lens in bifocals provides correct vision at a distance of about 12 inches, the distance at which you normally hold printed material. However, your PC screen is typically situated 18-24 inches away. Moreover, opticians usually place the near-vision lens below the long-vision lens. This design forces you to tip your head back uncomfortably to view the screen, causing strain to your neck and back.

Do you know that you can actually buy "computer glasses?" These are a type of bifocal designed specifically to provide sharp focus at the distance you sit from the screen. There is a disadvantage, however. You have to switch to your regular bifocals to read printouts or other documents.

LIGHTS OUT

Some people like to work in a light room. Others prefer working in a darkened room. The following paragraph makes a solid case for the latter. ·

The computer monitor produces its owns light and readability requires contrast. In other words, the darker you keep the screen, the better. Dim the lights, kill the overheads, and close the window blinds. (So much for a room with a view!) Illuminate your work area with a desk lamp and keep the light off your computer screen.

Working in the dark is generally easier on your eyes. Every time you look away from the screen, your pupils must adjust to the different levels of brightness in the room. In dim light, pupils relax and expand to let in more light, while they constrict in a bright room to diminish the amount of light. Reducing the amount of light in the room decreases the dark/light contrast so your eyes have less adjusting to do.

Two of the most common office complaints are irritated eyes and headaches. One major cause of these problems is glare from the computer monitor. Direct glare can be created by the monitor itself so turn down the screen's brightness and turn up the contrast. Also, make sure your screen is clean. Dust builds up quickly, making your screen hard to read.

Positioning the computer screen properly helps reduce optical insult. Indirect glare arises when the monitor screen reflects surrounding lights or windows. If you tilt your screen up, it mirrors ceiling lights. Turn the screen away from windows to reduce glare. If your monitor does not move, consider purchasing a tilt stand, which is fairly inexpensive and allows you to move your computer screen into a position that is just right for you.

In addition to the above techniques, consider buying a glare screen. These mesh glass sheets fit over your computer and reduce reflection. Be sure the one you buy fits your monitor and check to make certain it does not degrade the image of the screen.

KEYBOARD TO SUCCESS

Workers who spend long hours at keyboards sometime develop wrist and hand pain, and many medical transcriptionists develop carpal tunnel syndrome. The fault, dear readers, lies not in our keyboards but in ourselves — at least that's what some experts say.

How we use the keyboard may hold the key to avoiding discomfort and pain, carpal tunnel syndrome, and other cumulative trauma disorders (CTDs). Factors such as typing, posture, working without breaks, stress, and even certain hobbies can contribute to the development of CTDs. Reforming your keyboard habits can often solve wrist problems.

The most common CTD is CTS (carpal tunnel syndrome), a form of compression neuropathy. The QWERTY keyboard (the one you see before you each time you put your fingers to the keyboard) was created in the 1860s. It actually was designed to slow down typing on keys that tended to clump together in the original manual typewriters.

Development of computers and laser printers alleviated the key-clumping problem, but the keyboard remained the same. No one seriously considered changing the keyboard format because, although it was admittedly inconvenient and inefficient, typists were accustomed to the old format and they could type faster because the keys no longer clumped. In addition, typing speed was further enhanced because it was no longer necessary to remove one's hands from the keyboard to change typing paper, move the carriage return, or make manual corrections. Not a second's break! It is easy to understand how such unrelenting pounding on a hard keyboard can destroy wrists.

TAKING A BREAK FROM CUMULATIVE TRAUMA DISORDERS

Simple stretching and relaxation exercises can help prevent CTDs. Try each of these for ten seconds every hour:

- Gently massage the palms.

- Press the palm down to stretch top side of forearm.

- Press the palm up to stretch the underside of forearm.

- Rotate the neck from side to side.

- Wear wrist splints to avoid supination of hands.

One product that is currently getting a good deal of attention is the Handeze Glove. This type glove is made up of special material called Med-A-Likra. This material reacts to each movement, producing an automatic massaging and energizing effect. The more you work, the more you massage. At first the gloves feel like support hose or Isotoner™ gloves, but after keyboarding for awhile, the gloves make your hands feel great — as if they had been massaged thoroughly. There is no restriction in keyboarding ability because the gloves are fingerless. These gloves retail for around $20.

- **Therapeutic Appliance Group**
  Box 339 Woonsocket
  RI 02895
  800-457-5535

NEW TOOLS FOR MEDICAL TRANSCRIPTIONISTS SUFFERING FROM REPETITIVE STRAIN INJURIES

For decades, medical transcriptionists worked in unbelievable situations with unworkable equipment, e.g., desks that were too high, typewriters (many of us started on manual ones) and chairs that fell apart at the slightest attempt to make ourselves more comfortable. Since the advent of ergonomics in the 1980s, there have been many advances to alleviate and prevent CTDs (cumulative trauma disorders) — work-related injuries that result from many hours of repetitive tasks, which places great stress on the nerves and muscles of the hands.

Some of the newer product lines designed specifically to prevent CTDs include alternative keyboards. According to the March 22, 1993 issue of *Advance*, these keyboards are radically different, ranging from keyboards that bend at 90 degree angles or in three parts, or use the Dvorak configuration rather than QWERTY. The strangest looking ones don't even use keys, but are "chordic." Like a court stenographer's dictation machine, certain keys stand for combinations of letters or functions. Some designs even place fingers in "wells," rather than on keys, to select letters by back-and-forth movements.

DataHand offers padded handrests with individual finger wells that operate switches.

- **DataHand**
  Scottsdale, AZ
  602-860-8584

MIKey is a fixed keyboard with 12 function keys arranged in clock-face pattern.

- **Dr. Alan Grant**
  Chevy Chase, MD
  301-933-1111

The **Comfort Keyboard** is broken into three pieces, which can be rotated in any direction. It incorporates familiar key arrangements.

- **Health Care Keyboard Co., Inc.**
  Menomonee Falls, WI
  414-703-0170

THE EMF FLAP

Some health concerns have to do less with pain today than with illness tomorrow. One potential problem in particular stands out -— electromagnetic fields (EMFs). EMFs are a form of radiation emitted by computer monitors and many other electrical devices. Some researchers argue that repeated exposure to EMFs can cause cancer, birth defects, and other health problems. The idea isn't without controversy, however, and all scientific facts aren't in yet. If you remain worried, however, about potential hazards of EMFs, you can take several precautions:

- Try to stay at least an arm's length from your monitor. EMFs decrease rapidly with increased distance.

- Avoid sitting near the sides or rear of computer monitors. Most units emit higher levels of EMFs in these areas than from the front.

- Use monitors designed to emit low EMFs. This isn't an option for most people. To find these monitors, check with computer dealers or look through manufacturers' product literature. Also, watch for reviews of monitors in computer magazines.

FIVE EXERCISES TO PREVENT INJURY

- **Neck glide**: Glide your head back as far as it will go, keeping your head and ears level. Doing it correctly creates a double chin. Now glide your head forward and repeat three times.

- **Wrist flex**: Hold your right arm out, fingers pointed up. Take your left hand and gently bend your right hand back towards your forearm. Hold five seconds. Repeat on the other side.

- **Finger fan**: Hold your hands out in front of you, palms down. Spread your fingers apart as far as you can. Hold for five seconds, then make a tight fist. Repeat three times.

- **Upper/lower back stretches**: *Upper stretch* — raise your hands to your shoulders. Using your arms, push your shoulders back. Keep your elbows down. Hold for 15 seconds. Repeat three times. *Lower stretch* — lower your head and slowly roll your body as far as you can toward your knees. Hold for ten seconds. Push yourself up with your leg muscles and repeat three times.

North Coast Medical, Incorporated sells everything a medical transcriptionist needs to ensure a safe and comfortable working environment. You can get a variety of wrist rests for keyboards, mouse pads, lighting, chairs, foot rests, lumbar supports, protective and strengthening products for your hands. They also carry an interesting product called *TheraPutty*™, a silicon rubber compound that promotes increasing range of motion, hand closure, tendon gliding, and hand strength. *TheraPutty* comes in different consistencies and costs around $4. You can order a sample kit of all eight putty resistances for $24.95. Contact North Coast for a catalog.

- **North Coast Health and Safety Products**
  800-821-9319

ERGONOMIC VIDEO

Medical transcriptionists spend many hours a day at the computer, but few people know the correct way to sit at the workstation, use the keyboard, or look at the monitor. As a result, some computer users develop bad habits that can create physical problems such as eye strain, back pain, and pain in arms and legs. There is a new instructional videotape designed to help people avoid common physical problems related to working at the computer. It is a 30-minute videotape titled *Staying Fit at the Computer*.

Staying Fit at the Computer was developed by a noted Ph.D. and expert on health in the workplace. It offers relaxation and stretching techniques, posture tips, vision exercise, and information on proper body mechanics for the wrist and arm. Video guidelines and exercises can help computer users develop healthier work habits, prevent repetitive strain injury, reduce eye strain and enhance performance and productivity.

REFERENCE BOOKS

Every medical transcriptionist's office should contain copies of references ... and more references. They are essential and well worth the investment. There are numerous medical reference books on the market today, available through a variety of publishers. Gone are the days when the only reference book for MTs was *Taber's Dictionary*. Do not, we repeat do not, scrimp on these. Williams & Wilkins and W. B. Saunders Co. have entire libraries of medical reference books as well as electronic reference resources.

My reference library contains more than 100 books, many of which are medical references by specialty. All are essential for my work as a home-based medical transcriptionist. I update these reference frequently — some each year; the others, never later than three years or whenever updates are available.

Other essential references for the medical transcription library include grammar and punctuation references, a good collegiate dictionary, medical dictionary, anatomy book, and abbreviations, acronyms and symbols book. You'll also discover many other books that will prove helpful in your specific work.

Be sure to attend seminars, conventions and trade shows and visit the book vendors in attendance. You will see more books than you know what to do with. Once upon a time there were so few books it was easy to choose; you just bought one of each. Today there are hundreds of good references, and it will make your choice much more difficult. Purchase those that will meet your specific needs and keep them conveniently at hand.

For a list of some of our favorite reference books, check the reference books section at the back of this book. In addition, to obtain an excellent and comprehensive medical transcription reference list, contact the American Association for Medical Transcription, 800-982-2182.

Several publishing houses also specialize in books for the health care field. To obtain a list of titles available, contact our recommended book publishers listed in the reference section at the back of this book.

UTILIZING CONSULTANTS

Like all professionals, transcriptionists sometimes need the help of experts outside their field. These may include a lawyer to review contracts, an accountant/tax consultant, computer specialist, insurance agent, graphic designer, etc.

When possible, obtain personal recommendations for consultants from business associates. You may also call specific professional associations for referrals or find consultants listed in the yellow pages of the telephone directory. Contact potential consultants regarding their consulting procedures and fees. You may want to interview them. If you do not feel comfortable with a consultant, do not hesitate to seek another.

When consulting with specialists, do not expect them to make your decisions for you. They will make intelligent recommendations based on their knowledge and experience, but decision making related to your business is ultimately your responsibility.

When working with consultants, be open about your knowledge level of the subject and insist that explanations be in language you understand. If you do not understand something, ask for clarification. Remember, it is no disgrace to acknowledge that you are uninformed in this particular subject. That's why we hire consultants.

We suggest that you attend seminars, which are educational and also give you access to experienced professionals with whom you can speak — a type of informal consultation. Also, subscribe to publications that have Question-and-Answer columns that offer advice on issues and problems related to your business.

WORKSHOPS AND SEMINARS

Workshops and seminars are some of the most powerful self-improvement and professional development tools available today. They offer a refreshing change of pace from routine work — even if for only a few hours — and spending time in a stimulating, idea-filled environment is a motivating experience. It is also a great place to network.

Hundreds of millions of dollars are spent each year on professional training conferences. These events are excellent professional opportunities, especially when you plan ahead:

- **Write out your expectations before the event**. Think about conditions that currently affect your work environment. What skills you would like to learn? Make up a list of ways you would like the conference to help you and keep the list in front of you during the meeting.

- **Obtain information and plan conference activities ahead of time**. If you have decision-making authority over your attendance, or if you haven't yet committed to attending, ask the seminar sponsor to give you a detailed outline of seminar presentation materials, presenters' names and information about their experience and expertise. Study the outline and speak with past attendees. If one conference isn't right for you, chances are another will be.

- **Aim for comfort**. Dress flexibly. Wear light, loose-fitting clothes and carry a sweater or jacket. Layering is wise because air-conditioning in some facilities is uncomfortably cool or downright cold; other times, it's stifling.

- **Make action notes during the conference**. As you listen to the speakers, divide your note pad into two columns. In the left-hand column make notes about the speakers' comments; in the right hand column, jot down "to-dos" and ways you can apply the information and ideas presented. These notes will be valuable to you later on.

- **Get to know other conference participants**. Every conference you attend provides an opportunity to meet your colleagues, learn about their businesses and accomplishments, and share mutual concerns. Share with others your expectations as well as your successes. Be prepared to LISTEN. Meet as many people as possible, exchange business cards, and establish a personal network that you can use in the future. It will prove invaluable.

- **Get to know the conference leader**. While you may not be able to spend a great deal of time with conference speakers, they probably have some free time before and after conference sessions. Leaders expect participants to talk with them informally during these periods. Don't hesitate to explore a topic in more depth with the speaker or ask to discuss it during a break. Conference speakers have a wealth of information about topics they present.

- **Discuss the conference with others when you return and offer your impressions**. They will appreciate your sharing your time and valuable information.

- **Be prepared to implement what you have learned**. Start an idea file, keep one or two ideas in front of you at all times, and take the steps necessary to put these to work. The knowledge and ideas you bring back from each conference will help develop your skills. Exercise these skills and your seminar experience will pay big dividends to you in the months and years to come.

BEWARE OF EXPERTS WHO AREN'T

When I started as an IMT, there were no experts to whom I could turn. As with everything else I have done in my life, my experience came from "The School of Hard Knocks", i.e., if Plan A fails, go on to Plan B. I spent hours in the library trying to gain insight into the steps I needed to take to achieve my goals. At that time, most of the books available were published in the 1970s when typewriters were king.

Then there was the government bureaucracy to deal with. Those of you who have navigated this territory probably understand the depths of frustration I experienced trying to get information about zoning laws and tax regulations. Translated in typical government double-speak, public information was generally oppressive.

The end of the 1980s was a time of self-discovery and an "I want it now" mentality. Schools sprang up promising would-be medical transcriptionists a full-fledged medical transcription training program in an unrealistically brief period of 3-6 months and a job at the end of the program paying a grandiose $35,000-a-year medical transcription salary.

Currently there is a proliferation of books and seminars on how to start home-based businesses. Working at home is a viable business option in the 1990s and it seems everyone wants a piece of the action. Be forewarned: not all how-to books and seminars are equal.

Before you buy how-to books or attend how-to seminars, check promoters/authors' credentials. Is the "ultimate book on Victorian home restoration" written by someone experienced in Victorian construction, or is his expertise limited to wallpapering a bathroom? Did the author of *You Too Can Work at Home and Become a Bazillionaire MT?* ever actually own and operate a home-based medical transcription business? Has that seminar coordinator on starting a home-based medical transcription service ever typed a medical record report or owned a successful medical transcription home-based service, or was she only employed as a marketing rep for a computer company? Did that educator for the *Get-Rich-Quick School for Medical Transcription* ever work as a medical transcriptionist and become certified, or was her experience limited to legal secretarial work for a medical malpractice attorney?

Much misinformation is disseminated by so-called "experts." These people purport to know what is best for **us** and our profession even though they have no firsthand experience in actually running a successful home-based medical transcription service. Our profession is very specialized — unlike any other in the world. What works in our businesses doesn't necessarily hold true for other businesses.

ACCOUNTS AND SUPPLIES

When you acquire accounts, you will find that there are a variety of forms and formats you can work with. Individual accounts frequently have specific formats and sometimes their own paper supplies.

You can also use desktop publishing techniques, which are available in programs like WordPerfect, to create letterhead if there is an issue with your client supplying paper, (i.e., one of the IRS independent contractor definition guidelines). If the client does supply you with letterhead, be sure to return it if the business relationship is terminated.

If you are self-employed but your clients provide the paper, consider purchasing your own. In addition to denoting your independent transcriptionist status, you will also have another business expense to write off at tax time. Explain the rationale to your client. You may have to factor this expense into the rate you are charging for your services.

Hospitals often use tractor-fed, continuous feed paper preprinted with their name and logo, but many are now switching to plain paper documents generated through laser printers. Some clients have the transcriptionist modem files to their transcription department so they can be printed on their laserjet printer. Others may ask that you print the documents at your worksite on plain paper with their hospital format and deliver the documents. They may also request the documents on disk along with the hard copies. Doctors' offices usually provide letterhead for letters of consultation.

Paper for chart notes varies. Some transcriptionists prefer continuous feed, peel-off, or "sticky-back" paper for chart notes. Chart notes can be set up easily with the patient's name and date, body of report, and physician's signature line. They can be cut with a paper cutter and returned to the doctor/clinic office, peeled off, and placed in the patient chart. This eliminates handling charts and removing and replacing chart note sheets.

This paper can be purchased by the roll or sheet, for tractor-fed or laser printers. It is available with or without perforations. That without perforations offers somewhat more flexibility, allowing the transcriptionist to cut it wherever the chart note ends. Companies that sell this type paper — in continuous rolls and laser sheets — are listed below.

- **Script-Ese**
  800-553-7711

- **Briggs**
  800-247-2343

- **Pat Systems**
  800-543-1911

- **RayPress Corp.**
  205-254-3731

- **Specialty Business Forms**
  800-445-5875

Radiology departments have special forms and formats, but many are converting to laser printed forms that are easier to use. Many radiology departments have their own dedicated *radiology information systems (RIS)* which incorporate all patient demographics. The transcriptionist only has to type the body of the report, which is printed out in the department or wherever routed. In RIS systems such as these, patient demographics are entered into a computer when the patient registers for the procedure. Physicians love this because they no longer have to dictate all the patient ID information, requesting physician, x-ray report, etc.

With the RIS system, transcription is done online and can be completed onsite or through remote transcription connected by modem to the RIS. Transcribing is in real-time over the phone line. As the transcriptionist types, the information systems department in the hospital can monitor the document on the screen as the transcriptionist actually inputs information. This type technology brings us closer and closer to real-time transcription, which offers an almost instantaneous turnaround time.

Pathology departments also have individualized formats and these formats may vary from client to client.

If the client has no preference regarding format, prepare a generic format, i.e., block letter style, standard H&P, discharge, operation, consultation, etc., for their consideration.

When establishing a working relationship with a new account, come to an agreement regarding format to be used. This helps prevent misunderstandings. If the account staff prefer a specific format that is currently in use, they may make copies of chart notes and letters for you to use as references. However, they may decide to take this opportunity to update or make revisions to existing formats. They may even ask your opinion regarding formats.

If you are picking up tapes of dictation from a doctor's office or a clinic, check to see if the tapes have been scanned. If not, request a list of names on which the doctor has dictated.

Unscanned dictation tapes are a risk to transcriptionists. If a doctor claims to have dictated a report on a patient but no transcribed report is available, the transcriptionist may be accused of losing the dictation. Generally, when a patient is seen in a doctor's office, the receptionist will check off or line out the patient's name after the appointment. The appointment book page can easily be photocopied for you.

You can check patient names off as you transcribe and return the list to the office with the transcribed reports. If there are names not checked, the doctor's office staff can easily see that he or she still needs to dictate on those patients. If a log is not provided, I suggest you create your own log for reference and billing. List the subjects/names that were on the tape that you transcribed. (For more information, see section on transcription logs.)

In many offices, appointments are logged on computers, making it easy for staff to provide you with a printout of the day's patient register. This list will also assist you with correct spelling of patient names. Doctors are notorious for not spelling names and sometimes they even forget to give them! In those situations, note any discrepancies. Leave a blank for the patient's name with a note ("name not given"). Office staff will solve the mystery by locating the patient's chart. After picking up dictation tapes, be sure to confirm your turnaround or delivery time and dates, as well as the name of the office contact person who assists you with confirmations and details. Request a list of medical staff physicians (physicians list) to assure proper name spelling.

Hospital dictation should be handled the same way. A printout of patient name, medical record number, and physician name/identification number should be transmitted to you along with the dictated tapes. If computer printouts are not available, the hospital can provide you with the A&D (admission and discharge) sheets. These are generated daily on all patients admitted and discharged from the hospital.

You must have this information to transcribe the reports correctly. Hospital records require that the patient's name and medical record/identification number be present on each page of the record. Upon completion of transcription, these sheets can be returned with the transcribed tapes, or whatever you negotiate with your client.

ALERT! ALERT!

Erasing tapes after completing transcription can be risky. Some transcriptionists never erase tapes, even if asked to do so. They leave this responsibility to their clients. Other transcriptionists erase tapes upon request, following meticulous procedures to avoid potential problems. If you choose to erase tapes, the following guidelines will be helpful.

Never erase a tape of dictation until you have printed or transferred completed reports by modem. We all have horror stories to tell about the tape that got erased, the report the computer ate, etc. I keep a little colored basket/bin labeled "tapes to be transcribed" on the right of my desk and a different colored basket labeled "already transcribed" on the left side of my desk. When I have completed my work for that account, or that day, and the reports are printed out and secured in the delivery portfolio, I finally erase the tapes and include them in the envelope.

For accounts handled by modem, I first back up all reports onto floppy disks as my insurance; then I transmit the reports to the hospital, modem to modem. When my computer tells me the transfer is complete, I then erase all the tapes. If for some reason the transmittal did not go through and the hospital did not receive my reports, they are still on the floppy disk, and I can easily transmit again.

If you are downloading work off a digital system, you have completed the job and it is gone from your system, it can be recaptured. Usually the digital system will hold the signed-off jobs for 24-72 hours. If you find that you have accidentally deleted a report and you need to re-transcribe it, you can call the client and ask to have that job reassigned to you if it is still in the holding/suspension mode. This happens!

Aren't computers wonderful! We have been transcriptionists long enough to remember when state-of-the-art electronic typewriters wiped out entire tapes of transcription, which then had to be typed again. That was an incredible waste of time! For the most part, computers have solved that problem.

Always check with your clients beforehand to determine if they prefer that you erase your tapes or simply return them rewound.

If working with digital systems through telecommunication, always identify the job number, which will be somewhere on your transcription log or somewhere on the report that you are transcribing, so the dictation can be recaptured by that job number if necessary.

Telecommunications

*"Nothing, I am sure, calls forth the faculties so much as being
obliged to struggle with the world."*

—Mary Wollstonecraft Shelley

Telecommuting is sending completed work to a client's computer via modem. Modems allow your computer to connect to telephone lines and transmit data to and from other computers or online services. Online services can range from a local bulletin-board service, or BBS, to a large international data center such as Prodigy and CompuServe.

Telecommuting eliminates pickup and delivery time and expense. You must have a modem and the client must have compatible software and a modem to receive the work.

REASONS TO TELECOMMUTE

Natural disasters: As a result of the 1994 earthquake in Southern California, commuter gridlock sometimes lasted for five hours. Employees for The City and County of Los Angeles were encouraged to work out of their homes two to three days a week by leasing equipment from the County.

During recent disastrous floods in the Midwest and hurricanes in Southern Florida, entire regions were able to communicate their needs immediately through telecommunication. It was their only link with the outside for long periods of time.

In Washington D.C., because of extreme weather conditions and hazardous commuting conditions, government employees were sent home to work. If they had not been able to telecommute, many employees would have missed work, forcing government agencies to shut down.

During all of the above natural disasters, the first computer information networks — online services like Prodigy, CompuServe and America OnLine — were heavily and beneficially used. At this point in history there is no question that whether we're faced with overwhelming natural disasters or balmy days of routine living, online services and telecommunication offer many positive benefits.

Environment: Telecommuting has a positive impact on the environment in terms of reducing air pollution by cutting back on commuter traffic. Many cities across the U.S. are imposing environmental ordinances that are mandating workers work from home at least two or three days per week in an effort to reduce air pollution.

Time, Productivity, Dollars: Tremendous amounts of time are saved and productivity is greatly increased when workers telecommute. Employers report an increase in productivity of 12%-20% per employee, estimated to be a savings of $6,000-$8,000 per employee per year.

Office Space and Equipment: Telecommuting is kind to employers, too. With employees or independent contractors working at home, there is no need to invest company dollars in office expansion and added staff. In addition, smaller departments can be run more efficiently, making the company more competitive, and there is less managerial stress with fewer on-site employees and tasks to manage.

Flexibility: Businesses and individuals enjoy increased flexibility in performing their work.

Computers, fax machines and emerging telephone services are all developing in the same direction — to give us more control over where, when and how we conduct our work.

WHO ARE THE TELECOMMUTERS?

Telecommuting is best suited to people who like to work, who don't mind working alone, and who enjoy combining home and business activities. Those who have made the switch successfully praise the telecommuting lifestyle and its life-enhancing qualities.

In 1997, it is estimated that approximately 18 million Americans are home-based workers, and more than 10.5 million are telecommuters. According to all sources, these numbers will continue to increase. In California, telecommuting is more highly evolved than in most parts of the country as a result of regulations imposed by the Clean Air Act. For the first time in California's history, there are large numbers of displaced white-collar workers seeking meaningful employment. Many are using their professional knowledge and skills to establish home-based businesses. They are "going solo." Many are telecommuters.

TelNetwork, an Oakland-based association that researches the impact of telecommuting, recently estimated that at least 90,000 people in the San Francisco Bay Area alone now telecommute, and that another 700,000-1,000,000 commuters might be able to telecommute one to three days a week.

Air quality legislation, a more in-line work force, greater comfort with technology, and the dropping costs of high tech products are all fueling the growth of telecommuting.

> *"Even if you're on the right track, you will get run over if you are not moving fast enough."*
> —Will Rogers

TELECOMMUTER — THE PROFESSIONAL

Telecommuting is now established as a formal job description. More than ten million Americans are telecommuters.

More and more health care facilities are negotiating off-site work arrangements to reduce overhead expenses, taking into consideration that telecommuting has proven to significantly increase quality and productivity. The same transcription services that once boasted they used only in-house transcriptionists are now aggressively recruiting skilled off-site MTs throughout the world. According to Link Resources, the number of people telecommuting will reach 14 million by the end of the decade.

Occasionally telecommuters do encounter resistance from those who aren't comfortable with such arrangements. But despite occasional skeptics, the trend toward telecommuting represents a large — and probably unstoppable — shift in workplace priorities.

As medical transcriptionists shift to telecommuting, we are more adaptable to industry shift because ours is a profession of individuals who can work on our own and require little face-to-face contact. There are prerequisites to successful telecommuting, however.

The downside to telecommuting can be loneliness and overwork. You may work extra hours to prove your dedication and the worth of your service. You may tempted to stop working, wander from your desk and start doing something not related to your work. Keep focused. And if you find yourself cruising the refrigerator during working hours, take a brief walk elsewhere instead.

You must have an "end of the day" routine or you may find yourself wandering back into your office and working again. Tell yourself "DON'T GO THERE!"

TRANSCRIPTION ANYWHERE

More and more health care facilities and transcription services are utilizing skilled off-site transcriptionists at satellite locations to meet the ever increasing demand for transcription of dictation. The dictated data must be moved rapidly to resources that are the most available and cost-effective. The development of digital dictation has revolutionized the industry and more recently rerecord technology has been introduced. This allows transcriptionists to access dictation and download at a higher rate of speed than real time, thus cutting down on telephone rerecord costs.

There are now systems available, such as Dictaphone's STRAIGHT TALK system, that offer cost-effective solutions to high speed rerecording. This equipment can be programmed for the home-based MT to download dictation at any given time, and transcription can begin as soon as rerecording begins. This means no more waiting for cassettes to fill up or for the entire transmission to conclude.

INTERNET

Internet is the mother of all computer networks. It is actually a collection of networks with shared software standards. The system allows millions of people in business and academia around the globe to communicate. More than 15 million users are on the Internet network and the numbers are growing rapidly. Several hundred libraries worldwide have added their catalogs to the system. Full text data bases will likely evolve from this.

The beginning stages of a multibillion dollar user electronic highway are in place and it is anticipated that this highway will do for the flow of information what the first transcontinental railroad, and later the interstate highway system, did for the transportation of goods and people. Unlike those earlier communication networks, however, whose costs were supported by government, it appears that the costs of our multibillion dollar information highway will likely be borne by private enterprise.

From medical images and billings for physician services to movies and telecommunication, the electronic highway promises to transform the flow of information from a paper chase to almost instantaneous retrieval.

Internet services and data bases are so bewildering that software is being developed to specifically search for desired information. The overwhelming majority of revenues we get by the end of the decade will be from services and products that have not yet been invented.

To keep up with the digital revolution, there are many references we recommend reading. You may have heard of *Wired*. This is one of the first publications to actually capture the excitement of the merger of computing, communications and media that is changing every aspect of our lives from business to politics and education to entertainment. Call or write for information on this publication.

- *Wired*
  P. O. Box 191826
  San Francisco
  14119-9866
  800-SO-WIRED

ONLINE GLOBAL COMMUNICATIONS

There are many resources available for learning to navigate the internet but one of our favorites is *NetPractice, A Beginner's Guide to Healthcare Networking on the Internet*. NetPractice is a self-instructional guide designed to give health care professionals a no-nonsense approach to navigating on the Internet. It doesn't try to overwhelm you with a conglomeration of Internet services but lays a foundation for the most common and practical uses of the Internet. Contact Opus Communications for more information.

- **Opus Communications**
  Fulfillment Center
  P.O. Box 9214
  Waltham, MA 02514-9214
  E-mail at customer_service@opuscomm.com.

THE SEVEN-SECOND COMMUTE

The number of telecommuters is growing dramatically. In the year 1990 there were two million telecommuters. In 1994 there were 7.8 million telecommuters, and in 1997 there were more than 10 million. It is predicted that by the year 2001 there will be 30 million telecommuters. By the year 2010 a quarter of a billion people will be telecommuters, according to Link Resources.

Employers are finally realizing that where work is concerned, *the important thing is the individual and the quality of the work he or she produces*, not the location where the work is produced.

For many years, large transcription services have boasted that their work is completed by only the most qualified transcriptionists. Some brag that they use only "in house" MTs. These individuals supposedly work in a controlled environment where confidentiality is a priority, use the best technology to produce excellent transcription in prompt turnaround time, etc., etc. Some of the large services offer employee benefit packages and incentives. These perks used to be available only to those working in the office, but now these same services are promoting their employment packages to home-based MTs, to work as at-home employees with benefits or as independent MTs. This opens up great opportunities for home-based medical transcriptionists.

Large services have done an "about face" since our last edition of this book. They once suggested — either openly or indirectly — that independent transcriptionists were a threat to medical record confidentiality, but my experience has found that to be absolutely untrue. I have had the opportunity to transcribe reports in the acute-care hospital setting, as a transcription manager for a service, and as a home-based transcriptionist. Of these three environments, I found the home-office to be the most confidential.

Think about it. In the hospital setting the medical transcriptionist is the first one to see the patient's medical record, but she is certainly not the last! While the patient is in the hospital, that record passes through the hands of approximately 75 health care professionals — doctors, nurses, lab and medical imaging technicians, therapists, social workers, discharge planners, utilization reviewers and others. In medical records departments, the patient's record is seen by chart assemblers, coders/abstractors, and other medical personnel. And what about accounts receivable? In my experience, the transcriptionist is not a major risk factor in issues of patient confidentiality.

I live on a rural mountain top, a 5½-hour driving distance between me and the nearest transcription service. I'm a skilled, experienced, highly qualified transcriptionist. I, too, have a controlled office environment, confidentiality is a priority, my technology is up-to-date, and I provide great turnaround time.

This is the age of moving information through telecommuting and working where we choose. There is no reason why a person should have to sacrifice time and energy to commute hours on end just to get to a job, or get a job done! Transcription services that offer benefits can now have the best of both worlds. They can utilize qualified MTs who will gladly be a part of their team through telecommuting. With sophisticated technology at our fingertips, we can process data faster than Superman can fly to the top of a tall building, from anywhere in the world to anywhere else in the world — from where we are.

My work and lifestyle as a home-based transcriptionist suit my needs. I do commute thirty seconds every day to get to work, but I begin work when I like, and my schedule is flexible. I enjoy breathing the fresh air atop this mountain and gazing down at a beautiful lake. In this setting, I am able to work longer and with less stress. My work is done in a controlled office environment. My reference library is up to date, and my computer technology is state-of-the-art. I have my own clients and service them through telecommuting. I also do work for a larger service when my own client load slows down. My professional life and my personal/family life are kept completely separate.

The work does have its ups and downs and many times it's feast or famine, but that's true in a large service as well. Ultimately, a career is what you make it. I choose this home-based independent working situation as do thousands of others. With modems and fax machines we are able to receive patient information, job numbers, and admission and discharge logs.

RIDING THE WAV

With digital phone systems and rerecord devices now available, we can access dictating systems and offer incredible turnaround to our clients, just like the "big guys." And look what is coming now . . . the WAV. Soon WAV file technology will be an everyday medical transcription word . . . someone in New York will be reading what I am currently typing . . . that's what happens when we ride the WAV!

PREPARING TO TELECOMMUTE

Whether you're planning to talk to multiple businesses across the nation or simply connect to local clinics, technical requirements are essentially the same: a personal computer at your end hooked to a modem attached to a phone line. Whomever you're telecommunicating to will need the same equipment. Each computer configuration is a little different, but here are some suggestions for an "ideal" setup and the reasons for each recommended component.

- **The most current PC you can reasonably afford.** A 486 or Pentium class PC with at least 16 megabytes of memory and Windows loaded would be a minimum desirable configuration. It's a fact that you can run WordPerfect for DOS on an old AT with 640K of memory, but the main advantage a Windowed-machine gives you is multi-tasking or background processing. This means you could be sending or receiving files or faxes in the background while processing documents, spreadsheets or other items at the same time. This may seem trivial, but if you're spending five to ten minutes sending or receiving, that can add up to over 300 hours a year!

- **An external, high speed, data/fax modem.** *External* because it frees you from being locked into a specific computer. *High speed* because it minimizes your line charges and increases efficiency. *Data/fax* because sooner or later someone will need to fax you a hard copy or you will need to fax a hard copy to them. (Remember, you'll need a fax software package to utilize the faxing capabilities of your fax/modem).

A 33.6K bps modem costs around $99. You can get higher speed 56K bps external fax/modems for as little as $159! In addition, newer modems are more reliable and more compatible with other systems.

- **A *common* communications package. DON'T** use some hokey piece of software your brother or friend gave you for "free." Check the market you'll be talking with: what do they use? *PC Anywhere? Carbon Copy?* A combination? These two products (and *ProComm Plus*) have a distinct advantage over others in that they are easy to set up and can talk to most anything else. That means if you have PC Anywhere but the clinic has Carbon Copy you can still communicate. If possible, stick with the commonly used products. Check the references and resources in the back of this book.

> NOTE: If a business insists on a specific software package you don't have, ask for a copy of their software and adequate licensing documentation. Often, the license they've purchased will allow for your use of the software, too. Conversely, your license will often allow you to load the product on both your home PC and that of another host computer.

- **If you have substantial online time, a separate phone line for your fax/ modem.** If your time online is short, this may not be necessary, but if your phone has various options like call waiting, etc. you might experience connection interruptions. Check with the phone company to see what impact, if any, such services could have on your data transmissions.

Whenever possible, remain independent of the remote business. Sometimes, however, the business will require you to work online. In this situation you dial the business and do your work on *their* machine. Although your body is home, your transcription is in their office. There are two disadvantages to this scenario:

1) Most transcriptionists can out-type even the fastest phone line connection.

2) You are at the mercy of communications lines and hardware at the business site. If either fails, you're out of work until repairs are made.

Remember, too, that all communications packages provide dial-back capability. This means you can call a business that is long distance and the business's modem can dial your modem back to establish the connection. You benefit because that telephone call is on their dime (or dollar!), not yours. In addition, it gives them more security because they control outgoing calls from their modem.

Get to know your computer. Books like *DOS for Dummies* are a quick way to gain basic knowledge about your computer and telecommuting.

THE MODEM

To telecommunicate you must connect your computer to a phone line. For that capability, your system must incorporate a modem. In essence, a modem is a small electronic telephone. It can be installed either on a card inside your system unit (internal modem) or outside the unit, hooked up to a communications, or COM, port (external modem).

Your modem accepts data you input via your keyboard and translates that data into bits and bytes, which the modem then transmits across phone lines. After another computer or online system has received your telephoned transmission, its modem translates these bits and bytes back into readable form, and your telecommunicating begins.

Internal modems cost less than external modems, but whenever possible buy an external modem. External modems are easier to install than internal modems. You don't have to remove the cover from your PC and squeeze another circuit card into a tight-fitting slot. Most important, you will not have to reverse the process if the modem is set up wrong the first time you install it. If an external modem needs service you just unplug it! Removing an internal modem requires much greater effort.

Another advantage of external modems is their indicator lights, which are located on the front of the modem's case. These lights are computer status indicators and are great troubleshooting aids. After a short time, you will be able to tell which lights should be on, or blinking, during transmissions.

Internal modems are not helpful at all when something isn't working right, and some computer techs tell us they are discovering that internal modems are rough on the computer's hard drive and eventually cause failures more often than external modems.

The greater the baud rate, the faster information is sent over the phone line . . . and the higher the price of the modem. However, just because your modem may be a 33,300 baud, it doesn't guarantee that your data will **always** be transmitted at that speed. Data is transferred according to the availability of phone space through the lines, so during peak hours of the work day your modem may automatically bump down to whatever baud rate it needs to get the data through the line.

If you are anxious to try out your modem after installing it, contact a friend who has a modem and experiment. Connect with him/her and practice using the chat mode. Practice exchanging files, uploading and downloading. Sending a file is to **upload**, to receive a file is to **download**.

THE TELECOMMUNICATIONS PROGRAM

A telecommunications program is software that controls the connection between your computer and some other remote computer system or online service. Some online services such as *Prodigy* or *America OnLine* provide special software.

To call another computer system you need to know the following about the other system:

- The phone number to call

- Any password or log-in procedure the other system requires

- The baud rate (for example, 9600 bps, 14,400 bps)
  (Most new computer software will search your system and set up parameters automatically.)

- Number of data bits (usually 7 or 8)

- Number of stop bits (usually 1)

- The parity (odd, even, or none)

Software programs for modeming vary in price but, generally, they perform the same functions. Do some comparison shopping before making your final decision. Pro-Comm Plus is one software program that does the job for about $80.

FILE ARCHIVE (COMPRESSION) UTILITY

Archiving utilities squeeze one or more files into a single file, which occupies fewer bytes than the original file(s) did. For this same reason, these archiving utilities are also called compression utilities. There are several reasons why it is wise to use a utility for compressing and decompressing all files being transferred. Fewer bytes means less transmission time, often one-half to one-quarter the time required to transfer the uncompressed file(s). This speeds up your transfer time and keeps long-distance telephone expenses down. I use PKZip and PKUnzip, which can be downloaded from computer information services and bulletin boards. The following chart lists a few of the most popular compression utilities with notes on how they compare to one another:

ARCHIVE EXTENSION	ARCHIVE/ DECOMPRESSION UTILITY	COMMENTS
myfile.ZIP	PKZIP.EXE/PKUNZIP.EXE	By far, most common and powerful
myfile.ARC	ARC.EXE/XARC.EXE	Often used in commercial software
myfile.ARJ	ARJ.EXE	Only one utility needed
myfile.LZH	LHA.EXE	Also one utility

I recommend getting PKZIP/PKUNZIP; it is by far the most widely used, and in my opinion, the most versatile. You can download the latest version of PKZIP/PKUNZIP from PK Ware BBS.

- **PK Ware Bulletin Board Service (BBS)**
  414-354-8670

Whichever archiver you get, put it in a directory on your hard disk that is part of your MS-DOS path; that way, you can invoke an archiver utility from any other directory on the drive.

> *"Science and technology revolutionize our lives, but memory, tradition and myth frame our response. . . . The dialectic between past and future will continue to form our lives."*
> —Arthur M. Schlesinger, Jr., 1986

SERVICING CLIENTS THROUGH TELECOMMUNICATION

In the old days, hospitals mailed tape cassettes and waited several days for reports to be returned. Through telecommunication, digital dictation systems allow the transcriptionist or service to dial in and transcribe off the system, send files back via modem, at which point hard copies are printed at the facility. Turnaround is decreased to HOURS instead of days and weeks.

Telecommuting can be utilized to access dictation through the telephone system with digital dictation and using a modem to transfer or deliver transcription over the phone to another computer.

Computer bulletin boards (BBs) are also accessed through telecommunication. The Federal Drug Administration (FDA) has a computer bulletin board, as does the Small Business Administration (SBA). Both are very helpful resources for home-based businesses.

On the following page is a list of the most popular Bulletin Boards (BBs).

BULLETIN BOARDS (BBS)

SERVICE	ACCESS NUMBER TO CALL	COMMENTS
CompuServe	800-848-8199, or 800-848-8990 (Ohio - 614-457-8600), and ask for a local access #.	Largest information carrier, owned by H&R Block. Provides 24 hour access.
GEnie	800-838-9363 or 800-638-8369	General Electric Information Services.
Delphi	800-544-4004, or 800-365-4636, Enter. Wait a few seconds for menu to appear, type JOINDELPHI.	Best buy for business use. First BBS to offer online encyclopedia.
Prodigy	800-822-6922, ext 205 for start-up kit.	Custom software required. More costly than some; pretty pictures, pretty slow. Easy to navigate.
America OnLine	800-827-6364 for start-up kit.	Custom software required.

Servicing clients from the home office through telecommunication is now very popular and very cost-effective. It eliminates wasted time and travel expenses in pick up and delivery, and expensive courier fees required for rush jobs. With telecommunication, a two- or three-minute phone call transmits your transcription across the street or across the country. The cost for this type of service is a modem, software and a telephone call.

Currently, using modern technology and telecommunication, it takes me ***three hours*** to do what it took me eight hours to do ten years ago! My clients benefit from this improved service, and so do I — with less stress, increased productivity, and greater profits.

> *"Using modern technology and telecommunication, it takes me three hours to do what it took me eight hours to do ten years ago!"*

WHAT IS PRACTICAL FOR INDIVIDUAL CLIENTS

Telecommuting isn't always practical for physicians' offices, especially in remote areas. With health care policies and impending government reforms, many physicians are gearing up to implement a variety of cutbacks and reduce overhead expenses. We anticipate that one of the first cutbacks will be clerical and transcription services.

If you plan to market your services to physician accounts, be prepared to pick up and deliver cassettes, for this will probably be the most cost-effective plan for one- or two-client offices. Other doctors will prefer cassettes because, although a dial-and-dictate system might work well in their office, they do not have time to dictate in that setting. They are doctors who frequently use a hand-held recorder and dictate chart notes wherever they happen to be — in the examining room during or after a patient's exam; in their car on the way to the hospital or on their way home; in the recovery room after performing surgery; at home after dinner; or at the park while watching their kids or walking the dog. Their time is precious and they squeeze dictation duty into their busy schedules whenever and wherever possible. For these doctors, cassette tapes continue to be ideal.

Telecommuting and dial-and-dictate systems are very effective for hospitals and larger clinics where there is shared financial responsibility. These facilities are able to contract with remote services, use home-based medical transcriptionists who can connect directly to their dictation systems via modem, and even home-base their own employees.

TELEPHONE CHARGES

As a telecommuter you are responsible for telecommuting phone charges, and one of your biggest expenses will be long distance charges. If your potential clients are long distance, carefully weigh the cost of telephone charges against what you will earn. For current clients, consider rerecording or using your digital system during less costly off-peak telephone hours.

If you are interested in telecommuting with a service, look for a reputable service in your area that hires home-based telecommuting medical transcriptionists. If you are fortunate enough to find a good company locally, you will avoid the expense of long distance phone bills.

If you are hired by a service as a home-based employee, the service should provide you with tools to perform your duties for them. This should include their paying one-half of your social security payroll tax, covering costs for your computer, printer, toner, phone, paper, transcriber, and other necessary supplies.

If you contract with a service as an independent contractor, you should supply all of the equipment necessary to perform services for them — including the cost of accessing dictation.

RESEARCH PHONE SERVICES

If you are preparing to service long distance clients, you should definitely research long distance phone carriers. There are hundreds of long distance phone carriers (in California alone there are over 110 long distance carriers). Ask one or more long distance providers to do a traffic analysis of your phone calls. Check on special phone discounts, WATS lines, Circle Calling, etc.

Investigate telecommunication resource and management companies that specialize in recommending and implementing long distance, local data and other telecommunication services to customers. These companies research and find phone carriers for clients at a lower cost than companies can obtain on their own. With this service you benefit from cost savings, administrative benefits, and ongoing telephone line management and monitoring services. These companies also negotiate with many carriers in order to offer clients services that provide high quality service at the best reduced rates.

For a list of the five largest long-distance telephone carriers, send a self-addressed, stamped envelope and $2.00 to TRAC.

- **Telecommunications Research Action Center (TRAC)**
  P.O. Box 12038
  Washington, D.C., 20005

TELECOMMUTING FOR REMOTE SERVICES AND CLIENTS

To locate services that use telecommuters, investigate ads in trade journals and publications. If you are interested in working for a remote service, you will be asked to submit a resume of experience. After reviewing your proposal, they may ask you to transcribe a tape so they can review your transcription quality. Often they will simply have you modem the transcribed documents back to them. Other services will mail a tape to you and ask you to mail your transcribed documents back. If the company decides to use your services, they may require a trial period during which you will be given a limited amount of work. Some companies also require on-site training.

Many remote companies require that you dial into their dictation system and download onto tapes, then transcribe and modem the files back to them. (The service will provide you with instructions for setting modem parameters to send and receive files).

Now technology available to home-based transcriptionists is becoming much more sophisticated. Systems such as PC Dart allow the transcriptionists to download dictation into his or her computer, which eliminates tapes altogether. And, the transcriptionist can begin transcribing during the downloading process.

Be forewarned: Remote service downloading of dictation onto cassette tapes can be very time-consuming. However, the alternative — transcribing over telephone lines — would be far too costly.

Utilize time wisely while you are rerecording by organizing the office as you monitor the rerecord process. Update reference materials and finish other clerical tasks that you generally don't have time to do when transcribing. If you are working full time at least 40 hours per week transcribing, you will probably appreciate this "extra" time.

Some rerecord units can be set to automatically dial into the service system and start the recording process (even while you sleep). Many systems now have technology designed to download at a higher rate of speed, thus reducing your rerecord time. Other rerecord networks require you to key in numbers to begin and end each dictation. Rerecording is time consuming and you may lose some dictation quality/clarity in the process.

A reputable service will have quality standards which are usually outlined in the contract you enter into with them. If you do not meet their standards, for instance, if your error ratio is too high, it is standard procedure for them to impose a penalty or cut the rate of pay you agreed upon.

When working remotely for a service, remember to follow through on your commitments. Keep an open mind about upgrading systems and improving your efficiency. Be professional when accepting constructive criticism, and encourage feedback regarding your work.

If possible, before accepting work, try to visit the service in person to get a feel for their organization and the people you will be working for. Some services **require** that you arrange to visit their facility and participate in a training session before you begin working for them. Never hesitate to ask questions. Remember, you are an independent transcriptionist and are responsible for YOU, INCORPORATED.

TRANSCRIPTION SERVICES THAT USE HOME-BASED TRANSCRIPTIONISTS

- ARCO Transcription   619-576-3120; 619-576-3131

- Dictation Plus   800-743-PLUS

- Digital Dictation, Inc.   800-888-5295

- ECS (Electronic Communications Systems)   619-287-2000
  4760 Mission Gorge Place, Suite B   Fax: 619-287-2139
  San Diego, CA 92120

- EDIX   800-944-PLUS

- Secrephone   800-523-5335

- Signal Transcription   800-999-6639

- Transcriptions International   800-466-4326

- Transcriptions, Ltd. (A MedQuist Company)   800-233-3030

DOs AND DON'Ts FOR ONLINE COMMUNICATION

Make sure that both your modem and telecommunications software are set up correctly for the BBS or online system you are calling.

- Never disconnect your modem from a BBS or online service without correctly exiting the system, unless you absolutely must do so. Such abrupt exiting can damage a system.

- Use the highest baud rate possible when downloading data to reduce your on-line charges; *however,*

- Don't use a high baud rate when talking to another user in real-time on an on-line service; often the higher speeds are billed at higher rates, and you almost certainly type more slowly than your modem can transmit anyway.

- Use an automated program to download message headers and messages from CompuServe and other services; reading such messages online can run up big phone bills.

- Don't download program files from bulletin boards with which you are not familiar; such files may hide computer viruses.

- Install a separate telephone line for your modem if you can afford it. It frees up your regular line so that you can talk and type at the same time.

- Don't configure your modem to use the same COM port as any other device in your computer system, such as a mouse.

- Make sure your modem is connected correctly to both your computer and your telephone line.

TELECOMMUTING LINGO

- **Messaging**: Talking to others through the use of electronic mail.

- **Conferencing**: Talking to another in real-time. Your words appear on another user's monitor as you type them on your keyboard.

- **Uploading**: You transmit a file from your machine to a client or BB.

- **Downloading**: You transmit a file from a client or BB to your machine.

EXPRESSING YOUR EMOTIONS VIA TELECOMMUTING

When you "message" or "conference" online with other computer users, you sometimes want to express an emotion or attitude that may be difficult to convey in words on a computer screen. That's why a special system of expressions has developed among online telecommuters. These "*emoticons*" (emotion icons) use standard characters in set patterns to express specific emotions. When you look at an emoticon sideways (with your head turned to the left), it looks like a face in a particular expression.

For example :-) is an emoticon for happy. (It looks like a smiling face, right?) And :-(is an emoticon for sad. There are many different emoticons, including some that are completely off the wall. Plain bracketed comments also serve as emoticons to some users: when you see a <g>, it is shorthand for "grin" and it means the user is just kidding. Pretty cool, eh? <g>

Performance Improvement

QUALITY VERSUS QUANTITY

*"In personal and professional pursuits,
I demand of myself an ever higher
standard of excellence."*

—Beatrice Gage

Much has been written in the past several years about quality versus quantity. Should we sacrifice the quality of the report in order to produce more transcription in a given day? The consensus has been a definite "No."

This certainly holds true for the home-based medical transcriptionist. If the quality of your reports suffers, the patient may suffer, your client may suffer, and so may your income. It is impossible to maintain accounts or procure new ones if your product quality is poor. The world of medical transcription is a very small one, and word does travel about the quality of one's work.

This author has worked for two large transcription services, one that provided an in-house proofreader and one that did not. The service with the proofreading staff sent out A+ quality reports, while the latter did not. The latter was more interested in format than content, and the firm had difficulty retaining accounts for any length of time.

During my tenure with the first firm, I learned more than I ever had about medical words and usage. It held me in good stead when transferring to a second firm and eventually establishing my home-based business.

ERRORS IN THE MEDICAL RECORD

As professionals, we want our transcription of the medical record to be as accurate as possible for the sake of patients and our clients, but being human, we do make errors.

Sometimes a transcription error will occur through no fault of our own. Other times, it will be decidedly our mistake. No matter where the fault lies, it is important to learn from the mistake and find ways to prevent the same error in the future.

Most dedicated professionals strive for perfection in work as well as in personal life. In truth, we realize that perfection is unattainable except for small slices of life, but even small slices of perfection whet our appetite for more. As a group, we medical transcriptionists tend to be workaholics who thrive on challenge and look forward to the day when innovation by man and/or technical beast solves the problem of errors. Until that time, we persevere.

As medical language specialists, we must keep in mind that the English language, as well as the language of medicine, is still evolving and new words are added every day. Discovering new words is an exciting and worthwhile experience. Skilled transcriptionists never stop learning.

Perfection may not be attainable, but transcriptionists must always strive for knowledge, understanding, innovation, and creative ways to improve our product while remaining adaptable to changes in our profession. We must be objective and able to accept criticism. We must learn to work with and through fellow transcriptionists and other health care professionals. After having sat through a grueling and tedious dictation, there is no greater satisfaction than to sign off a report with my initials, knowing that I have done my very best. It feels very much like perfection.

THE FINE ART OF EDITING

Unless the dictating physician was also an English major in his premed days, most medical reports you transcribe will require some form of editing. Editing can be as simple as changing plurals to singulars, correcting punctuation (semicolon instead of a period), or correcting a medical inconsistency (changing metatarsal to metacarpal).

A useful resource book for answering questions regarding editing is the *Style Guide for Medical Transcription* published by the American Association for Medical Transcription. In 1982, Vera Pyle, CMT, addressed the issue of how and when to edit in an article published in the *Journal of the American Association for Medical Transcription*. The article is reprinted in the *Style Guide*.

Vera Pyle is quoted as saying, " In editing we do not go charging in, doctoring up reports in an aggressive way, in an intrusional way. It has to be done so subtly, so delicately, so carefully, that we get a favorable response from the author. We must be so involved with what we are transcribing that we know what is going on and can detect something that is dictated that does not make sense, that does not flow, that does not add up. We must listen with an educated ear, with an intelligent ear, so that we can produce an accurate, intelligent, clear document, always remembering the fine line between editing and tampering. "

On the subject of when *not* to edit, Pyle asks, " What about those who are inconsiderate of us? What about those who mumble? What about those whom we can't help because we don't know what they mean? If you know what they are trying to say, you can help clarify the dictation. If you don't know, that is the time to transcribe verbatim; it's our only recourse. "

Editing has changed considerably during the past fifteen years. In the United States, many changes are a result of the influx of foreign-born physicians, who are popularly referred to as ESL or English-as-a-Second-Language physicians. Although most of these doctors are very conscious of their accents and do an exceptional job dictating, there are others who have not quite mastered the intricacies of English, especially in differentiating between past and present tenses and noun and verb usage.

As a medical transcriptionist, you must have a good grasp of the language, not only of English but of medicine, to equip you for some very complex editing challenges.

According to the *Style Guide*, it is important that you retain the dictating physician's style. We have no right to impose our style on the report. As a good rule of thumb, edit grammatical, punctuation, spelling and similar dictation errors as necessary to achieve clear communication. Edit slang words and phrases, incorrect or verbal inconsistencies and medical inconsistencies. Edit inaccurate phrasing of laboratory data.

Physicians also tend to talk with colleagues when dictating and sometimes make inadvertent, derogatory comments about the patient, which, of course, should not become part of the medical record! Never include informal, inappropriate statements in the transcribed medical report.

PERFORMANCE IMPROVEMENT

Developing good quality in your medical transcription business is essential to your success and survival as an independent transcriptionist. Continuing quality improvement (CQI) should be an ongoing process in your business. Developing quality guidelines should be established at the onset of business. AAMT has established recommended guidelines for such quality control (see example).

KEEPING ONE STEP AHEAD OF THE HEADHUNTERS

Medical transcription companies merging is hot news on the Internet. Recently there was a post stating that this is good news for MTs working for services, home-based MTs and independent MTs.

I guess it's good news if you want to work for someone else. Personally, there are MTs who prefer to remain "*independent.*" The latest merger means a work force of over 2000 MTs throughout the US. The merger will also mean better bargaining power with health care corporations in negotiating contracts for less. The bigger the bargaining power, the better the price.

This is just another example of why the IMT must keep pace with industry trends and technology, because when the dust settles, and work is being done for fewer dollars, in less time, with fewer people, only the *creme de la creme* will be skimmed from the top of the bucket. The most technically savvy and knowledgeable, not only in medical transcription but in all aspects of professional and business management, will survive.

As health care corporations continue to acquire physician practices, clinics and outpatient centers, they will incorporate and manage their cost centers as well. As managed care continues to negotiate capitated contracts with these health care organizations, physicians will be required to cut operating costs to maintain a place on the provider list. This means that MTs servicing individual physician practices may lose clients because those clients can no longer afford their services, or because this expense has been absorbed by a larger cost center which is negotiating cheaper rates elsewhere. Health care headhunters are already including a "medical transcriptionist" category in their marketing material.

Independent medical transcriptionists should focus on real-time (meaning, "happening now") business management practices. The medical transcription industry and technology are evolving more rapidly than ever before and to keep pace, independent medical transcriptionists must look at 1) how we do business and how we can do it better, 2) increasing our knowledge and 3) promoting our professionalism.

TAKING A PROACTIVE APPROACH WHEN RENEGOTIATING CONTRACTS

At the start of any professional relationship with a client, the parties involved commit themselves to certain promises. This is done through agreement and is documented in a contract. During contract negotiations it is important to discuss policies and procedures on all items that will be incorporated into the contract. Once a contract is signed, both parties are expected to live up to the terms of the contract.

Regularly review how you are doing business and servicing your clients. This is important so you thoroughly understand what does and does not work for you and your business. Frequently one party or the other wants to change one or more terms or conditions in the ironclad contract. What should you do when faced with the need to change a contract? Renegotiate . . . wisely.

A valid contract involves *mutual consideration*. A term used to explain consideration is "quid pro quo," meaning *"this for that."* When renegotiating a contract, the parties are required to come up with new consideration in order for the revised agreement to be equally binding. Here are some cues to aid in successful renegotiations.

- **Keep in touch with your client**. Frequently touch base with the client to review any problems that arise and keep notes in your contract file. Also document activities so that new policies can be written into the contract.

- **Offer something new.** Offer something of value to the client that is not already in the deal, i.e., your new technology and ability to provide more efficient "quality" service, i.e., discount for quick pay, rate break for volume of dictation, etc.

- **Be creative and flexible**. When situations change and there is a need to renegotiate the deal, recognize that the other side's wants and needs may have changed from the time the contract was initially negotiated. Be sure to include these in your renegotiation considerations.

- **Use a cooperative approach.** Remember that cooperation, creativity and flexibility play an important part in your success with clients. Both sides need to realize that they are negotiating with feeling people. If you are initiating the renegotiation of your contract, your approach should convey a sense of cooperative teamwork so the client does not feel you are an adversary or merely trying to escape your commitments. Likewise, the facility needs to cooperatively reciprocate, maximizing goodwill and reputation to make you feel like a winner. Ultimately, of course, a truly successful relationship will depend on the cooperation of the facility staff. In renegotiation, both sides should feel they have received more than they gave up.

- **When terms are finalized, have legal counsel review the contract before signing.**

NOTE

It is important to remember that the Internal Revenue Service does not recognize a written agreement as verification of your status as an independent contractor. Contracts and agreements only provide details and terms of your services with the client. Even if your contract states that you are acting and operating as an independent contractor in providing your services to the client, this has no effect on IRS determining whether you are an independent contractor or an employee.

THE POWER OF SHARING EXPERIENCE

We are living and working in an ever-changing communication age. Old conventional ways of gaining knowledge about our profession and marketplace through professional organizations are not as effective as they once were. Many professional organizations are no longer able to hold the interest of members, for whom they were developed to serve.

Throughout history, there has been a tremendous amount of information to be gained from collective, tribal sharing of information and experience, and that continues to be true today. In modern times, many of us have grown up working within and serving relatively homogenous social, business and organizational groups with a fairly narrow, inward focus. For many decades, the knowledge and professional contacts gained in this manner were adequate for professional growth. However, in the past few years some organization members have discovered they are learning more from one another, as well as from many other sources, than from presenters at association meetings.

As independent transcriptionists and business owners, our professional needs have gone beyond what is offered by inbred, narrow-minded, myopic organizations that are not keeping pace with worldwide business trends. More often, the linkages we need to gain knowledge about professional practices, business management, and marketing are not with the people who are like us but with dissimilar stakeholders who complement us in unique value-adding ways.

Homogenous groups always risk becoming self-absorbed. It is critical to the success of our business, and as independent medical transcriptionists, to continuously address new issues and process diverse views. Today, we need to invest our valuable time in a network of resources. An internally focused association too often inhibits this process.

People need new ideas and new methods if they are to achieve their goals. In health care, with the physician shift from "boss" to "team member," there is greater involvement of nurses and other allied health professionals at medical conferences. In fact, most conference audiences are composed of mixed groups of health care professionals.

The world of the CME (continuing medical education), CEU (continuing education units) is rapidly becoming the CPE (continuing professional education).

As an independent medical transcriptionist, the more diverse your communication experience, the more positive the effect on your business. As a solo business you should seek out new, updated information and resources on managing your business, accessing and marketing on the Internet, dealing with difficult personalities, quality and productivity enhancements/standards, risk management, negotiating skills, self-improvement, finances and record keeping, long-range planning, and other relevant topics. There are specialized groups that provide seminars on many subjects that will enhance the operation of your business, and for which you can receive CPE (CEU).

THE "NET SET"

Although the World Wide Web cannot yet substitute for good old face-to-face networking, the base of online medical transcriptionists is steadily growing throughout the world. The Net was not meant to be monitored or moderated by one personality over the other, and merely because one is found online does not necessarily make him or her an expert. Rather, the net should be utilized as a resource to communicate with other professionals, provide support for newcomers in the field and to share knowledge, experiences, bits and pieces of miscellaneous information and opinions, agreeable or not. What works for one may not work for another, for our careers are shaped by many factors — education, training, experience, attitude, personal preference, technology, work environment, social arena, etc.

A recent Internet trend is for individual MTs and organizations to set up their own online Websites. You will find Websites for Health Professions Institute, AAMT, MTIA, AHIMA and many other health care and business networks. Associations are beginning to take advantage of the Internet to promote conference programs, which will save organizations a tremendous amount normally spent on marketing and reaching a greater target market. At the same time it will provide the Internet visitor with additional educational opportunities they probably would not have been aware of otherwise.

Even more important is the immediacy of the Web. For educational programs, registration can be completely automated, the program schedule detailed before your eyes, and information provided about CEU available, product exhibitors, host city amenities, hotel reservations, airline schedules and prices, and more. For information on other conferences just do a search for "conferences." Log on and take a look!

CREATING YOUR OWN WEBSITE

Perhaps you are interested in creating your own Website. If so, create a site that will compel visitors to return again and again.

- **Make it interactive.**

- **Promote participation from "visitors."**

- **Keep it simple.** Visitors prefer to read through information quickly. Don't make them wade through large blocks of text or wait for large amounts of information to be downloaded onto the screen. This frustrates your audience and they may not return. Having a "tool bar" on every screen helps ensure easy navigation around the site.

- **Target your information.** Offer a menu of information by subject matter so visitors do not have to spend time scrolling through all your data. A well-designed site will lead them to the specific information they are seeking.

- **Keep the page current.** Update information continually. Fresh information encourages repeat visits.

- **Strive for consistency.** The "look" of a Website makes a statement about the sponsor. Develop site architecture that makes the visitor's experience seamless, intuitive and effortless. Be creative but make sure your resources are accurate. Consider offering "sneak previews" of information, products and trends. Make your Website a place where visitors will enjoy a unique experience. Since it is easy to put up-to-the minute information on the Web, make your site "the place" for the latest-breaking industry news.

- **Respond to Website visitors.** Offer an e-mail component to your site to help visitors get answers to questions they may have.

- **List your site in appropriate online directories and search engines.** Remember to include Website promotion in your printed material. Add it to your letterhead. Mention it when networking with colleagues and other contacts.

- **Track Website hits.** Establish a method of tracking "hits" to see how many visitors your site is getting.

The cost of a Website varies depending on the complexity of the architecture. Paying for a Website is much like building a home. There is a one-time cost to lay the foundation and put up the frame. Additional improvements increase costs. You can change the content of a site whenever you need to. Updates may be at half the initial cost.

Internet advances and worldwide business trends will seriously impact all professionals in the years ahead. These authors have been working independently since before "home-based," "solo," "SOHO" or even IMT or the Internet were recognized. We have seen and continue to see tremendous change in this industry. We have worked in the acute-care setting, in the service setting and independently. We choose to remain independent.

What does the future hold? Will our independence be threatened? Will organizations attempt to employ or contract only with companies that have multiple transcriptionist employees? Will independents be faced with legislative changes and legal battles over restraint of trade? One thing is certain, if and when that time comes, we will fight for our right to work independently; we hope we will not be fighting alone. Both now and in the future, we pray for a strong professional organization supporting our cause.

AAMT QUALITY CONTROL FOR MEDICAL TRANSCRIPTION

- Medical transcription services within (or for) the health care organization are performed and supervised by qualified medical transcriptionists.

- Designated equipment is utilized effectively, skillfully, and efficiently.

- Patient identification and demographics are verified.

- Dictator identification is verified.

- Appropriate format is followed.

- Appropriate medical terminology is used, and English language rules are applied.

- Current reference materials are used appropriately and efficiently to facilitate accuracy, clarity, and completeness.

- Visual proofreading and spellchecking (and electronic spellchecking, if appropriate) are performed.

- Inconsistencies, discrepancies, and inaccuracies are recognized and appropriately revised, edited, or clarified, without altering the meaning of dictation or changing the dictator's style. All remaining inconsistencies, discrepancies, and inaccuracies are flagged for dictator review or brought to the attention of supervisory personnel for appropriate action to assure accurate completion of the document.

- Appropriate personnel are consulted regarding dictation that may be considered unprofessional, frivolous, insulting, inflammatory, or inappropriate.

- Appropriate risk management personnel are consulted regarding unusual circumstances and/or information with possible risk factors.

- Quality and productivity standards and deadlines are met.

- Appropriate measures are taken to protect the confidentiality and security of the record.

- Administrative procedures are followed (e.g., copy distribution).

- If amendment or revision of the record is required, appropriate policies and procedures are followed, with corrections or revisions made according to established medicolegal guidelines.

- Document storage, security, and retrieval guidelines are followed.

- Random quality control review is performed by a qualified medical transcriptionist.

Performance improvement standards require that documents produced must demonstrate continuing efforts to improve the process and content of patient-care documentation. The quality issue means that documents must be accurate in content and presentation, ensuring that patient confidentiality and privacy are protected throughout the documentation process, dictation, transcription and storage. Documents should be well organized and succinct, and reflect a commitment to professionalism and quality.

Monitoring quality should be done by independent medical transcriptionists as well as in-house transcriptionists. Quality checks should include correctness of grammar, patient identification and errors. Develop a quality audit program for your business. During times of low volume, randomly select twenty-five reports for review. Your CQI program could contain some of the items listed below.

- Enhancement with productivity software

- Turnaround time

- Quality management procedures

- Continuing education

- Technology and computer security

INCENTIVE PROGRAMS

A well-written incentive plan covers quality and quantity while monitoring results. Before incentive plans, quality of work was frequently poor. Incentive plans motivate employees and encourage top-quality work. If the quality is not there you will not be in business long, and if you work for a service as an independent, you may suffer a reduction in your rate of pay if your error rate is substantial.

PRODUCTIVITY AND TURNAROUND

Productivity software is computer software enhancements such as keyboard shorthand programs or basic macro commands. There are several programs like this currently available, and they make it easy to quantify improvement and reduce labor and keystrokes. Also, they create an atmosphere of excitement and have the added benefit of improving quality while decreasing transcriptionist fatigue.

The choice of productivity software should be made after surveying what is available, talking to users, and comparing prices and customer support. Adapting to this software takes time — usually about two weeks — so be sure to allow extra time for that in your schedule. You may want to modify your workload during this learning period, taking less work than usual.

Evaluate your productivity figures after two weeks and periodically thereafter, weekly or biweekly, to see how the program has benefitted your productivity in dollars and time. A logical time to do this is at the end of a billing period.

With productivity software you must also monitor your documents by proofreading on a regular basis. A spellchecker will not pick up expanded short-forms that are incorrect. For example, if the patient's name is Pat, she may end up as "paroxysmal atrial tachycardia" if "pat" happens to be your short-form for that term.

CONTINUING PERFORMANCE IMPROVEMENT MANAGEMENT

Consider updating reference materials, macros, and updating and/or changing formats regularly. Perform quality audits of your reports and look into upgrading your computer technology.

Perform ongoing audits on your documents and consider developing a formal report of your audit procedure. This is essential if you are to provide ongoing improvement and enhancements to adequately meet the needs of your clients.

AUDIT LOG SHEET

Month Audited: _____

DATE	MT ID	DOCUMENT TYPE	NO. PAGES	POINTS	TYPE ERROR
					Rev: 1/98

Medical record entries are only as accurate as the people who write, dictate and transcribe them. As businesses and service providers learn about continuing quality improvement procedures (CQI), they will expect them to be implemented in daily activities. We must always try to do the job right the first time, focusing on the benefits of timely, accurate and complete documentation and the effect it has on patient care and our professional lives. Errors, of course, will occur from time to time for a variety of reasons, including doctors who mumble crucial words that transcriptionists hear incorrectly or not at all. When errors are found, the recorded entry should be corrected as soon as possible.

TIME MANAGEMENT

Here are some tips for managing your time and productivity.

- Organize and prioritize your responsibilities. Use a notebook, calendar or a "to do" list. At the end of each day write down the next day's activities.

- Give yourself deadlines. If you estimate how much time you need to complete a task, you're more likely to finish it on time. Block out time on your calendar.

- Determine your peak productivity period. Try keeping an hour-by-hour log of activities for a few days. You may discover you are particularly productive during certain times of the day.

- Make beneficial use of commuting and waiting time. Carry a cassette recorder or note pad with you to record ideas and thoughts that pop into your head.

- Take some daily quiet time. Set aside a period of each day for uninterrupted concentration, planning and thinking.

- Don't procrastinate.

- Combat clutter.

- Make efficient use of your telephone time.

By using your time more efficiently, you may improve your productivity. It's definitely worth the effort.

FLAGGING AND LEAVING BLANKS IN A REPORT

To safeguard the integrity of the reports you transcribe, never second-guess what a physician means. If something is unclear, don't hesitate to flag a report and ask for clarification. If in doubt, leave it out.

Be sure to leave enough blank space for the word or phrase to be inserted later. Make a copy of your "flags" for your records.

If you are working for a hospital account, ask for their quality assurance standards. If they have none, explain your standard editing procedure and use your best judgment on individual cases, always keeping in mind that your goal is to type the most accurate medical report possible.

You will occasionally encounter words that you have never heard before. Even the best transcriptionist has this problem, so don't feel bad. If you cannot find the term in your reference materials, flag the report.

Physicians sometimes get right and left mixed up. One minute they may be dictating an operative report on the right femur, only to switch to the left femur later in the report. Clearly, such a report should be flagged.

There are times when physicians are interrupted during their dictation and do not complete the report. Always be sure to flag that report as incomplete and keep a record of it on your transmit log sheet.

Avoiding second-guessing is especially important for laboratory data. Transcriptionists must understand the normal ranges for all laboratory work so they can detect inconsistencies when they appear.

Sticky-notes are a blessing. Simply flag questionable reports where a word, phrase or number would have been typed and make a notation of what you heard so that the word, phrase or number is brought to the attention of the dictating physician.

Some software systems also have flagging capabilities.

If you have consistent difficulty with a certain dictating physician because of accent, poor tape quality, or poor dictating habits — dictating while eating, dictating from an erratic car phone, etc. — talk with the transcription supervisor or medical records director. Most accounts are willing to work with the outside service to ensure integrity of the medical record and a satisfactory working situation for the transcriptionist.

Don't leave too many blanks, however. This will suggest a deficiency on your part. If you find yourself in this position, you should reconsider whether you have the background experience or are adequately qualified to take work at this level of technical difficulty.

ONCE UPON A TIME BEFORE COMPUTERS

Before the computer, reports were transcribed with pen and ink. Multiple copies were duplicated by hand. Next came the manual typewriter, followed by the electric typewriter, typing first and second drafts, multiple carbon copies, ink erasers, and that wonderful invention, "whiteout."

The computer has certainly changed our way of doing things, and editing is now as easy as hitting a few command keys. The computer industry has responded to our needs by giving us abbreviation, spellchecking and dictionary software. These are wonderful tools to aid us in quality control.

Remember, though, that your spellchecker is only as good as your computer dictionary, which should be updated on a daily basis. Also be certain that new words added to the dictionary are spelled correctly. The same applies to macros and abbreviations. And most important, proofread your documents. Remember that a spellchecker cannot proofread your document for inconsistencies or omitted words.

When working for hospitals, it sometimes seems that medical records personnel are more concerned with format than content. Be sure to spend time with your hospital account contacts, and don't be afraid to ask questions. Discuss and come to agreements on quality assurance guidelines and details of format to be used.

We recommend that transcriptionists just learning to use computers find a programmer who understands the work of a medical transcriptionist, or ask a medical transcriptionist who is familiar with formatting to program the formats into your software. This will save you much time and aggravation and prevent your having to constantly experiment with formatting.

When working for individual physicians, their formats may not be a "statement of professionalism." Do not hesitate to point out that a different format may indeed be more representative of their professional image. It may also save them unnecessary expenses and win you a client for life.

Each physician has his or her own style of dictating and may use pet phrases or terms that cannot be found in any medical or English language dictionary. Keep the lines of communication open with those clients. If they consistently misspell a medical or English term which you know to be incorrect, don't hesitate to communicate that to them.

If a client continues to doubt your information, a good way to handle the situation is to take your reference material to the office for review. More often than not, your candor will be appreciated. On the other hand, the client may continue to insist that you type it "their way," in which case you have two options. You can do what the client demands or you can simply walk away from the account. The choice is yours, a decision not easily made nor to be taken lightly.

Risk Management and Insurance Protection

*"The Lord gave us two ends — one to sit on and
the other to think with. Success depends on
which one we use the most."*

—Ann Landers

In every business there are risks that must be managed, and the medical transcription industry is no exception to this rule. There are risks for every small business. Just think a minute about the hundreds of things that most business owners must worry about. Some concerns are predictable and can be eliminated or controlled to some extent:

- Volume

- Salary costs

- Taxes

- Overhead

- Equipment and supply costs

- The price you charge for services offered clients

Other risks are unpredictable and largely beyond your control:

- Competitors actions

- Changing technology and trends

- Effects these the above actions and changes have on your market and your clients

- The economy and its impact on your client base

Other events can also directly affect your day-to-day operations, reduce profits and result in unexpected financial losses serious enough to cripple or even bankrupt your business. You have probably already considered the most obvious risks, such as fire or injury, and have bought insurance to protect against them. But there are hundreds of other losses and liabilities that every small business faces, many of which are overlooked or ignored.

Large corporations often employ full-time risk managers to identify and analyze possible exposure to loss or liability. The risk manager takes steps to protect the firm against accidental and preventable loss and to minimize the financial consequences of unpreventable or unavoidable losses. As an independent business owner, you can't afford the services of a risk manager, even part-time, so you must take on that responsibility.

WHAT IS RISK MANAGEMENT?

Risk management consists of the following:

- Identifying and analyzing events that may result in loss

- Choosing the best way to deal with each potential loss

Let's discuss ways to help you identify, minimize and, in some instances, eliminate business risks.

Identifying exposure is a vital step to risk management. Until you know the scope of possible losses, you won't be able to develop a realistic strategy for dealing with them. Unless you've experienced a fire, you may not realize how extensive fire losses can be. For example, you may experience the following:

- Smoke and water damage

- Damage to your personal property and to the property of others that is left on your premises (e.g., data processing equipment you lease or client's property left with you)

- Business lost during the time it takes to return your business to normal

- The potential permanent loss of clients to competitors

Take a close look at each of your business operations and evaluate where losses might occur. For each exposure identified, determine how serious the loss might be and what that loss might cost.

Many business owners use a risk analysis questionnaire or survey, available from most insurance agents, as a checklist. In general, most questionnaires and surveys address the potential for these losses:

- Property losses

- Physical damage to property

- Loss of use of property

- Criminal activity

- Business interruption losses

- Indirect losses — Although insurance provides money for repairing or rebuilding property damaged, most policies do not cover indirect losses, such as income that is lost while the business is interrupted for repairs.

Business Interruption Insurance reimburses policyholders for the difference between normal income and the income earned during the shutdown period. During this period not only is income reduced or cut off, but business expenses such as taxes and loan payments continue. Frequently, interruptions in business also trigger extra expenses such as those incurred when subcontractors must be used to complete previously contracted work for clients. These expenses put an added strain on finances at a time when little if any income is being produced. Don't forget to protect your business against loss of income and unusual expenses that may result if indirect loss forces you to close temporarily.

- Liability losses

- Court decision (lawsuit charging negligence)

- Violation of contract provisions (a contract that makes one party responsible for certain kinds of losses)

- Public liability (injuries or loss to others)

- Key person losses — What would happen to your business if an accident or illness made it impossible for you to work? It is important for you to prepare your business for survival before you become disabled. Carefully evaluate the following questions:

    1) What impact would your absence have on your business such as volume, productivity, costs, etc.?

    2) How will you reassign duties to cover this period?

    3) What extra costs will you have to incur for a replacement to cover the operation of the business?

    4) How long will it take before the replacement is trained and productive?

    5) What would your source of income be?

    6) Who will continue your business? What if the person is not qualified or is a minor?

    7) If a will is not in place before your death, will the business close, or will someone inherit it?

    8) If your life-savings are invested will the family be able to use it wisely?

    9) What will the surviving family's source of income be?

The answers to the previous questions can be determined with the help of your business planner, attorney, accountant and insurance agent. Let them help you develop a risk management plan for your business.

As you can see, a business may face several types of risks and exposure. You must decide upon the risk management measures that will best protect your business.

• What can be done to prevent or limit exposure to risk?

• What techniques can be used to ensure that funds will be available for unavoidable losses?

LIMITING EXPOSURE TO LOSS — AVOIDING RISKS

One principle of loss prevention and control is to avoid activities that are too hazardous. For example, although exposure to loss from fire can seldom be eliminated completely, the risk can be reduced by installing smoke detectors and fire alarms and by having fire extinguishers readily available on the premises.

Insure business vehicles rather than take the risk of canceling collision coverage; or hire a delivery company, thus transferring the risk to the local delivery service.

TRANSFERRING RISK

The most common method of transferring risk is insurance. By insuring your home and car you transfer much of the risk of loss to the company that issued the policy. You pay a relatively small insurance premium compared to the risk of not protecting yourself against the possibility of a much larger financial loss.

With business insurance as with personal insurance, only you can decide which exposures you absolutely must insure against. Some decisions, however, are already made for you:

• Those required by law

• Those that others require, such as operating an insured business vehicle (required in some areas)

- Few lenders will finance property acquisition or construction unless it is adequately insured and the lender named on the policy as having an insurable interest.

ESSENTIAL COVERAGES

Four kinds of insurance are essential: fire, liability, automobile and workers compensation. In some areas and in some types of business, crime insurance is also essential.

THE ROLE OF THE INSURANCE PROFESSIONAL

The professional independent insurance agent has been trained in risk analysis. She or he is familiar with insurance coverages and financial strategies available in your state and with regulations that govern them. With this expertise the agent can point out exposures you may overlook. The agent can suggest a menu of risk-management strategies and amend a basic policy to suit your needs by adding special coverages and endorsements. The resulting policy will be custom tailored to your business's unique protection needs.

You may not be aware of other services that insurance companies provide to the policyholders:

- Legal defense — liability insurance usually includes legal defense

- Rehabilitate — Workers' Compensation/disability policies may offer rehabilitation services and in some cases, retraining

- Claim management services for loss analysis

INSURANCE PROTECTION

Safeguard your business with insurance. A home-based business is a significant investment. To be adequately covered for potential losses, you will probably need increased insurance coverage.

To protect business equipment in your home, you may need a special rider on your homeowner's policy. Even this, however, will generally not provide full replacement cost reimbursement, but only for the depreciated value of equipment at time of loss. Therefore, some home-based professionals invest in a personal property policy, which may require a hefty deductible but does reimburse at replacement cost values.

Don't depend on your homeowner's policy to meet all your personal needs in a crisis. You will also need some type of disability insurance. After all, your fingers are your life. How will you survive if you are suddenly unable to use them?

In the past, it was difficult to find a disability insurance carrier who would provide a policy for home-based workers, but fortunately, this is changing. There are now insurance companies that recognize home-based transcriptionists and are meeting our needs.

Contact your insurance agent to discuss your present business coverage, if any, and evaluate possible additional coverage. Be prepared to provide a written description of your business for your insurance carrier.

Your insurance agent will assist you in obtaining appropriate protection from potential hazards resulting from your business operations.

STANDARD INSURANCE COVERAGE FOR SELF-EMPLOYED BUSINESSES

- Fire, theft, and casualty damage to inventories and equipment

- Business interruption coverage

- Fidelity bonds for employees (if applicable)

- Liability for customers, vendors and others visiting the business

- Worker's compensation and worker's disability insurance

- Group health and life insurance

- Business use of vehicle coverage

- Business life insurance

- Disability insurance

- PC and software insurance

   . . . and also consider . . .

- Errors and Omissions

CREATING AN INVENTORY LIST

It is a good idea to make an inventory list of all home furnishings, business furniture and appliances, including model numbers, prices and purchase dates.

Photograph or videotape each room including interiors of cabinets and closets. Keep the inventory list, photographs and/or videotape in a safe-deposit box (tax-deductible) or some safe place outside your home. This will speed up the collection process should you ever need to file a claim with your insurance company.

GROUP INSURANCE POLICIES

Health insurance is very expensive and individual policies tend to run higher than group rates. You may find a bargain in a group policy through a professional organization. As an organization member, you may obtain the coverage you need at attractive group rates.

INSURING AGAINST CATASTROPHE

As micro-businesses, we take pride in possessing the newest in technology, not only to be competitive but to make our working hours less stressful. Most of us have the latest turbo computer, the latest software and peripheral programs, laser printers, fax machines, digital dictation equipment; standard, micro- and mini-transcribing machines. In just a matter of a few minutes, this could all go up in smoke, quite literally. It is reported that the two disasters most responsible for the demise of a home-based business are fire and water damage. However, most of us live with the added threat of earthquakes, tornadoes and hurricanes.

If you were to be caught in such a disaster, would you have the means to rebuild your business? The National Fire Protection Association states that 30% of all businesses that experience a major fire go out of business within a year; and 70% fail within five years. Those are frightening statistics.

Now is the time to evaluate your business and take steps to ensure that you would be capable of rebounding after a catastrophic loss.

• **Insure your business equipment and records adequately.** Take out a separate business policy that covers general liability and the **full** replacement cost of equipment and furnishings, including computer hardware and loss of your home office. Verify that insurance coverage that specifies "replacement" means **"full replacement value."** Also make sure operating a business out of your home does not invalidate insurance coverage.

• **Document valuables adequately and safeguard records.** Document your possessions including serial numbers, purchase dates, and prices, and file receipts and detailed descriptions as proof. Periodically send an updated copy to your attorney or a relative in another state, or store it in a safe-deposit box.

• **Back up computer data and safeguard files.** Back up computer data regularly and store copies of data files in an alternate site or in a safe-deposit box. This is cheaper and more efficient than special data-loss insurance, and you won't lose valuable information.

• **Use UL certified transient voltage suppressors on your computer and other business equipment.**

• **Safeguard office equipment and records on-site.** Arrange furniture and equipment to guard critical items and records against leaks, floods, crashed windows, heavy vibrations or earth tremors.

• **Clean, organize and maintain your office.** Regularly pick up and toss those mounds of paper, the ones you think you can't possibly throw away because you might need them someday; or keep them and just call it "kindling."

GET WITH THE PROGRAM

Good risk management and good insurance management are achieved through good planning. A lifetime of work and dreams can be lost in a few minutes if your insurance program does not include certain elements. To ensure that you are adequately covered, take these steps:

- Recognize the ways you can suffer loss.

- Follow the guides for buying insurance economically.

- Organize your insurance management program.

- Get professional advice.

RECOGNIZE THE RISKS

The first step toward good protection is to recognize the risks. If you have costly equipment in your business, obtain special insurance covering loss, damage, or business interruption resulting from not being able to use the equipment.

HAVE A RISK MANAGEMENT PLAN

Have a definite plan that defines the objective of your business.

- Write down a clear statement of what you expect insurance to do for your firm.

- Select an agent to handle your insurance.

- Do everything possible to prevent loss.

- Don't withhold information about your business and its exposure to loss from your insurance agent.

- Don't try to save money by underinsuring.

- Keep complete records of your insurance policies, premiums paid, losses and recoveries.

- Have your property appraised periodically by independent appraisers. This informs you of your exposures and allows you to prove what your actual losses are if any occur.

GET PROFESSIONAL ADVICE

Insurance is a complex and detailed subject. A qualified agent, broker or consultant can explain the options, recommend the right coverage and help you avoid financial loss.

Some small business owners look upon insurance as a sort of tax. They recognize it as necessary but consider it a burdensome expense that should be kept to a minimum. But used correctly, the potential benefits of good insurance management make it well worth your study and attention.

THE ERRORS AND OMISSIONS CONTROVERSY

In the first edition of IMT, we urged you to consider investing in an errors and omissions liability policy. However, after lengthy discussions with medical transcriptionists, attorneys and other business professionals, we feel this coverage is not a necessity. If you are just starting your business, the last thing you need is to spend $600 to $2000 per year on a policy that does nothing but cover the attorney fees should you be sued. In addition, most policies have caps of one to two million dollars.

While there have been a few cases in which medical transcriptionists have been sued, such cases are rare. If you contract with a physician who does not carry his own malpractice insurance, your risk for a lawsuit is increased; however, according to legal consultants, lawsuits are often initiated and targeted toward parties who have large assets (that translates "lots of money") such as the doctor, hospital, etc. Logically speaking, a larger medical transcription service would more likely be named in a lawsuit. For a single independent transcriptionist, it's unlikely.

In investigating the issue further, the authors sought advice from insurance brokers, underwriters, and lawyers, who advised against this particular type of insurance coverage at the present time. In most cases, insurance brokers weren't even sure what it was, why we would need it, or where we could get it! The feeling of these professionals was that with insurance being as costly as it is today, one is wise to spend money on insurance that is really needed and that is required by law — not on something you will probably never need.

In the process of consulting with an attorney for some business advice, the authors were presented with a six-page contract from the attorney that included his fee schedule. At the top of one page was a disclaimer: *"I DO NOT CARRY ERRORS AND OMISSIONS INSURANCE."*

If an attorney does not feel the need to carry this coverage, why should we buy it? In the opinion of many experienced transcriptionists, this type of liability insurance is not necessary. Perhaps those who promoted errors and omissions insurance overreacted to unsubstantiated fears; perhaps they were ultra conservative; or perhaps they were simply greedy for the revenues that increased insurance premiums would produce. In any case, most medical transcriptionists feel that if the physician's signature is on the bottom line as required, it is the doctor's responsibility to read the transcription for accuracy and completeness. This is the position of health care regulators as well.

In talking with insurance underwriters, an errors and omissions policy basically provides coverage for attorney fees. IT DOES NOT PREVENT YOU FROM BEING SUED BY SOMEONE.

Instead of errors and omissions insurance, we suggest that all independent medical transcriptionists take measures to safeguard themselves against the trickle-down effects of lawsuits that could result from errors in dictation. When negotiating a contract with a new client, include a WAIVER OF LIABILITY clause (see two examples below). A waiver is the surrender either expressed or implied of a right to which one is entitled by law.

Ask your legal adviser to review the contract. By addressing this issue, your clients will appreciate your professionalism. If they do not, reconsider whether you want them as clients.

Within our industry, there is a definite need for discussion, clarification and definition of errors and omissions liability and other contract issues. It is the responsibility of every medical transcriptionist to help develop clearly defined and acceptable professional practice standards.

EXAMPLES OF LIABILITY WAIVERS

All technical terms and words shall be proofread and spellchecked. However, the parties agree that final responsibility for proofreading the transcript lies with the above named client. Client, therefore, agrees to waive any liability which might otherwise be asserted against (your business name) excepting breach of this contract. In addition, client agrees to indemnify and hold (your business name) harmless against any claims which might be asserted by third parties arising out of the performance of this contract."

. . . or . . .

It is my policy that computer-authenticated or artificial signatures generated by means other than actual dictating physician's signature are not endorsed by me. Therefore, the doctors should proofread the transcription for document content, accuracy and quality control. This means that they will accept the liability of the transcription and I will not purchase errors and omissions liability insurance.

In your contract with clients, also consider stating the following:

I DO NOT CARRY ERRORS AND OMISSIONS INSURANCE.

NOTE

Laws and procedures change frequently and are subject to different interpretations. Always contact a lawyer for specific legal advice. We have researched legal issues to the best of our ability, but it is your responsibility to make certain that facts and general information contained in this book are applicable to your situation.

PREVENTING D.P.S. (Deep Pocket Syndrome)

Because of the important services they provide, MTs, IMTs, MTSOs and the medical transcription profession are vital components of specific health care provider systems and of the general health care culture as well. As health care systems change so, too, will the role of medical transcription professionals.

The health care system continues to decentralize many services, including technology, support staff and programs, by outsourcing to contract services. The integrated local health care system is very patient-focused, sensitive to patient concerns, patient perspective, patient wellness, patient education and patient satisfaction. To meet patient needs and control costs, critical health care pathways and systems are being established to monitor appropriate use of resources and selection of technologies that provide information and service in the fastest, safest manner at the least cost.

Outsourcing of some medical transcription services has been occurring for years, but today's explosive outsourcing levels, which have surprised many health care professionals, is good news for independent medical transcriptionists. In a survey published in *Medical Records Briefing—Special Report* (January 1996) almost 66% of hospitals surveyed contract out transcription to independent contractors, transcription services, OR BOTH. This information continues to confirm what we have long been aware of: Independent medical transcriptionists are in demand, and those who maintain competency and professionalism will have successful careers.

There are many ways to determine competency. In medical transcription, certification, documented ongoing continuing education, and performance improvement and other quality assessment mechanisms are all ways of measuring competency. For the independent transcriptionist, competency results in success and survival in a very competitive marketplace. If you are not competent, you won't keep old clients or get new ones. It is just that simple.

Maintaining competency will depend upon many factors besides just your education, training and fund of knowledge. Staying competent means addressing problematic areas within your business and reducing your professional liability through good day-to-day management. Begin by developing quality and productivity standards for your business based on your professional qualifications. For example, if your skill and experience are limited, your transcription output will also be limited. Therefore, you should set your quality and productivity standards at realistic levels and seek out clients whose needs will match your current potential production level. Given your level of expertise, it would be a mistake to set standards too high or market your services to hospitals or other highly sophisticated and demanding areas of medicine.

Develop a plan to evaluate and improve performance. Monitor quality comprehensively and continually within every aspect of your business: transcribed documents, service to clients, confidentiality, technology security and turnaround. Once problems areas are identified, implement methods to solve the problems, monitor them for effectiveness, and make adjustments as necessary.

If you discover weak or potential high-risk areas within your business, utilize the services of an appropriate consultant — accountant, lawyer, insurance agent, or experienced IMT. Dedicate yourself to being the best transcriptionist ever with the best service anywhere. Never forget that your competency is your best protection against liability.

LIABILITY INSURANCE

Liability is an issue in health care as in all professions, but is liability insurance really necessary for the medical transcriptionist? We believe it is not.

We recommend that you carefully evaluate any source that promotes liability coverage for medical transcriptionists. In our decades of experience as medical transcriptionists, we have never known nor heard of one incident in which a medical transcriptionist has been sued. We have heard *rumors* about such lawsuits, but no one has ever validated these rumors by presenting documentation of specific lawsuits or industry case rulings. Facts and facts alone are what we need. We cannot make wise decisions without evaluating the facts.

Rumor does not justify running out and purchasing a million dollar liability insurance policy. Of course, if we all run out and purchase liability insurance there will be an enormous bank of funds which will surely encourage somebody to initiate a lawsuit because there is insurance to pay for it! In such a scenario, who would get the lion's share from this new deep pocket? Insurance companies and lawyers.

Information from legal consultants indicates that lawsuits are often targeted toward individuals, groups, or facilities that have substantial assets, great sums of money or hefty insurance coverage. In investigating this issue further, the authors sought advice from insurance brokers, underwriters and lawyers, who recommended that we medical transcriptionists spend our money on insurance that is necessary or is mandated by law.

Currently, independent medical transcriptionists carry a variety of insurance coverages; some are essential; others, practical but optional: auto insurance (mandatory in most states), health insurance, life insurance, homeowners/renters insurance, personal liability insurance, business insurance. Depending on coverage, total insurance premiums can add up to thousands of dollars per year. To add professional liability insurance would cost an additional $250 to $2000 per year. Budgetary considerations cannot be ignored.

Then, too, if medical transcriptionists were to purchase professional liability insurance, we would also need to purchase errors and omissions coverage, which, if our sources are correct, is basically enough insurance to pay your lawyer's fees in the event of a lawsuit. To afford this type of coverage, we estimate an IMT would have to earn $100,000+ a year! Medical transcriptionists don't make that kind of money.

One professional liability policy currently being promoted has "limits of liability" of $1,000,000 each incident and $3,000,000 aggregate. These limits of liability are one-third that expected of the MD, DPM, DDS, and all other licensed allied health professionals.

It is important to differentiate between medical transcriptionists and the above licensed professionals, which are 1) ACCREDITED HEALTH CARE PROVIDERS, 2) LICENSED through state medical boards, and 3) CREDENTIALED to practice. They have direct patient-care contact as well as health-record documentation responsibilities.

1. **Accredited Health Care Provider.** This category includes health care professionals such as physical therapist (PT), occupational therapist (OT), registered nurse (RN), certified registered nurse anesthetist (CRNA), medical doctor (MD), doctor of osteopathy (DO), doctor of dental surgery (DDS), doctor of podiatric medicine (DPM), and many others. All are professions that have been accredited by their state medical associations and the American Medical Association through application and/or approval of education and training programs and have been given the status of allied health care provider.

2. **Licensing.** The recognized health care professionals we have mentioned above and other recognized allied health professionals are, for a fee, licensed to practice in their profession through their state licensing boards (in California, the Board of Consumer Affairs; in New York, the New York Board of Medical Licensing, etc.) The license is generally for two years. Along with this license, they must document their continuing medical education units with their State licensing board. There is a reporting mechanism for complaints and for monitoring professional practice.

3. **Credentialing**. Physicians and recognized allied health professionals must be credentialed and privileged to practice in a number of health care settings, mainly acute care and managed care. They must apply for privileges through an extensive application-and-review process. They must document their activity from the time they enter their medical training to the time of their application for appointment, with no lapses in their experience unaccounted for. An extensive background check is done by requesting references from medical schools, teaching institutions regarding postgraduate training, all professional references and prior work settings, licensing, drug enforcement agencies (where applicable), etc. This credentialing process is a very time-consuming procedure that could take weeks to months to complete before an applicant is notified that his/her application and request for privileges has been approved.

In comparison, medical transcriptionists do not have direct patient-care responsibilities and are not recognized as allied health professionals. We do transcribe the patient's medical record and make every effort to produce an accurate document, but we cannot vouch for medical record accuracy. Only the physician, after reviewing his or her transcribed report, can do that. Therefore, why would we need liability coverage?

The "burden of responsibility" is central to any liability issue and where medical records are concerned, the physician's signature is still "where the buck stops." This is the accepted standard in health care, recognized through the health care regulating, accrediting and licensing bodies. Hospital surveyors will ask a physician if he reads the transcribed reports he dictates. If the physician answers "no" or "not always" the surveyor will remind him that he — not the transcriptionist! — is legally responsible for the content of that document. The burden of responsibility lies with the dictating physician when his signature is on that document.

Speaking with physicians regarding medical transcriptionists' purported need for professional liability insurance raises a lot of eyebrows and comments like "That is ludicrous!". . . "Ridiculous!". . . "Someone is hoping to dip into deep pockets!" More important, these doctors affirm that the accuracy of the health care records they dictate and which are subsequently transcribed is their responsibility.

It is interesting to note that the Joint Commission for the Accreditation of Hospitals (JCAHO) accreditation does not require a facility to carry liability coverage on

289

health care practitioners credentialed to practice within the hospital setting. Some state regulating agencies do, but only for those groups noted above.

According to Link Resources, by the year 2000, 50% of the work force in this country will be working from home, as an employee of others or self-employed. The insurance industry, which is satisfactorily meeting IMT insurance needs today, is well aware of this trend and will, we believe, anticipate and meet our future insurance needs.

WAIVER OF LIABILITY AND INDEMNIFICATION CLAUSES

All independent medical transcriptionists should be proactive in protecting their business and personal interests from the trickle-down effects of lawsuits. When negotiating a contract with a client, address liability issues and consider including a Waiver of Liability Clause or an Indemnification Clause (client agrees to hold you harmless against any claims which might be asserted by third parties arising out of the performance of this contract).

In addition, contact your insurance agent to discuss your present business coverage and evaluate possible additional coverage. Professional independent insurance agents have been trained in risk analysis and are familiar with insurance coverages. Your insurance agent should be able to assist you in obtaining appropriate protection from potential hazards resulting from your business operations.

COMPUTER SECURITY

In past years a computer system was an information reporting tool and sometimes a long term planning tool. Today, information technology has penetrated virtually every aspect of business operations and is an integral part of corporate service. It empowers companies to provide customers with timely, accurate information, which clients have grown to expect. Information technology enables companies to provide new levels of customer service and gain a competitive advantage.

Today's marketplace is information driven. If you lose your information, you lose your competitive advantage. However, information security specialists concur that security depends on people more than on technology. They note that employees are a far greater threat to information security than independents.

Therefore, it follows that improving security depends on changing beliefs, attitudes and behavior of individuals and groups.

PROTECTING YOUR INVESTMENT

Every year millions of dollars of computers and computer equipment are stolen. You can protect yourself and your business by insuring your computer and regularly backing up your data, but there is little you can do to prevent an actual theft. Most desktop PC makers offer a Kensington Lock-like feature on their computers that stops unwanted users from booting up your system, and some manufacturers offer cable locks for securing a notebook or desktop to the desk. But what's to stop someone from stealing the desk, too?

Absolute Software (800-220-0733) has put viruses to good use by creating a user-friendly variety that tracks stolen PCs, much like the Lojack auto theft retrieval device. The company's CompuTrace TRS tracks down crooks when they hook up your stolen machine's modem to a telephone jack. CompuTrace TRS dials the modem to Absolute Software's headquarters to reveal the location of the guilty party, and Absolute Software officials notify the authorities. CompuTrace TRS runs in the background and disables your modem's speaker to ensure that the cons are clueless to when they are about to give themselves away.

Swap-Crypt from SCM Microsystems (408-370-4888) makes your PC's files and directories unreadable and useless to the PC thief. The Type II PC Card Encryption Card codes the original file to a temporary file, permanently deletes the original file, and then renames the temporary file with the name of the deleted file. Each file or directory can have five-character passwords and uses SCM Microsystems's One Time Pad encryption technique (patent pending).

Just think of the marketing possibilities! It will be exciting to tell clients of both new and old accounts about the new antitheft features you have added to your service, and clients will be favorably impressed with your knowledge of current technology and your commitment to maintaining patient record confidentiality.

BELIEFS AND ATTITUDES

Copying software without authorization is a felony. Nonetheless, some users have the attitude that it does not matter. The Software Publishers Association (SPA) training video *It's Just Not Worth the Risk* presents the issues involved in copyright infringement and warns that sooner or later software thieves will be caught and their careers devastated.

ANTIVIRUS TECHNIQUES

Currently there are a number of antivirus techniques available through vendors of antivirus products. As a personal computer user, you should have a practical, working understanding of computer viruses and how they can damage your PC. You can then evaluate the various antivirus products and decide which will best address your computer needs.

THE TARGET

The sole purpose of viruses, trojan horses, logic bombs, stealth viruses, and the myriad other malicious codes being unleashed upon the PC community is to wreak havoc on computer systems and programs. A representative of the National Computer Security Association (NCSA) in *Fighting The Virus Bulletin* stated, "There currently are anywhere from 2200-3000 known viruses worldwide. Between 50-60 new viruses appear each month and it has been this way for the last 18 months. There have been some months where the total has reached as high as 90 and the low has been around 25."

Techniques currently available that protect the PC environment from various virus exposures can be broken into two categories: software techniques and hardware techniques. There are three main software techniques employed within a number of vendor antivirus products:

1) Antitamper/integrity check

2) Signature scan

3) Use of activity monitors

Some antivirus products use combinations of the above. As with any other product, do your homework and talk with experts before purchasing.

The *advantages* of the antitamper/integrity check are these: the program and data files can be protected; no prior knowledge of the assailant is required to detect the change in the programs; and any change will be flagged. The *disadvantages* are the following: the technique is time consuming; the program must go through every program/directory to generate/check the checksums; and the checksum files themselves can become targets of attack.

The signature scan technique scans for specific code combinations, which may indicate that a virus is present. The *advantages* of this technique are these: a virus can be detected prior to execution of the program; the signature will identify the type of infection; and by identifying the virus the user may be able to reverse the damage of the infection or remove the virus.

The *disadvantages* of this technique are the following: it is time consuming; the software must search every file looking for all known signatures; constant software updates are required to keep up with new viruses being created on a daily basis; as the number of signatures increases, the possibility of false alarms also increases; and the detection of a virus means the infection has already occurred.

The activity monitor is different from the previously mentioned techniques in that the software is loaded in the background and monitors system activity. If the application software executed an operation the monitor considers suspicious, the monitor will alert the user of a possible virus attack. The *advantage* of this technique is that it can detect and neutralize propagation. The *disadvantage* is that it can be bypassed. Because the monitor program resides in memory itself, it also may be subject to attack.

HARDWARE TECHNIQUES

Four types of hardware techniques are currently available. They include boot-up protection, command monitor, sensing, and sector-by-sector protection. The first two techniques do not involve protecting the actual physical drive. They set logically on the PC bus, which is the main information highway from the computer CPU to the peripheral cards. Access to the PC bus is through the PC card slots in the machine. (A PC usually has eight slots for cards).

The last two techniques are physical drive protection techniques. They fit logically between the HD controller card and the physical drive. Boot-up protection is a hardware board that plugs into a PC bus slot and operates logically on the PC bus. This board prevents a boot from a floppy drive, thereby eliminating a major source of infection.

INFORMATION SECURITY BASICS

When users are asked about security they often say, "Well everyone seems to tell us to change our passwords, and that's about it." However, information systems security is more complex than a simple catch-phrase. Various computer crime techniques are called *sabotage, piggybacking, impersonation, data diddling, super zapping, scavenging, wire tapping, trap doors, trojan horses, salamis, asynchronous attacks and logic bombs, data leakage, simulation, viruses and worms.* Human errors, accidents or omissions are estimated to account for 50-80% of the annual dollar loss in computer data information destruction. Criminal hackers, although flashy and attractive to the news media, actually account for a small percentage of all harm to computers.

Investing in effective security policies and ensuring proper training are important factors to computer security.

PREVENTION

Security measures cannot totally eliminate all human errors and accidents, but they can reduce the likelihood of such events by using several techniques:

- Eliminating access

- Providing audit trails

- Emphasizing accountability for actions

- Showing how important data is to the business

WHO ARE THE CRIMINALS

An American Bar Association study in 1984 found that 75% of computer offenders were insiders who had authorization to access data they mistreated. Employees were the third most costly threat to information security.

Because of the preponderance of insider "data diddlers," outsiders are probably an overrated threat. In the 1988 Internet worm case, a graduate student caused an estimated $96 million dollars of damage by introducing a program that replicated itself throughout the network and brought thousands of computers to a halt. One of the resources used by criminal hackers (a term that originally referred to dedicated programmers but now is used loosely to refer to anyone who tries to gain unauthorized access to computer systems) is public bulletin board systems (BBS). Hackers have shared a variety of illegally obtained information such as details of corporate security measures, dial-up-port telephone numbers, passwords, and even stolen credit card numbers for long distance phone calls.

HOW TO DISCOURAGE HACKERS

To make it more difficult for hackers to steal valuable information from computer records try the following:

- Turn your modem off when the office is closed.

- Protect passwords and access codes. Don't distribute that information to people.

- Disconnect units with internal memories after hours.

- Don't forget that digital copiers, laser printers and fax machines have internal memories that can be accessed by hackers.

- Read the security control sections of manuals that come with these units.

- Store sensitive data on disks rather than in the computer's hard drive and remove the disks from the computer drives at night.

SOFTWARE THAT COMBATS MALICIOUS CODES

Logic bombs, worms and viruses are among the most interesting forms of infosec attacks. Logic bombs are routinely and secretly inserted into programs. They check for conditions such as date of presence of the programmer's name on the payroll. Worms and viruses are programs that reproduce. The effects can include obscene messages on the screen, bizarre effects, e.g., having all letters on the screen drift slowly to the bottom of the screen like leaves in autumn, or random data modification, new errors in spreadsheets and outright data destruction (wiping out your hard disk).

NETWORKS

Another threat of growing importance in industrial espionage is telecommunications networks. Local area networks (LANs), which have been installed at a growing pace worldwide, are vulnerable to easy eavesdropping using "off the shelf" "sniffer" software available for about $1000 in stores but also available free on the Internet and from underground BBS.

SOME FINAL THOUGHTS ON COMPUTER SECURITY

Antivirus software is and has been effective in the detection and removal of malicious codes infecting PCs and networks. These software solutions minimize the amount of damage from both the cost perspective and the loss of information perspective; but antivirus software only identifies the infection the user *already has*. Users must continuously update their antivirus software in order to keep up with the seemingly unending release of new viruses. Software solutions, while providing a limited level of effectiveness against viruses, requires users to actively monitor their systems. Newer systems have virus scanware that is activated when you boot up your computer.

Viruses released today are more sophisticated than viruses released in the 80s. They are now polymorphic viruses that continually mutate and create new signatures. They are viruses that target the actual hardware level of the PC, and they also appear at a much faster rate — fifty to sixty new viruses per month. This means, when looking toward the future, that software solutions alone may not be able to stop or detect all new viruses appearing on the market.

Currently there is no way a user can be certain that software is providing effective antivirus protection. The only way users will know why their software did not work is when something terrible happens. In order to maximize your protection, it is recommended that a top quality scanning software be used to check files for obvious known infections before activating hardware protection.

Experts agree that education is the key element to all computer crime prevention. It must begin in the earliest levels of school, continuing through high school and college and into the workplace. It has been said that when revealing your password causes the same emotional response as pulling your pants down in public, we will be on the way to better computer security.

A very important point is that prevention is a form of insurance. Just as most organizations spend money on insurance policies to cover losses after an accident, you should spend money to prevent accidents before they occur. This approach is all the more sensible given reports of difficulties in collecting even coverage that was paid for.

THE UNLICENSED SOFTWARE POLICE

There is a significant amount of unlicensed software use occurring throughout the industrial workplace, including the health care industry. According to the Business Software Alliance (BSA), 26% of all software in use in the United States is pirated, accounting for vendor losses of about $2.9 billion dollars.

The BSA, an international organization, is funded by companies such as Adobe, Apple Computer, Autodesk, Bentley Systems, Lotus Development, Microsoft, Novell and Symantec. Since its inception in 1988 it has filed more than 600 lawsuits worldwide against suspected copyright infringers. Through public policy and education, the BSA seeks to control software piracy.

Making a copy of a software product is relatively easy, and frequently, people think of it as a victimless crime. However, no sector of the computer-using community is exempt from the Copyright Act or is protected against the unauthorized duplication of software. The BSA reports that the health care industry is particularly prone to this copyright infringement and has instituted an investigation of these crimes. The majority of tips regarding software piracy are received through the complaint hot-line.

The BSA operates 35 complaint hotlines around the world for callers seeking information about copyright matters or wishing to report suspected incidents of unauthorized copying of software. If you have concerns about software or want information about the Copyright Act, call the following number:

- **888-NO-PIRACY**
  (in the United States)

MAINTAINING FAX CONFIDENTIALITY

FAX machines are very effective in transmitting stat reports required for patient care. In order to maintain confidentiality of patient records and decrease professional liability, the following guidelines are recommended:

- Locate the fax machine where access is limited and monitored at all times.

- Always use a fax transmittal sheet (cover page). Transmittal rates are determined by the amount of information on the sheets transmitted, so keep your fax cover page as simple as possible.

- Verify the recipient's fax number before transmitting transcribed material.

- Call ahead to notify recipient that information is being transmitted via fax.

- Identify the recipient on your fax transmittal sheet, and indicate the number of pages transmitted.

- Maintain a log, or copies, of information transmitted via fax machine. Many fax machines automatically record and print a copy of fax activity including date, time, and fax number accessed.

- Consider inserting a sentence on the transmittal sheet that states: "These documents are for the eyes of the receiver only."

- Stamp or write the word "COPY" on each sheet transmitted, so it will not be mistaken for an original document.

Protecting patient privacy remains our main concern as professional medical transcriptionists, whether we're an employee or are self-employed. When contracting our services to hospital accounts, most of us have been asked to sign nondisclosure agreement clauses, which state that if the confidentiality of any report is violated, our services may be terminated immediately.

By California law, health care professionals are required to maintain confidentiality of patients' personal and medical records. We are legally bound to limit discussions of patient information to health care professionals only for patient care purposes. We cannot legally discuss patient information with family, friends, insurance representatives, private investigators, pastors, newsmen, attorneys, etc.

When a medical report is faxed to either a hospital account or a physician's office, we do not know who is receiving that information on the other end. Could it be a family member of the patient whose report is being transmitted? If you think this could not happen, then you better think again. The pathology department of a hospital transmitted a biopsy report via fax to the surgeon's office. The diagnosis: terminal cancer. Imagine the shock of the physician's receptionist when she took the report from the fax machine and realized the patient in the report was her mother. It was an insensitive way to be informed of a loved one's brief life expectancy.

Although we cannot stand by each fax machine as reports are transmitted, there are steps independent home-based medical transcriptionists can take to minimize the threat to patient confidentiality. Each faxed report should include a cover sheet that includes the following:

TO: **FAX NUMBER:**   **DATE:**
FROM: **FAX NUMBER:**
NUMBER OF FAX PAGES:

Most fax machines include a "confirmation" feature that prints out everything you have faxed including phone numbers, time of day, and date.

Every faxed medical report should also include a disclaimer such as:

> *"The information contained in the transmission accompanying this notice is confidential and protected by the physician-patient privilege. It is intended only for the use of the individual or entity identified above. If the reader of this message is not the intended recipient, you are hereby notified that any dissemination or distribution of the accompanying communication is prohibited. The physician-patient privilege is not waived by the parties sending the accompany documents. If you have received this communication in error, please notify us immediately by telephone, collect, and return the original message to us at the above address via the United States Postal Service."*

You can have a rubber stamp made for this purpose and stamp it either at the bottom of each report or along the top. Keep in mind that although a report may be faxed, an original report must also be sent to the physician or hospital.

CONFIDENTIALITY AND THE CELLULAR PHONE

Everyone in the health care field is concerned about patient confidentiality. How many of you are transcribing for physicians who dictate their reports from car phones? We would venture to guess that 90% of you are. You might want to inform your doctors that there are scanners on the market designed to monitor car phone conversations. Imagine someone sitting in their living room listening to a history and physical, an operative report or a discharge summary being dictated on a neighbor or relative. No one is safe from the technobots, neither MTs nor MDs.

AUTOAUTHENTICATION

Autoauthentication has long been an issue of concern to health care professionals. Although many facilities have practiced auto authentication for years, recently, new and significant concerns regarding this practice have arisen. The problem involves the process of obtaining timely, accurate and complete patient-care documentation; authorship and authentication.

We differentiate authorship and authentication as follows:

- **Authorship:** The process of identifying the responsible health care practitioner who has released a health care entry for use. The identification process occurs in writing, by dictation, with keyboard or keyless data entry.

- **Authentication:** The voluntary, secondary process of confirming the content of the health care entry. Confirmation occurs by written signature, identifiable entry, biometric identifier or computer key.

The above definitions convey the differences between authorship and authentication and also address the responsibility of the health care practitioner who is documenting.

In autoauthentication, doctors are routinely assigned an identification number for dictating. A file card with their written signature indicates they "authorize" their electronic signature, and they must also key in their assigned number for autoauthentication.

The key issue is whether hospitals have adequate systems and appropriate policies to monitor and control document authentication by physicians — not by transcriptionists.

> ## NOTE
>
> In every authentication situation physicians have the option to review and personally sign transcribed documents. Physicians can also specify at the beginning of dictation if they feel it is particularly complex and should not be electronically signed.

The JCAHO requests that health care providers develop proposed scoring guidelines for documentation with second party intervention, with the provider demonstrating 98% documentation accuracy in cases where second party intervention was obtained prior to implementing authorship. JCAHO and Medicare Guidelines of the HCFA, of the U.S. Department of Health and Human Services (HHS), require that signatures, electronic or otherwise, be done by the practitioner and not be delegated.

It is the position of the American Association for Medical Transcription (AAMT) that the HCFA and JCAHO guidelines that permit the use of electronic signatures by physicians and other caregivers and require that signatures electronic or otherwise be affixed by the author of each entry *not* be delegated to anyone other than the physician who dictated the material.

Medical transcriptionists can attest to the quality of their transcription, that it is complete and is as correct as possible based on dictation provided, but we cannot attest to the accuracy of the dictation itself, including but not limited to the identity of the dictator and of the patient, dates given, history and treatment recorded, and the physician's conclusions. Only the direct caregiver can attest to the accuracy of patient-care documentation.

The patient should be a primary concern to all parties when signature policies are established because the patient's medical record will be a primary source of his or her future medical care. It will, of course, also be the primary source of documentation for legal, reimbursement, and statistical purposes. Thus, the accuracy of the patient record is appropriately the responsibility of the health care provider. Therefore, we believe it is not appropriate for health care providers to delegate persons other than physicians the authority to affix signatures that authenticate documents.

AUTOAUTHENTICATION — AN ACCIDENT WAITING TO HAPPEN

Hospitals are facing severe shortages and cutbacks by most insurance programs, especially government-sponsored programs like Medicare. Time is of the essence. The faster a chart is completed, the faster the institution will be paid by the insurance carrier. In eliminating the need to confront doctors about signing charts and/or completing their records, many hospital administrators have begun to implement autoauthentication, even though such programs are discouraged by many regulating agencies.

This shortcut is certainly an added liability to medical transcriptionists and is one we should not be asked to assume. We all know that most doctors hate dictating almost as much as they loathe reading their dictation. As seasoned veterans in the war of words, we know, too, that the quality of dictation is often lacking in clarity. Dictating stations are invariably located in recovery rooms, emergency rooms, and physician lounges, where it is not uncommon to hear the cries of a screaming child awakening from anesthesia, the sounds of CPR in progress, or the latest Hillary Clinton joke. We also know that while dictating, doctors have an affinity for chewing gum and/or food, taking big gulps of liquid, yawning, snorting, burping, whistling, singing, playing musical instruments, talking to peers, and even snoring! By adding the phrase "DICTATED AND AUTHENTICATED" after the dictating physician's name, we are attesting to 100% accuracy in the medical record. We should not, indeed we cannot, do that. How can we verify that the patient was in stable and satisfactory condition upon arrival in the recovery room or that medication was administered to the patient? We weren't there. The only person who can, and should, attest to the accuracy of transcribed physician dictation is the physician himself.

Medical transcriptionists must not give in to those who urge us to cooperate with autoauthentication, arguing that there is no risk. **There is risk — to our individual services and to our profession — and the risk is great**.

AAMT POSITION SUMMARY*

Medical transcriptionists are medical language specialists who transcribe dictated patient reports. They interpret and edit raw data and dictation as completely, clearly, consistently and correctly as possible. Medical transcriptionists can attest to the accuracy of their transcription; they cannot attest to the accuracy of the dictation on which it is based. Patient care and well-being are at risk if health care providers do not give proper attention to the content of the patient record before the provider's signature is affixed. The provider's signature communicates accuracy of record content that only the provider can give. Thus, delegation of authority to affix signatures is inappropriate and should not be allowed.

This position summary was adopted by the AAMT House of Delegates, August 4, 1993.

CONFIDENTIALITY

Consultation and documentation are the twin pillars of malpractice prevention. Like all sensible approaches to risk management, good documentation is also good clinical practice. Integrally linked with consultation and documentation is confidentiality, which is also of central importance to quality patient care and malpractice prevention. The medical record is relied on heavily in the investigation of potentially compensable events and lawsuits. Often, medical malpractice suits can be eliminated or mitigated through accurate documentation, medical record security, and adherence to a policy of confidentiality regarding patient information.

Every transcriptionist needs a basic understanding of risk and how to manage it. In the health care field the patient record is the medium of exchange. Our business is information and this information becomes a permanent part of the patient record. We must take into account in our business strategy the significance of the information that we move in our business; how fast we turn it around, our work capacity, and the quality of the work.

The movement to electronic information is taking place in two specific segments. One segment is on the financial side. To promote standardization of the medical record, health care reform is proposing that each health care facility be able to access a record of all health information for any given person. We believe such a level of access is an intrusion of patient privacy. The inability of computer systems to communicate is perhaps the greatest vanguard of privacy individuals have. Thus, the development of a standard record will have serious confidentiality and privacy implications.

It is up to those working in the health care field to determine how much privacy we are willing to risk for an automated health care system. Those setting standards for automated patient records must realize there is more at stake than just confidentiality issues. The electronic medical record will also be used by attorneys, for peer reviews, and during other proceedings.

AHIMA has established a position paper on disclosure of health information. They maintain that health records, regardless of the media in which they are maintained, are the property of health care providers, but the health information contained in the records belongs to the patient. Disclosure of health information must be handled prudently to protect the patient's right to privacy.

The issue of confidentiality is a hot topic today. In our business, maintaining confidentiality is of utmost importance. Those of us in the health information field have a responsibility to help guard health information. A breach of confidentiality, invasion of privacy, and defamation of character can have major legal and financial implications. We all know that humans err, and no individual or facility can fully guarantee confidentiality. A breach can occur from within or without a facility, and the system is especially vulnerable as a result of the communication technology we use. Now, more than ever, we must attempt to establish guidelines that will help us provide a program for confidentiality protection.

Guidelines for facsimile transmission should be established, and access procedures for files and users should be protected. We can start as follows:

- Determine state and federal regulations, agency standards and local precedents affecting confidentiality and release of information.

- Identify all manuals and computer sources of patient-specific information within the business and retention methods.

- Establish safeguards for appropriateness of information retention.

HOW TO MAKE TOUGH DECISIONS

Be aware that you cannot control the outcome of a decision. All you can do is control the decision-making process. Start by identifying your wants and needs, and jot them down on paper — even if they appear to be contradictory. Rank things you want and need in order of importance. If some items are contradictory, ask yourself, "Which would I choose?" Gather all the information necessary to make the decision. Look at your alternatives, consequences, advantages and disadvantages. Be as objective as possible, and don't let your emotions interfere with the decision process.

Determine how much risk you are willing to take, and once you have done this consider the following strategies:

- Choose the safest alternative — the one that can't fail.

- Pick the option with the best odds for success. Select the alternative with the most desirable outcome — despite the risk.

- Eliminate any option that might present a loss you won't be able to live with — despite high odds for its success.

- Picture how you would deal with negative consequences.

Outsourcing (Subcontracting)

*"In golf and in life, it's the follow through
that makes the difference."*

—Anonymous

As your business grows and you add new clients, there will be ebbs and flows in the volume of dictation. This fluctuation occurs for a variety of reasons, and although low volume probably creates greatest concern, high volume can result in problems, too.

Sometimes a hospital or clinic's transcription department is short-staffed and must contract with a service to process overflow. If you take on such an account, you may be delighted to have the extra volume of work and added income but find yourself unprepared and unable to personally fulfill the transcription demands. You need help to meet your deadlines. The solution lies in backup transcriptionists with whom you can outsource work when the need arises.

Through networking, you can easily accumulate a list of transcriptionists in your area who will take on overflow transcription. These are generally individuals who have full-time jobs but enjoy moonlighting occasionally.

Many independent transcriptionists also use outsourcers (subcontractors) to cover them while taking days off or vacations, and outsourcers are lifesavers in the event of illness or other emergency.

EVALUATING OUTSOURCERS

After developing a list of potential outsourcers, your next step is to request resumes and review those submitted to you. Always interview the best prospects as if you were employing them for a major company. Some professionals like to interview at this time; others prefer to wait until after reviewing "test tape" transcription.

"Test tapes" are a common practice with larger transcription services and are an excellent tool for accurate evaluation of a potential outsourcer's technical skills. Send test tapes to all transcriptionist candidates and review the tapes carefully when they are returned. You will know immediately if the transcriptionist's skills are not up to your standards or if the candidate is trainable. If the work is satisfactory, you will schedule an interview, or a follow-up interview, with the applicant.

It is important to be selective in your choice of outsourcers. Remember, it is your account and your reputation that are ultimately on the line. Regardless of who actually transcribes, the end product is your responsibility so make your outsourcing decision wisely.

Before delivering work, verify that the outsourcer has adequate and appropriate transcription equipment, and make it clear that the working relationship is on an as-needed basis. If completed work is satisfactory, let them know. If not, briefly explain why and then locate a more skilled outsourcer.

It is also important to be certain that you are not the only source of income for outsourcers. Like you, they are independents and fall within the same guidelines as "independent contractors," so you should ask them to sign an outsourcer agreement.

Transcriptionists' work styles are as different as their personalities. When interviewing, it is important to determine a potential outsourcer's technical skill level, work style, workplace, and attitudes. If the work you release through your service is to be uniform and of consistently excellent quality, outsourcers will have to conform to your standards. Some transcriptionists find this difficult; others find it impossible. You will eliminate many future problems by being aware of, and avoiding, a transcriptionist who is unwilling to forego an old style and conform to your standards.

PAYING OUTSOURCERS

You will pay your outsourcers so much per line or page, and keep a percentage for yourself. Be sure that your percentage covers your administration time.

It is wise to have enough cash reserve to pay your outsourcers on a regular basis, usually once or twice a month, even though it may take longer for your accounts to pay. It is difficult to keep good transcriptionists if they never know when they are going to get paid. Even if your accounts do not pay you promptly, you still have an obligation to your outsourcers.

TERMS OF AGREEMENT

The terms of agreement between you and your outsourcer can be spelled out in a contract, which might include performance, equipment/supplies, pricing/ payment, communication with clients, non-compete clause, scope of work, termination, etc. There is a sample contract included in the appendix of this book. Have the contract reviewed by your attorney.

When working with outsourcers, schedule ahead of time, well in advance of the actual outsourcing work date. Outsourcers have other personal and professional commitments, frequently work with more than one transcriptionist, and usually have calendars that fill up as quickly as your own. Advance scheduling gives you more flexibility in selecting an outsourcer and helps prevent last minute frustration.

Communicate periodically with outsourcers and potential outsourcers to verify their continuing availability and to discuss any status changes.

WHEN YOU ARE AN OUTSOURCER

Newly independent transcriptionists frequently work as outsourcers while establishing their business and building clientele. Even after they are well established, many independent medical transcriptionists continue to accept outsource assignments when work is slow.

If you decide to take on outsource work, carefully consider all factors involved. Be sure to discuss job requirements in full and verify payment arrangements. If you disagree with the work plan or have questions, suggestions or requests, speak up before signing a contract.

OUTSOURCER UNDERBIDDING

Unfortunately, outsourcers have been known to "go in the back door" and "underbid," or, as some put it, "steal" accounts from others. This is generally considered unethical, but it happens.

If you are the outsourcer, resist any temptation to underbid. Respect the service you are working for and maintain professional transcription standards. The transcriptionist who resorts to unethical practices usually ruins his or her professional reputation and finds a career as an independent short-lived.

OUTSOURCERS AND THE IRS

Those who use outsourcers must complete an IRS Form 1099 on each noncorporate subcontractor to whom you pay more than $600, and these must be mailed by January 31st to the subcontractors, with a copy to IRS and the State Franchise Tax Boards where applicable, along with Forms 1096 and 596, by February 28th. If you outsource/subcontract your services, you should expect a 1099 from the service you worked for.

OUTSOURCING ISN'T FOR EVERYONE

Outsourcing on a wide scale has drawbacks, and we do not recommend it for every independent transcriptionist. It is rarely appropriate for new independents, and experienced transcriptionists do not always find outsourcing a suitable option.

Outsourcing requires a great deal of administrative control, a level of responsibility that many independents cannot manage. It requires relinquishing a substantial percentage of standard fees, which many cannot afford.

If you choose to work with outsourcers, you will be responsible for the quality of your transcription and for the quality of their transcription, which must meet your standards and those of your clients. As a quality control measure, you will spend many hours distributing work, proofreading and verifying that work is done to specifications. Other responsibilities will increase, too. You will spend more time billing and paying bills, handling additional telephone calls, maintaining more complex public relations, and dealing with a greater number of unanticipated problems.

If you work with more than one outsourcer, you may find that you are spending the majority of your day administrating instead of transcribing. You must schedule pickup and deliveries, sort and arrange the work load for each day, estimate and know how much volume each outsourcer can handle.

You will provide formats and samples for new accounts, help with transcription difficulties, and when the outsourcer does not follow through or complete assigned work, be prepared to pickup the pieces until the job is completed. Soon you may discover that you are managing a "transcription service" and have lost the freedom and flexibility of independence.

Overcommitting is always a risk in outsourcing. If outsourcing with one transcriptionist works well for you, you may be inclined to accept greater volumes of work and outsource more frequently, which may present difficulties for you and your subs.

Spurred by enthusiasm for increased business, you may develop an inappropriate dependence on outsourcers. Likewise, outsourcers whose service is used frequently may grow to depend on your overflow for their primary source of income. If your volume drops off or you lose accounts, you will be responsible for breaking the news to the outsourcer, which is a very unpleasant task.

On the other hand, if your volume suddenly expands by leaps and bounds, you may find yourself with inadequate people-power to meet deadlines. Or you might lose an outsourcer and, even with standard levels of work, be unable to fulfill your commitments.

The Independent Contractor

"The secret of happiness is not doing what one likes,
but in liking what one does."

—Logan Pearsall Smith

INDEPENDENT CONTRACTOR

A person hired to perform a service with responsibility for the end results of the effort. The hirer has no control over the independent contractor's methods of performance or details of work such as one would have over an employee's labor.

On the surface, the definition of an independent contractor seems simple, but in working-world reality, it is actually quite complex. Our government has established very specific rules and regulations regarding who and who cannot legally call themselves independent contractors. Even with rules, however, there are gray areas, and some "independent contractors" have found themselves in legal limbo. Others, of course, are in hot water because they have made no attempt whatever to follow the rules. Don't let this happen to you.

Anyone desiring to be an independent contractor should clearly understand the following four points:

1. Government rules determine if a worker is an independent contractor. The IRS and state laws determine whether a worker is an independent contractor or an employee — not the written or oral agreements between you and the person you contract with. A contract in a file is not proof of an independent contractor relationship.

2. Workers are employees unless the hiring firm can prove otherwise.

3. Independent contractor status has nothing to do with job titles or type of work. Two people can do exactly the same job. One can be a true independent contractor, and the other can be an employee. It all depends upon how the hiring firm treats each worker.

4. One mistake can cause an independent contractor to be converted into employee status. Independent contractor status is not static. Any action by the hiring firm or its employees to control independent contractors can convert them into employees.

> State and federal rules concerning independent contractors come from two sources: direct legislation and court decisions.

Court decisions or legislation may significantly alter the validity of this information. It is wise to periodically consult an attorney or other tax professional who monitors independent contractor rulings.

The key issue in determining whether or not a worker is an independent contractor is this: Who has the right to control the worker and how the work is accomplished. If a hiring firm controls the means by which work is done, the worker is automatically an employee. If the hiring firm can exercise control only on results of the work, the worker can be an independent contractor. It is the right to control, not the actual exercising of control, that is important.

The hiring firm cannot control an independent contractor's work. If it does, the worker's legal status will automatically be an employer-employee relationship and the hiring firm will be liable for employment taxes and benefits.

The hiring firm does have the right to exercise control as to the results of the work; it can provide job specifications to the independent contractor.

A hiring firm can only terminate independent contractors if it breaches the contract or if completed work is unacceptable. If a hiring firm claims the right to fire a worker at will, the worker's legal status usually is an employee.

BENEFITS TO INDEPENDENT CONTRACTORS

• Personal flexibility

• Being your own boss

• Business expenses are tax-deductible

BASIC CHARACTERISTICS OF INDEPENDENT CONTRACTORS

• Hired on a job-by-job basis

• Operate as a separate business

• Offer their services to the general public

• Hired to perform a specific task with no ongoing relationship or obligation by the hiring firm

> Independent contractor status has nothing to do with job titles or type of work. Two people can do exactly the same job. One can be a true independent contractor, and the other can be an employee.

HOW FIRMS BENEFIT BY HIRING INDEPENDENT CONTRACTORS

Firms that hire independent contractors benefit in significant ways. They avoid responsibility for the following:

- Social security taxes or Medicare premiums

- Workers' compensation insurance premiums

- Unemployment insurance (1997 state and federal rate for new businesses is 4.2% on first $7000 of wages, up to $294 per employee)

- In some states, employment training taxes

- Health insurance and retirement benefits

- Long-term employee commitment

- Liability for the worker's action (with exceptions)

- Dealing with labor unions and their accompanying demands for union scale wages, benefits, and hiring/firing practices

RISKS TO THE INDEPENDENT CONTRACTOR

- **No disability or workers' compensation insurance**
  If the independent contractor is injured, they cannot collect disability or workers compensation insurance.

- **No unemployment insurance**
  Independent contractors are not eligible for unemployment insurance.

- **Can be held liable**
  Independent contractors can be held liable for their actions, instead of being protected by the hiring firm or its insurance coverage.

- **May develop tax troubles**
  Independent contractors must pay quarterly income tax and Social Security self-employment taxes (in 1997, 15.3% on first $65,400 net taxable income) — a big shock to those who do not plan ahead. When you add federal income tax (15%-33%) and state taxes, the total tax bill can be huge. If independent contractors spend that money elsewhere before tax time, they can get into significant trouble with the government.

INDEPENDENT CONTRACTING AND THE TWENTY COMMON LAW PRINCIPLES

When the IRS audits a company and spot-checks for fraudulent independent contractors, it relies on these twenty "common law" principles:

1. No Instructions
Contractors cannot be required to follow instructions to accomplish their tasks.

2. No Training
Contractors rarely receive training to perform a task.

3. Service can be rendered by others
Contractors can hire others to do the work for them.

4. Own work hours
Contractors set their own work hours.

5. Nonessential work
Contract work is not essential to the company.

6. No day-to-day working relationship
Most contractors do not have a day-to-day relationship with their employers.

7. Control of assistant
Contractors can hire, supervise and pay assistants independent of their employers.

8. Time to pursue other work
Contractors should have enough time to pursue other work.

9. Job location
The contractor decides when and where the work is done.

10. Order of work set
The contractor has control of the sequence of tasks that lead to finishing the job.

11. No progress reports
Contractors are not required to submit interim reports to employer.

12. Paid for the job
Contractors are paid for the job, not for the time spent doing the job.

13. Working for multiple firms
Contractors should have time to do work for more than one employer.

14. Business expenses
In most cases, contractors should pay their own expenses involved in doing a job.

15. Own tools
Contractors usually furnish their own tools.

16. Significant investment
Contractors' investment in their trade must be significant enough to make them independent of employer's facilities.

17. Services available to the public
Contractors must show they make their services available to other employers.

18. Potential profit or loss
Contractors are liable for any expenses and liabilities they may encounter in performing their jobs.

19. Limited right to discharge
Contractors cannot be fired at will so long as they produce a result specified in their contract.

20. No compensation for noncompletion
Contractors cannot be paid for partial completion of a job.

Failure to satisfy all 20 principles may result in an Internal Revenue Service audit on the past three years with the business owner penalized for each misclassified worker, whether they were deliberately misclassified or the misclassification resulted from an honest mistake. One mistake can easily cost a business $25,000.

The 20 common law factors described above were developed by the IRS. There are at least five other government agencies in California involved with determining whether workers are independent contractors or employees:

- Employment Development Department (EDD)

- Workers Compensation Appeals Board

- Immigration and Naturalization Service

- U.S. Department of Labor

- Labor Commissioner

These governing agencies will vary from state to state.

Like the IRS, all these agencies consistently agree upon one key determining factor: In a true independent contractor relationship, the hiring firm has no right to control the work of the worker.

However, each agency has developed its own "factor list" to show right to control. For the most part they parallel the IRS factors. Here are the most important factors common to all these agencies:

1. Hiring firm does not have the right to control the worker

2. Type of work is not the hiring firm's primary business

3. It is not a continuing relationship

4. Payment is made by the job

5. Worker has own tools

6. Worker cannot be fired at will

7. Worker determines job location

8. Worker has a distinct occupation or operates a separate business

The U.S. Department of Labor uses a six point "Economic Realities" test to determine if a worker is an independent contractor. Reference: *Employment Relationship Under the Fair Labor Standards Act*, Publication 1297, U.S. Department of Labor.

SIX FACTOR "ECONOMIC REALITIES" TEST

1. Work should not be part of the hiring firm's regular business

2. Working relationship should have a degree of non-permanence

3. Worker should have invested in equipment, materials, or assistants

4. Hiring firm should have no right to control work

5. Opportunity for profit or loss exists, depending on the worker's managerial skills

6. Work should require initiative, judgment, or foresight to successfully compete with others

Regarding homeworkers, the IRS and California have ruled that homeworkers are statutory employees if the hiring firm gives them specifications, provides them with materials or goods, and requires them to return the finished goods to it and the following conditions exist:

1. Substantially all work is performed personally

2. Worker does not have substantial investment in facilities

3. Work is not a single transaction

4. Worker does not offer services to the general public

5. Worker does not keep records

6. Worker sometimes uses hiring firm's facilities and equipment to perform the task

7. Worker is paid hourly

THE BOTTOM LINE

You must look at **all 20 common law factors** to form a total picture. Do not rely on any one factor. Aside from determining which factors are the most important, examine the factors that you cannot meet and ask yourself why? Work on meeting all of those factors before you classify yourself as an independent contractor.

You must be willing to be an entrepreneur and take business risks (make a profit or loss on jobs), assume liability if the work is faulty, hire assistants, invest in your business, advertise, and be able to conduct business even after losing a client. If you are not willing to do that, then you cannot classify yourself as an independent contractor.

Educate yourself. In California there is an Independent Contractor Package designed to make it easier for independent contractors to comply with government requirements and plan for unexpected illnesses, injuries, or unemployment. This package is available through the state chamber of commerce and through some local chambers.

- **The California Chamber of Commerce**
  P. O. Box 1736
  Sacramento, CA 95812-1736
  916-444-6670

For those outside California, locate your state's chamber of commerce in the resource section at the back of this book.

Chamber of Commerce
An association of businesspersons and merchants for the promotion of commercial interests in the community.

ADDITIONAL PROTECTION FOR THE INDEPENDENT CONTRACTOR

To protect itself, the hiring firm may ask you for the following items:

1. Contractor's business license

2. Contractor's fictitious name statement (if applicable)

3. Evidence of insurance (business liability coverage)

OFFICE RECORDS

Most transcriptionists enjoy transcribing, and independent transcriptionists sometimes wish they were free to concentrate entirely on that responsibility, focusing all their attention on producing the quality work that results in an excellent income. For independent transcriptionists, such a wish will never be realized because they must also carefully and conscientiously administer their business — organizing, restoring and retrieving, and taking care of accounts receivable and accounts payable. A well-organized office is essential to success.

To maintain accurate and organized records in your office, we recommend the following:

1. **Clients**
   A file for each client.

2. **Physician lists**
   If you are dealing with hospitals and large clinics, you must keep a physician directory. Each hospital has a directory of active staff physicians, consulting staff, courtesy staff, and temporary staff physicians.

   It is also a good idea to keep a directory of physicians from the area you are servicing. This can be obtained by copying the yellow pages of the local telephone directory, or by requesting a physician directory from the local medical society (not all physicians belong to medical societies, but most do). These lists should include not only the names, but addresses and phone numbers as well. You must keep the lists updated yearly as new physicians are added.

3. Daily work log sheets

Logging in jobs daily is very important if you are dealing with several clients.

This log can identify the work you take in daily by date, client name, minutes; and upon completion you can log the lines. We find a daily log reference invaluable, especially when the schedule is very busy and there isn't always time to transfer information to a ledger. We often catch up on paper work on weekends or in the wee hours of the morning before starting work the next day. Establish good daily logging habits in the beginning, and you won't regret it.

4. Service contracts

We have a file for equipment service contracts that are renewed yearly. If there is a problem with equipment, the information is readily available when calling for service.

5. Rolodex® - Business Cards

Keep these handy, and collect them from other transcriptionists at seminars, meetings, trade-shows, etc. Also collect business cards of book and equipment vendors, and any other appropriate contacts.

6. Continuing education

As a certified medical transcriptionist, you must obtain a certain amount of continuing education credits (CECs) to maintain your certification.

For each chapter meeting, seminar, symposium, there are certificates verifying the number of CECs obtained from attending. If no certificate is available, save your program and place that information in your file. Even if you are not certified, continuing education is important, so we suggest you maintain this file, because your ultimate goal should be to become certified in the future.

Your continuing education credits are also impressive to prospective clients and employers, and you can include this information on your resume or curriculum vitae. This helps to build credibility and to attract more clients.

7. Outsourcers lists

If you have occasion to use outsourcers, and even if you do not, it is still a good idea to keep a list of other self-employed transcriptionists that you can call upon if needed — to cover your vacation time, for emergencies, or for unexpected overflow. This list should be updated at least yearly.

8. **Calendar/meetings**

   Keeping a daily planner at your desk is very handy. You can pick these up at a local office supply store. The calendar can be filled in monthly, weekly, or daily, as you see fit, and is an ever-present reminder of your daily, weekly, and monthly schedule.

9. **Correspondence**

   Be sure to keep a file of your correspondence. You may not think this will be necessary, but the paperwork just seems to accumulate!

10. **Formats/transcription samples**

    Keep a file of your client formats and transcription samples. If you have several clients, it's usually a good idea to keep an individual file, or a binder with dividers for each client, to avoid confusion.

11. **Contracts/agreements**

    You should have copies of all contracts and agreements you enter into with clients, other services, and outsourcers.

12. **Word lists**

    From medical lectures, magazines, newsletters, and a variety of other sources, you will accumulate many new word reference lists. These lists will be handwritten, photocopied, and printed — not in book form. You'll want to keep these handy references in a readily accessible place. A file or binder is convenient. Maybe someday you will write your own word book but in the meantime, never throw away a word list!

LOG SHEETS

Every transcriptionist must keep a record of what was transcribed on any given day. If your software program offers the capability of constructing a daily log, all the better.

Why is a daily log necessary? Simply put, to increase efficiency. Here is a typical scenario: An account calls asking if and when you transcribed an operative report on Mr. Blank, which was supposedly dictated three months earlier. If you don't keep a daily log sheet, how are you ever going to find that work?

First, you check your computer files, which indicate that you did not transcribe dictation on Mr. Blank during the specified three month period. Your log sheet backs you up.

A sample of a daily log sheet appears on the following page of this book. It should include the name of the account, the date transcribed, number of tapes received and returned, and the total line count for that date. It should also include the patient's name, the dictating physician's name, type of report, date dictated, number of lines for that report, and any problems associated with the dictation.

Of course, a log sheet can be designed to fit your style and mode of work, but it is a necessary tool in the field of transcription. Many line count software programs include generated transcription report logs similar to the one shown on the following page.

TRANSCRIPTION LOG SHEET (SAMPLE)

Minutes of dictation _____   Total lines _____

Tapes picked up _____   Date _____

Page _____   Transcriptionist: H1

Account name _____

DATE DICTATED	CONTROL #	PHYSICIAN	PATIENT	REPORT	TOTAL LINES

RECORDS

In addition to retail books and forms, free or low cost reference materials are also abundantly available. Use resources at your local library or order government publications from the Internal Revenue Service (IRS), the Small Business Administration (SBA), the Department of Commerce, and your state resources.

SEPARATING YOUR PERSONAL AND BUSINESS CHECKING ACCOUNTS

There are three important reasons for opening a separate banking account for your business:

- It will provide you with a complete record of your income and expenditures for tax purposes, and at tax time, you won't waste hours separating personal from business expenses. Also, if you are ever audited by the IRS, the auditor will not be able to look into your personal finances.

- Using personal checks for your business expenses suggests that you are a small-time operation and your credibility may suffer. On the other hand, if your business checks are embossed with your business name and logo, you will enhance your professional image.

- It is much more difficult to unravel your business and personal finances if they are kept in the same account.

When opening your business checking account the bank will ask you for your business license and your fictitious name statement (if you have one), as well as your Social Security number. You should ask to have your check numbers start at 300 or above. This will give the image that you have been in business for awhile. This may be helpful because some suppliers are reluctant to extend credit to a new business that has no track record of reliability or success.

APPLYING FOR A BUSINESS LOAN

In order to qualify for a small business loan, you must provide the lender with information regarding your business. You will need a business plan describing your product or service, your target market, your financial projections, and your current financial statements.

The SBA (U.S. Small Business Administration) offers excellent references for the small business owner. One publication is called *ABCs of Borrowing* (FM-1). This publication covers what lenders will require, what type of financial information you will have to provide, collateral, the loan application and agreement, types of loans and much more.

The SBA also offers an extensive selection of information on most business management topics. All of this information is listed in *The Small Business Directory*. For a free copy write to SBA Publications.

- **SBA Publications**
  P. O. Box 1000
  Fort Worth, TX 76119

THE SMALL BUSINESS ADMINISTRATION (SBA) AS A BUSINESS ALLY

According to the National Association of Women Business Owners, 32% of small business owners are women; however, only 8-10% of women entrepreneurs receive SBA loans. Why the disparity? According to the National Association of Women Business Owners (NAWBO), ". . . personal or commercial bank loans are the number one type of short-term financing among all businesses, but credit cards are clearly the number one funding source for women. Most women probably have one or two cards and they see them as readily available sources of cash. They also don't have to supply the two years of financial statements required for most bank loans." Why are women having to turn to alternative types of financing in order to keep their businesses alive?

 A study by NAWBO indicates that attitudes and practices of loan officers are a significant barrier to many women seeking business loans. The NAWBO study noted that common complaints among women business owners include bank requirements for more assets or collateral and a longer business track record, and the banks' own limited experience in dealing with service businesses.

There are other reasons why businesswomen turn to credit cards. In the past, Small Business Administration requirements for obtaining business loans were too stringent and only the fittest survived the loan application process. All too frequently the process required many months of paperwork and meetings with lenders before approval could be obtained from the SBA. Most women business owners, frustrated with the interminable process and the lack of progress, turned to other sources — primarily credit cards — to finance their businesses

Until 1994, 90% of all loans given by the SBA were covered under the 7 (a) Guarantee Loan Program. The purpose of this loan was to assist the new or growing business with its financial needs. Eligibility was restricted to manufacturers with up to 500 employees; wholesalers with up to 100 employees; agricultural businesses up to $500,000 in annual sales; retail businesses with a maximum of $5,000,000 in annual sales; service industries with a maximum of $5,000,000 in annual sales; contractors up to $17,000,000 in annual sales; and special trade businesses with a maximum of $7,000,000 in annual sales. Proceeds from the loan were to be used strictly for working capital, acquisition of machinery and equipment, purchase of inventory, business buy-outs and start-ups, debt refinance, purchasing land and buildings, construction including land acquisition, improvements and renovations. To obtain a 7 (a) loan, collateral was needed such as mortgage on land, building and/or equipment, assignment of warehouse receipts, mortgage on personal property, guarantees and assignments of current receivables and assets of the business. This loan was for a maximum guaranty of $750,000. As you can see, most IMTs would not meet the eligibility requirements for securing such a loan.

SBA SMALL LOAN "LOW DOC" PROGRAM

In 1996 the SBA made available a Small Loan "Low Doc" Program to women business owners. The process is very simple. The applicant meets with an SBA advisor for screening at a local Small Business Development Center or at another organization designated by the SBA. After screening, a "pre-qualification" letter is issued. The applicant takes the letter to the lender of her choice for an SBA loan. The letter assures the lender that a loan made to the applicant will be guaranteed by the SBA up to a maximum of $250,000.

The "Low Doc" program is designed to reduce the paperwork and cost of providing loans of $100,000 or less and to increase the availability or such financing to small businesses. Emphasis is placed on the applicant's character and personal and business credit history rather than on traditional credit criteria. No predetermined percentage of equity injection is required.

SBA "LOW DOC" PRIMARY CREDIT CONSIDERATIONS

- Willingness to repay debts, as indicated by a good credit history; a cosignor may be considered if applicant has no credit history.

- The likelihood that expected earnings will be sufficient to pay obligations.

- With the requested financing, the business has a good chance of achieving success.

SBA "LOW DOC" LOAN APPLICATION REQUIREMENTS

In order to apply for an SBA loan you must provide the proper documentation. This includes the following:

- Personal financial statement: Within past 60 days current.

- Personal tax returns: Prior three years, all schedules.

- Credit report: Get your own copy free from TRW 1-800-682-7654.

- Company's financial history: Business financial statement (Balance Sheet and Profit and Loss Statement) — as current as possible, no older than most recent quarter end.

- Accounts payable and accounts receivable aging statements (same date as financial statement).

- Business tax returns: Prior three years, all schedules. If your business is a sole proprietorship, the business's "tax return" is your Schedule C in your personal tax return.

Find out the location of your SBA Administration Development Center (every town should have one). Before seeking loans from lenders, make an appointment with an SBA advisor to see if you qualify for one of their new programs. In addition to being an excellent resource center, these development centers are wonderful for networking. Most of them provide a resource library, which can be used for free, as well as monthly workshops, which are usually less than $10 each, on a variety of business topics.

Business funding opportunities are opening up for women in other areas, too. Two of the nation's largest banks are now embracing female business owners by aligning themselves with major women's business organizations. **Wells Fargo Bank** has teamed up with the National Association of Women Business Owners, a Washington-based group with 60 chapters, while **Bank of America** recently linked up with Women Inc., a Sacramento-based trade association.

Wells Fargo and NAWBO: Wells' loans are unsecured and require a one-page application form with no tax returns or financial statements. The minimum loan amount is $5,000. To qualify for a loan, women must have good personal and business credit, have been in business for two years and be profitable. For information, call 888-767-2444.

B of A and Women Inc.: Bank of America recently jumped into the market with its own lending program targeted toward women. B of A's alliance with Women Inc., which provides a variety of services and discounts to members, makes sense because both organizations share the goal of financially empowering women business owners. Women Inc.'s members benefit from a 50% discount on setup fees for new Advantage Business Credit loans up to $100,000. The bank also offers a one-page loan application.

- **Women Inc.**
  800-930-3993

A Note To Men: For our male readers, we certainly hope the previous section on business loans for women does not offend you. It is not our intent to do so. It is unfortunate that we even have to include this in the book, but the fact remains that for many years there has been an almost impenetrable barrier in the banking world that has kept a large segment of our society from participating. If we are to achieve true parity in the business world, we need a level playing field.

DECIDING WHETHER TO KEEP GROWING

For those who resolve the difficulties encountered in running a home business and enjoy its advantages, the ultimate challenge becomes controlling growth. Many healthy home businesses begin to outgrow their settings after a few years, at which point one must decide whether to give up the benefits of working at home or scale back and keep the business small.

At this juncture, some businesses outsource work in order to stay small. Others choose to expand into office space and hire employees. If you are successful in your business, be prepared to think about this because you will be faced with this decision sooner or later.

As an independent you have the opportunity to make a great deal of money, but you probably will not make an annual income of $30,000-$60,000 during the first two or three years. For a few, financial security comes soon, but it is rare.

The length of time it takes to become financially secure depends on the individual. For many, it is reached at the point when they are no longer spending excessive time using reference materials, and this usually takes a number of years. There is no way to hurry becoming a good transcriptionist — no crash course. Excellence takes time. Medical transcriptionists get paid for what they know as it relates to quality production. The more we know, the more we can produce, ergo, the more we get paid.

Many successful independents eventually discover they have more work than they can handle. Some enthusiastically decide to find other MTs to help them . . . and soon they have several people helping them. Because their business has a reputation for excellence, they must utilize ICs or employees who conform to excellent standards, and the overhead creeps up. Even more work is accepted and more helpers employed ... and then the process is repeated. Naturally, with all this work, increased deliveries must be scheduled, new equipment must be purchased and old equipment must be upgraded. The overhead climbs higher while the successful (although no longer so enthusiastic) MT's percentage of profits goes lower as she administers the business operations more and more and transcribes less and less. In addition, Uncle Sam always wants a bigger share.

When the time comes, carefully weigh the pros and cons of expanding. You may discover you had a lot more money when it was JUST YOU!

EXPANDING TO A MEDICAL TRANSCRIPTION OFFICE

If the idea and challenge of expanding your service beyond independent freelancing appeals to you, perhaps you should consider opening an expanded medical transcription office in a commercial area.

> NOTE: Although much of the information contained in this book will prove helpful to you in developing a successful medical transcription office, we do not address this subject specifically and recommend that you seek counsel elsewhere in this pursuit.

BURNOUT

Hopefully your business will soon grow beyond your wildest expectations, which is terrific if you are able to maintain a balanced life. However, beware if you discover the following symptoms: you are working your fingers to the bone; your eyesight is fading due to screen fatigue; your mind is filled with medical terms and nothing else; you can't sleep without your fingers and right foot moving; you are developing a wrist drop, a hunched back, and saying to yourself, "Is this all there is?" These are the first signs of burnout!

Perhaps it's time to learn how to erase old mental tapes and redictate new ones for your life. Work should not be your primary source of self-esteem, nor should it be used to escape from the outside world. When either occurs, burnout is inevitable.

Workaholism in our society today is rewarded. Corporations encourage employees to fill their off-time by traveling from one assignment to the next and attending self-improvement seminars. Workaholism leads to burnout.

Burnout is easy to spot. It occurs when one gives more than one has to give and there is nothing left. Frequently, the first signs of burnout are depression and an inability or unwillingness to get out of bed in the morning, by sleeplessness at night or waking every couple of hours, and wanting to eat everything in sight or nothing at all. Physical symptoms can be characterized by tightening of the jaw, neck, shoulders and chest; palpitations, ringing or buzzing in the ears, and a general sense of unease.

Once you are able to realize that there is a big world outside of transcription, which is meant to be enjoyed, you can start making some changes. The term "work" must be redefined. It is necessary to conclude that it is just a job and nothing more, an activity to be performed for a prescribed amount of time per day that allows you to pursue other interests. To many medical transcriptionists — and other professionals as well — being "unproductive" translates into "worthlessness." Have you ever felt that if you said "no" you would be replaced and if you did not do everything perfectly, you were not good enough? Beware burnout!

Remember, the main reason for becoming independent is to work smarter not harder. Of course one's best laid plans can fall by the wayside. After a few months at home, you might realize that you are working harder than ever before and definitely enjoying it less. There is always work to be done and you can no longer leave it at the office. Your clients are demanding more and more of you.

Many transcriptionists overwork because they are not making enough profit. If this is your situation, evaluate your transcription rates and if they are low, consider raising them.

Without work limits and lacking confidence to say "no," it is easy to fall into a workaholic rut. You fear saying "no" will send clients scurrying elsewhere, leaving you to pound the pavement in search of accounts.

It is important to set limits for yourself and do only what is acceptable to you. Start by really communicating with your accounts, telling them what you feel is practical and what is not. Tell them emphatically how much work you can take per day and that if they give you more, they cannot expect a fast turnaround time. Explain to them that when you decline to take work on any given day, it is because you are running behind and know you will not be able to make the delivery within the time limit already agreed upon.

The first time you use the NO word, your hands might be clammy, your brow beaded with sweat, and your voice no bigger than a squeak. You will probably be pleasantly surprised to find that instead of rushing out to find another service, the client will actually call you back the next day. By setting limits for yourself, your clients will respect you for your honesty. They will know what they can expect from you, and you will know what to expect from them. What a professional concept!

Following are ideas we have found useful in developing good work habits.

- **Know your performance style and accept it.**
  Independent contractors are usually very goal-directed and like to get work out as fast as possible in order to have time for themselves. Whether you are a person who likes to work from 9 a.m. to 5 p.m., do your best work at night or wait until the last moment, do it. Individual work patterns are neither right nor wrong. The power comes in acknowledging what works best for you as an individual and accepting it.

- **Be aware of your priorities and live by them.**
  It is easy to give everything equal priority; working, doing laundry, watering the garden, filing income taxes. Make a priority list every morning and attempt to complete the list in order of priority. Some days, you might be able to accomplish everything on the list and some days not, but the structure will keep you from feeling overwhelmed and panicky.

- **Discover your limitations.**
  No matter how much you try, you cannot do everything. Everyone has limitations. Be aware of how much you can comfortably transcribe in a given day. By knowing this and accepting it, you will have eliminated much stress from your life.

- **Build in time for yourself.**
  It is essential that we have balance in our lives: work, family, friends, and hobbies. Allow yourself time to play and enjoy this wonderful life and the fabulous people in it. Set aside one hour each day just for yourself. Go for a long walk, ride a bicycle, take a long, hot luxuriating bubble bath, read, or go out to dinner or to a movie with friends. When you know there is a block of time set aside just for you and only you, the day goes smoother and faster.

> *"The trouble with life in the fast lane*
> *is that you get to the other end*
> *in an awful hurry."*
> —John Jensen

Finances

> *"Money, which represents the prose of life, . . .*
> *is in its effects and laws, as beautiful as roses."*
> —Ralph Waldo Emerson

Setting up an independent medical transcription business requires an investment of time and money. In the beginning, your dollar investment need not be great, but it must be managed well if you want your business to survive. As your business grows, consistent and regular money management will bring you not only economic success, but professional respect, too.

FINANCIAL NEEDS AND CAPITAL INVESTMENT

A home-based business can be established with little or no start-up capital. Your business is a labor intensive business — you provide a service. Initially you will need only a modest monetary investment in facilities and equipment. The greater investment will be the labor involved; that is, the service you offer which you will personally provide.

You will need little in the way of office facilities, and you may provide your services in facilities provided by your clients — on-site, on the client's premises — where you have free access to computers, copying machines and other equipment.

Perhaps you have enough personal working capital to get started on a modest scale, but you may soon find that you do not have enough operating capital to pay expenses right away or draw even a modest salary while your business is growing. This is a cash flow problem to avoid if possible.

Many entrepreneurs do not recognize the need for up-front operating capital. They assume that income will begin to flow as soon as they begin their business. There are two serious flaws to this line of reasoning:

1. **Your business may not start with a rush.** Most new businesses get off to a slow start. It usually takes time to develop business to the point where income exceeds expenses. This is especially true for a home-based venture.

2. **Cash may not flow in immediately.** Even if you acquire clients quickly and business is very good, it will still take some time for collections, or cash inflow. It depends on your billing practices and the length of time it takes clients to pay. Let's assume you bill on the 1st of each month.

If you start your account on the 10th of the month, you will work 20 days before you can bill, and the client will likely take another 15 or more days to pay the bill. On a full month, from the date the billing period starts until the time you receive payment could be 45 or more days.

Some of your clients may deliberately delay payment to you to enhance their cash flow. Soon, you may have a great deal of "billed out" money owed to you ("accounts receivable"). You need to collect that cash in order to pay your bills.

Instead of using personal savings, you may choose to take out a loan to get started. Do a monthly cash flow projection to forecast the cash you expect to receive and disburse during your first year or two.

It has been said that the little guy who can least afford to wait gets paid last — even by the federal government. Be prepared for slow collections at first, until you become established and develop some collection leverage with your clients.

WATCH YOUR COSTS AND EXPENSES

Cost reduction is important and cost avoidance even better, especially for a start-up business. The typical mistakes made by many novices are understandable.

You start out in business with enthusiasm, cheered on by friends and relatives. With this solid base of self-assurance and confidence, you begin with great style: handsome new furniture, shiny new equipment, expensive stationery, loads of office supplies, and a few extra goodies you could not resist. Almost all of this expense is not absolutely necessary!

You can do as much business at a secondhand desk, using modest stationery. If you purchase a computer and word processing system, think twice before you invest $3000 in a copier. A fax machine might prove a better value for you.

USING A BUSINESS CREDIT CARD

I don't know about you, but every year at tax time I find myself inundated with little bits and pieces of paper detailing my business expenses. Well, I have found the perfect solution . . . the American Express Gold Card.

Two years ago, AMEX began offering its customers an end-of-year summary, detailing all transactions made on the card per year by categories, i.e., airline, travel, restaurant, merchandise, service fees, entertainment, health related, etc. I made the decision at that time to use this card only for business expenses. Don't get me wrong, I still save all my receipts. But, at the end of the year when I'm gathering and organizing financial data, it's so much easier to refer to my AMEX summary for itemizing tax deductions. Since almost all businesses accept the AMEX card, it is a very easy way to keep track of business expenses.

The annual fee for the AMEX card is $75/year, which is quite a bargain when you consider all the time spent, and time saved, getting paperwork ready for your accountant.

One special benefit to AMEX card users is a warranty extension on equipment. When using the AMEX card for equipment purchases, the company will double the warranty agreement. For instance, if you used your AMEX card to purchase a computer which came with a one year warranty, AMEX would extend the warranty for another year so the equipment would be covered for two years.

There is one major drawback in using the AMEX card, however. You must pay all charges as they are billed. There are no monthly installments. Therefore, before making any purchase, you must make sure you will have money in your business account to cover that expense when it becomes due and payable the following month. For more information regarding the credit card, call American Express.

- **American Express**
  800-635-5955

EQUIPMENT: LEASING OR RENTING VERSUS BUYING

You can rent most equipment needed for a business including computers, printers, modems, copiers, or fax machines. The rental agreement may be for a period as short as a single day or for a year or more. If your need for computer equipment is short-term, it usually costs far less to rent than to buy.

Renting can serve as a low-cost way of sampling various pieces of equipment. If you are unsure about the features you need in a computer system, fax machine or copier, short-term renting is a good way to evaluate new or different technologies. If you need to upgrade your equipment within the first year of business, renting will probably offer greater flexibility to acquire equipment.

When starting your business, you may have enough money saved to cover the first three months of your new venture, but that money may be needed for operating expenses — not for purchasing equipment. Even if you want to make an equipment loan from a bank, local bankers may be wary of lending money to your new business.

Rental agencies retain ownership of rented equipment. The renter merely pays for the privilege of using it for a period of time. During the period of the rental agreement, the rental agency is usually obligated to service the equipment if it becomes inoperable. When necessary, the agency is also responsible for replacing the equipment in a timely fashion.

The primary benefits of renting office equipment are conserving up-front cash payment, potential cost savings, and convenience. You pay only for what you use, and may save money by avoiding a large purchase price. Renting should also save time. Rental agencies often have fairly extensive inventories, so they can promptly deliver what you need.

For tax purposes, rental fees, like lease payments, are considered business expenses and are fully tax-deductible. You won't be bothered with complex records of fixed assets and depreciation calculations at tax time.

If you think you will need temporary equipment beyond a few months, determine the most economically advantageous rental period. Monthly payments for personal computer rentals typically hover between 8-11% of the average retail price of the equipment. However, payments can go higher. After eight months to a year of renting, your rental payments will total approximately what you would have paid to buy the system.

Many computer stores offer computer systems for rent. Don't assume that local dealers will be cheaper or more efficient than national chain stores. Prices can vary greatly, so shop for the best bargains.

Don't hesitate to ask questions. Does the quoted price include a complete system? For a computer, will the necessary cables, monitor, video card, or keyboard cost extra? Does the quoted price include delivery and installation of the equipment at the beginning of the rental period and its dismantling and removal when the agreement expires? Does installation service include loading software onto the hard-disk? Does the quoted price include normal maintenance and emergency services?

The level of service offered may differ from vendor to vendor. Do you get prompt on-site service or is the service limited to a technician guiding you through a troubleshooting routine over the telephone?

LEASING EQUIPMENT

When building your business, it is helpful to know how to acquire the equipment you need when you need it. Although you may not have cash or credit to buy equipment outright, you may be able to lease equipment and create an efficient and cost-effective office.

A lease arrangement, with affordable monthly payments applied to the purchase price of equipment, is a viable option for many business owners on a limited budget. At the end of the lease agreement period, the business owner may own the equipment.

Large corporations frequently lease all or part of their office equipment. Among other things, they appreciate the increased flexibility and the convenience of equipment and financing neatly wrapped in one payment package.

The main advantages to leasing equipment are financial. Even though leasing is usually more expensive than buying outright, the ease of tax-deduction from lease expenditures may be more desirable than purchasing and depreciating equipment.

NOTE

IRS rules and regulations change frequently, so check with your accountant for specific information regarding depreciation.

Even though you may have ready cash to pay for office needs, leasing offers the advantage of cash conservation. In the beginning, you may need or want to put some of your cash to work in areas that will help generate profit. Instead of buying equipment, you may invest in advertising — business cards, fliers, and space advertising. Leasing allows you to manage cash flow, paying for your equipment over time.

Leasing equipment also gives you a little more leverage with the vendor if a piece of equipment is a "lemon."

In addition, leasing also offers you greater flexibility in terms of payment plans and equipment updates. Because the computer industry is changing at such a rapid pace and new technology is offered with incredible frequency, leasing minimizes your risk of having to use obsolete technology. If your business needs change in mid-lease, you may be able to get more powerful equipment, with little or no financing penalty. However, this depends on the specific type of lease.

Fixed monthly payments over time represent some savings in real dollars, i.e., your lease payments are made in increasingly devalued (inflated) dollars. In contrast, if you choose to purchase your equipment outright, every dollar you recover through depreciation is worth less due to inflation.
Let's look at your leasing options.

- **The closed-end lease, or finance-lease**, allows you to actually purchase the equipment after the last installment has been paid. Generally the purchase price is either a percentage (often 10%) of the original price or a pro forma amount (usually $1). A closed-end lease is nothing more than a disguised loan.

- **An operating lease or open-end lease** offers you three options at the end of the agreement. You can purchase the equipment at its fair market value or blue book value. You can renegotiate and extend the lease, usually with new equipment. Or you can simply terminate the lease and the equipment reverts back to the lessor.

You must decide which type lease is best for you. If financing is your primary reason for leasing because you want to eventually own the equipment, the closed-end or finance lease may meet your needs. However, if your goal is to upgrade equipment conveniently and economically, your best bet is the open-end, or operating lease. Consult your accountant before making a final decision.

Be aware that you will be paying more by leasing your equipment than by buying it outright. Like credit card loans, you are paying for the privilege of paying over time.

There is a simple formula used by lessors for calculating the monthly cost of a lease, applying a "rate factor" to the purchase price of the equipment. For example, if the rate factor on a three-year finance lease at $5000 were 0.035 or $35 per $1000, monthly payments on this lease would be $175 or five times $35. The rate factor can vary slightly depending on other provisions in the lease, such as payment timing and end-of-lease purchase agreements.

When shopping for a lease, look for one in which the total cost is as close as possible to the equipment's purchase price. Expect to pay a 33% premium if you lease instead of buy.

With a finance lease, shop for the lowest rate factor. To get the maximum benefit from an operating lease, consider the economic life of the equipment and your projected need for equipment upgrades. The ideal operating lease is one whose term actually coincides with the economic life of the leased equipment (the point when the equipment ceases to depreciate any further). At this point you can purchase it at the lowest possible price. If the lease term also corresponds to the "useful life" of the equipment (expiring at just about the time you would be upgrading your equipment), it gives you maximum flexibility in renegotiating the lease for new equipment.

WHEN NOT TO LEASE EQUIPMENT

Internal Revenue Code Section 179 allows immediate deduction for up to $17,500 per year of equipment purchases. With this immediate deduction, you can reduce your income taxes and thereby keep more of your hard-earned cash. Section 179 requires that you use your equipment for five years, so if you plan on trading in your system in three years, you may have to pay the IRS taxes related to the unused portion of the five-year depreciation period. So, generally, you are likely better off purchasing equipment and deducting it under Section 179 instead of leasing the equipment and taking the deduction over the lease period.

In general, leasing makes the most sense when you buy expensive equipment. A $2000 PC won't be worth the effort and expense of setting up a lease agreement. When computers first became affordable for home businesses, the technology was changing rapidly — by the micro-minute it seemed. Just when you thought you had purchased the latest turbo-driven computer, it seemingly became obsolete overnight. Leasing computers at that point made sense. For a very small outlay of cash, one was able to keep up with expanding technology. Now, however, computers have become very upgradable and it is not hard to keep up with the Jones'. However, in any case, always check with your tax adviser for advice on purchasing vs. leasing in the context of your business situation.

There are other situations when leasing might not be a viable equipment option.

- You may not qualify. Some computer equipment lessors want to do business strictly with registered companies, preferably corporations with credit histories, and not with individuals.

- Some leases have riders that prohibit you from moving the equipment out of the state in which you received it. If relocation is a possibility within the next few years, leasing should be avoided.

- A leasing company lien may prevent you from selling the equipment before the lease has expired, even though, with a finance lease, you may eventually own the equipment.

You can't "prepay" a lease. Whereas most bank loans and mortgages allow the borrower to prepay without penalty, with leases you must pay your installments every month whether your business is thriving or floundering. This is generally no great risk to your business, but it is something you should be aware of.

PAYING YOURSELF

As a sole proprietor, how much are your services worth? Well, that depends on your gross receipts. As pointed out earlier in this book, you must save a portion of your gross income to pay such mundane things as self-employment (FICA) taxes, state and federal income taxes, health insurance, disability insurance and all business related expenses. According to most financial experts, your salary could be between 10-45% of your gross receipts. Being home-based medical transcriptionists, our overhead is fairly low once the large expenditures for equipment have been made. Therefore our percentage would be greater than that, say, of a building contractor who needs equipment and supplies and may be at the lower end of the pay scale.

Without question, it's tough to figure out your pay when you're self-employed. Take too little from the business and you begin to wonder why you ever kissed off that hospital job and its sweet biweekly paycheck. Take too much and your business may slowly go bust. That's why, according to most financial experts, it is better to err on the side of paying yourself too little. You can always give yourself a bonus at the end of the year.

One way to gauge your pay is to look at the age of your business. Independent medical transcriptionists just starting in business shouldn't expect to draw a paycheck from the get-go. Financial experts advise that first-year owners take just enough to cover personal expenses, keeping the remaining revenues for business expenses. In general, it takes six months of steady cash flow — a sign that your business is viable — before you can cut yourself a monthly paycheck.

For service businesses such as ours, a good rule of thumb is to divide gross income into thirds. One-third goes to pay business overhead, one-third goes home, and the other third goes for taxes.

Unfortunately, accounts payables sometimes exceed receivables. Those of us who have been in business for awhile understand the fickle nature of medical transcription. Come flu season or Joint Commission, we are inundated with work and find ourselves sitting at our computers fourteen hours a day, seven days a week. Then comes summer vacation, and it seems that no one is dictating. Always ensure that you have enough cash in the bank to cover expenses in down times.

When money piles up in your account, don't be lulled into thinking you can cut yourself a bigger monthly paycheck. If there's one thing you can always count on, it's unexpected expenses, and a little spare cash may mean the difference between making it through a rocky period or folding up your headset.

TAX INCENTIVES: BUSINESS TAXES

Smart home-based medical transcriptionists should learn all they can about different types of business taxes in order to take advantage of tax savings opportunities. In reality, this can mean the difference between success or failure.

Learning all about taxes is not an easy task. In fact, one independent transcriptionist colleague recommends that anyone considering self-employment should investigate this area first. She recommends, "Go to the nearest IRS office and ask for information regarding self-employment. That alone may make you return to your previous job pleading temporary insanity when you gave your notice."

A primary goal of any business should be to operate in such a way as to avoid (legally!) as many taxes as possible. Appropriate deductions may be taken for home maintenance and improvements, automobile expenses, telephone expenses, office and work space, and major purchases, as well as for items like safe deposit rental, stationery and business cards. As a business owner you can also take advantage of tax-deferred retirement plans and tax-deductible medical insurance.

This chapter is meant to give you a simplified understanding of tax law and practice. However, as stated before, it is imperative from the outset that you seek the counsel of an accountant who can guide you through specific tax issues and help you plan and implement strategies to minimize taxes.

Always bear in mind that being aware of how the tax system works, and paying only those taxes legally required, will be to your advantage. Knowing the facts about tax breaks will save you tax dollars, help you avoid unwise purchases, and guide you in better record keeping.

> NOTE: Tax laws change frequently. What holds true today may not necessarily be the case in future years. Consult your accountant about tax law changes that may affect your business.

TYPES OF TAXES

Remember the old saying, "In this life you can be sure of only two things — death and taxes?" Well folks, you can run but you can't hide from the IRS.

There are home-based medical transcriptionists, as well as other independently employed professionals, who have not filed a tax return in years. Many feign ignorance of tax law; some have convinced themselves they don't owe any taxes and, therefore, are not required to file; others have procrastinated filing a return to the point of embarrassment, fear and denial; and a few simply think they can outsmart Uncle Sam.

However, the majority of tax evaders are caught and penalized heavily for not filing a proper return when it was due. Today's IRS computer system is very efficient in cross-checking earnings records in detail.

For most people, tax evasion also takes a personal toll in terms of physical, mental, and emotional stress. The longer the evasion, the greater the tension. After a time, personal and professional relationships, as well as business activities, may suffer.

Business owners must pay taxes to federal, state, and local governments. The following are the most common types of taxes.

FEDERAL TAXES

Federal taxes that apply to sole proprietors, partnerships, and S corporations, and their appropriate tax forms, are listed below. For **free** forms and publications, call your district IRS office or write to the government printing office.

- **IRS District Office**
  800-TAX-FORM

- **U.S. Government Printing Office**
  Superintendent of Documents
  Washington, D.C. 20402

Or, particularly brave souls can call the IRS at the 800 number listed in the Government Pages of your telephone directory under "United States Government, IRS Forms."

- **1040** Individual Income Tax Return 1040C *Profit or Loss from Business or Profession*: This form is used to report the revenue, detailed deductible expenses, and resulting net income of your business.

- **1040ES** *Estimated Tax for Individuals*: This form is used to report quarterly best estimates of income tax you will owe for the calendar year, and to calculate amounts to pay quarterly.

- **1040SE** *Computation of Social Security Self-Employment Tax*: Your estimated tax payments will also include payment into your Social Security fund.

- **4562** *Depreciation and Amortization*.

If you have employees, you will also need to submit the following forms:

- **SS-4** With Circular E. This is the *Application for the Employer Identification Number (EIN)*: Circular E, the Employer's Tax Guide, explains the federal income and Social Security withholding requirements.

- **940** *Employer's Annual Federal Unemployment Tax Return*: This form is used to report and pay the Federal Unemployment Compensation Tax.

- **941** *Employer's Quarterly Federal Tax Return*: Use this form to report income tax withheld from employees' pay during the previous calendar quarter and Social Security tax that was withheld and matched by you, the employer.

- **W-2** *Employer's Wage and Tax Statement*: This form is used to report to the IRS and to your employees the taxes withheld and compensation paid to employees.

- **W-3** *Reconciliation/Transmittal of Income and Tax Statements*: This form is used to summarize information from the W-2 and is sent to the Social Security Administration.

- *Index to Tax Publications* (No. 048-004-01596-B)

- *Your Federal Income Tax* (Publication 17)

- *Tax Guide for Small Business* (Publication 334)

- *Starting a Business and Keeping Records* (Publication 583)

- *Business Reporting* (Publication 937)

- *Business Use of Your Car* (Publication 917)

- *Business Use of Your Home* (Publication 587)

- *Employer's Tax Guide* (Circular E)

- *Self-Employment Tax* (Publication 533)

- *Tax Information on Depreciation* (Publication 534)

- *Business expenses* (Publication 535)

- *Retirement Plans for Self-Employed* (Publication 560)

- *Information on Excise Taxes* (Publication 510)

- *Tax Withholding and Estimated Tax* (Publication 510)

- **U.S. General Services Administration**
  Consumer Information Center
  P.O. Box 100
  Pueblo, CO 81002

- *Financial Management: How to Make a Go of Your Business* (Publication 130Y)

- *Starting and Managing a Business from Your Home* (Publication 132Y)

FORM 1099 AND YOUR BUSINESS'S INCOME TAXES

If you work as a noncorporate independent contractor for hospitals, clinics or physicians and are paid more than $600 in commissions, fees or other compensation including payments to outsourcers, you should receive a 1099 form in February or March of each year. Form 1099 is like the W-2 form that employees receive. Copies are sent to the IRS, to the state taxing agency, and to you.

If you are a sole proprietor, you must report your 1099 income on form 1040, Schedule C, *Profit or Loss From Business or Profession*. Your business expenses are also recorded on this form. You should consult a tax adviser and read the book *Smart Tax Write-offs* to make sure you are taking all business expenses you are entitled to. You will also have to attach 1040, Schedule SE — *Computation of Social Security Self-Employment Tax*.

TAX DEPOSITS

Independent contractors must deposit three taxes each quarter:

- federal income tax

- social security self-employment tax

- state income tax

The deposits must be carefully calculated or the IRS and state taxing agency (Franchise Tax Board in California) will assess fines. As a self-employed individual, you will have to pay estimated taxes quarterly.

If in doubt about how much to pay, you should pay at least as much as you paid the previous year, and in most cases the IRS cannot penalize you for underpayment of estimated tax. When your clients pay you, be sure to set aside money for taxes, including self-employment tax (in 1997, 15.3% of the first $65,400 of income and 2.9% of the excess. If you have any questions, it would be wise to talk to a tax consultant or call the IRS.

- **IRS**
  800-829-1040

The three taxes are paid with two forms: the federal 1040 ES (for federal income tax and Social Security self employment tax) and California's 540 ES (for state income tax). Tax deposits are due on April 15, June 15, September 15, and January 15.

```
┌─────────────────────────────────────────────────┐
│                     NOTE                        │
│                                                 │
│  To avoid income tax penalties, you must prepay │
│  90% of the taxes owed for the current year or  │
│  the equivalent of 100% of your tax liability   │
│  of the previous year, or 110% if your previous │
│  year's adjusted gross income exceeded          │
│  $150,000.                                       │
└─────────────────────────────────────────────────┘
```

Independent contractors pay taxes on their net income, which is gross income minus business expenses. An expense must be "reasonable and necessary" for it to be deductible. Exact deductions vary for each type of business and are continually changing. When estimating your business expense deductions it is wise to remember that the expenses must be "reasonable and necessary." Generally, the more you can prove something was used exclusively for your business, the easier it is to prove it is a legitimate deduction.

If you don't use equipment, car, or other items exclusively for business, you should keep records which clearly detail tax-deductible use: specific equipment used, dates of use, time, and purpose.

SOCIAL SECURITY TAXES (FICA)

All self-employed people must file a self-employment form when the annual profit claimed on Schedule C reaches $400. At this point, the self-employed person starts to pay into a personal social security account at a rate specified by the government. In 1997 the rate is 15.3% of the first $65,400 and 2.9% on any amount over $65,400.

Social security benefits are available to the self-employed just as they are to wage earners. Your payment of self-employment tax contributes to your coverage under the social security system, which should eventually provide you with retirement benefits and medical insurance benefits (Medicare). To learn the amount in your account, contact the Bureau of Data Processing.

- **Bureau of Data Processing**
  Social Security Benefits
  Baltimore, MD 21235

Paying this tax can be quite a shock, especially for those of us who worked as employees in the past. When working as an employee, the employee and employer each pay half of the Social Security tax. That advantage is lost, however, when a self-employed medical transcriptionist becomes solely responsible for payment of the entire tax.

The independent does get a break though since half the social security tax may be deducted from the self-employed's gross income.

CHECK YOUR SOCIAL SECURITY RECORD

The Social Security Administration (SSA) has thousands of uncredited earnings reports totaling hundreds of millions of dollars. If three years pass, the statute of limitations may prevent otherwise eligible recipients from correcting a mistake in their earnings records, and their social security benefits may be reduced as a result. Check your earnings record by filing SSA Form 7004 with your local SSA office. This is a free service and one which all independent MTs should take advantage of, especially since we are paying **all** our FICA taxes.

EMPLOYER'S IDENTIFICATION NUMBER (EIN)

Partnerships, corporations, and sole proprietors that have employees are required to have an Employer's Identification Number (EIN). Sole proprietors without employees have the option of using their social security number or obtaining an EIN number.

The purpose of the EIN is to facilitate record keeping by the government. Failure to use the number on the appropriate form can result in a fine of $50 each time it is omitted.

An EIN is obtained by filing IRS Form SS-4, which is available from the IRS.

ESTIMATED TAX PAYMENTS — A HORROR STORY!

Taxes are withheld throughout the year from wages earned by employees. However, as a self-employed individual, you are responsible for making periodic payments of your estimated federal income tax.

A case in point: When one of the authors went into business, she was naive about tax law. At the end of her first year, she dutifully met with an accountant to discuss taxes. She was horrified when he informed her that she owed $14,000 in federal and state taxes on April 15th — all because she had not been making quarterly tax payments.

To avoid such a catastrophe, have your accountant set up a schedule of quarterly tax payments, which are due April 15th, June 15th, September 15th, and January 15th. These will include payment of federal income tax, social security tax or self-employment tax, and state income tax. This procedure will help you avoid a shock to your system and your checkbook when April 15th rolls around.

To avoid penalties in most cases, you must prepay at least 90% of the taxes owed for the current year or the equivalent of 100% of your tax liability of the previous year. You can request estimated tax payment forms from the IRS. As stated above, your accountant will also be able to give you the needed forms and advice, calculating the amount you owe each quarter.

STATE TAXES

Taxes vary from state to state, but most have an income tax. This tax is calculated on net income and is usually due at the same time you file federal tax returns. In some states, the tax is calculated on gross income, less certain qualified deductions.

Some states require employers to carry Workers' Compensation Insurance for all employees. Even though it is called insurance, it feels like a tax. The program can be managed by the state or by the insurance agent who carries your other business insurance. Contact your state administrators to research this issue.

HOW TO EARN $40,000 NET INCOME

Earlier in the book we talked about netting $40,000 per year. As you will recall, we also stated that in order to do so, you would need to **gross** $80,000 for that year. Net income is determined by deducting from gross income the allowable expenses of doing business. Following is a scenario showing estimates of typical business expenses and how they contribute toward "netting $40,000" from an $80,000 gross income.

NET INCOME CALCULATION

Gross income	$80,000
Less expenses	32,660
Taxable business income	47,340
Less self-employment tax	7,240
"Net"	40,100

BUSINESS INCOME TAX DEDUCTIONS

- **Automobile** $ 3,000
  (The greater of 31.5 cents per business mile or the business portion of actual expenses, which includes DMV, maintenance, insurance, gas and oil)
- **Office Supplies:**

Laser printer cartridges	750
Laser toner	260
Printer paper	460
Fax paper	100
File folders	30
Tape cassettes	60
Pens/pencils	50
Pencil sharpener	50
Appointment book	30
Dot matrix printer ribbons	310
Ledger book	50

- **Convention/trade shows**	1,200
- **Courier** ($15 per day)	3,900
- **Gifts to business organizations**	300
- **Dues & fees to professional organizations**	260
- **Education**	150
- **Entertainment of clients**	300

- **Insurance**

Health	1,270
Disability (incorporated businesses only)	1,580
Life insurance (incorporated businesses only)	2,500
Special rider for home business ($50 per month)	600

- **Cleaning person** ($30 per week)	1,560
- **Legal/professional fees**	

Computer consultant	300
CPA	200
Lawyer	500
• **Licenses/permits/fees**	
Business license	100
DBA	100
• **Service contracts**	
Digital systems	85
Transcribers ($250 each)	500
Fax machine	225
• **Mail box rental**	55
• **Outsourcers (Subcontractors)** (overflow)	1,800
• **Postage**	150
• **Print communications**	
Stationery	225
Business cards	50
Fliers	145
Brochures	225
• **Promotional costs**	225
• **Repairs to business equipment**	
Computer	225
Printer	500
• **Safe deposit box**	75
• **Subscriptions/reference material**	500
• **Tax preparation fees**	300
• **Travel for business only**	
Plane	750
Car rental	200
Auto storage	100
Parking	75
Meals	175
Tips	50
Telephone & fax	30
Hotel room	1,050
Laundry	75
• **Rent/lease expenses**	1,900
• **Depreciation (including Sec. 179 expense)**	2,500
• **Interest on business loan**	500

TOTAL EXPENSES   **$32,660**

Remember that these are just your business expenses. In order to determine your personal taxable income, you also need to consider your itemized deductions, personal exemptions, and your personal income from other sources, such as interest income, etc.

HOME-SWEET-TAX-DEDUCTION

As a home-based business owner, you qualify for tax deductions for your home office — either as a portion of your rent or as depreciation. The amount of the allowable deduction is based on the percent of the home used for business purposes. For tax deduction purposes, the home-based office must meet the following criteria:

• Clearly separated from family living space

• Used exclusively for business purposes

• Used on a regular basis for business purposes

• Used as your principal place of business or used as a meeting place for you to interact with clients.

Keep in mind, however, that any business deduction taken for depreciation of your home office reduces the tax basis of your home and normally must be "recaptured" when you sell your home. "Recaptured" means you will pay income taxes at your regular rate instead of at the lower capital gains rate on that portion of your home sale profit represented by your home office depreciation.

There are two ways to calculate the percent of your home used for business purposes:

• One method is to divide the square feet in the home by the number of square feet used for business purposes. Thus, if in a 3000 square foot home, 1000 square feet of space is used for business, 33-1/3% of applicable home expenses can be claimed as a tax deduction.

• The other method for figuring space is to count the number of rooms (if they are nearly equal in size) and divide the number of rooms used for business purposes by the total number of rooms. If one room is used in a five-room house, then 1/5 or 20% of the home expenses are legitimate home-use business deductions.

Either method is acceptable, so use the one that results in the best benefit to you.

A percentage of the expenses listed below can be deducted from income as business expenses:

• Rent

• Mortgage interest

• Insurance premiums on home

• Utilities including gas, electricity, and water

• Services such as trash and snow removal, house cleaning, and yard maintenance expenses

• Home repairs, including labor and supplies

The TOTAL amount of the following expenses are also tax-deductible.

• Decorating, painting, and remodeling costs for the part of the home used solely for business purposes.

• Telephone — all long distance business calls and charges for extra business related services.

WHEN THE HOME OFFICE DEDUCTION IS NOT THE BEST OPTION

According to stringent IRS rulings, any home office that qualifies for the deduction must be a distinct space that is specifically used for business. If you qualify for and take the deduction, when you subsequently sell your home, you may be forced to shell out income tax on the business portion of your gain instead of rolling all the profit into a reduction of the tax basis of your new home.

Here's how the IRS sees it: If a taxpayer claims a deduction for an in-home office, he or she has changed that portion of the property to a commercial tax status. So in the year the taxpayer sells the property, the business portion may not qualify for the much easier rules that allow rollover of the gain from the sale of the residential portion. Depending on your individual tax situation, you may want to plan ahead concerning the sale of your home and make sure it's considered a 100% residential property by claiming no home-office depreciation deductions. You should follow a similar strategy when planning to take the once-in-a-lifetime, post-age-55 exclusion of any capital gains taxes on the sale of your principal residence.

AUTOMOBILE EXPENSES

The legitimate business use of a car can generate significant tax deductions for small-business owners. Commuting is not deductible, but other business travel is: picking up and delivering work, client meetings, trips to the post office, trips to office supply stores, etc.

Keep a mileage log in your car to document business use is still a smart idea. In addition to keeping a log book, keep the first and last repair bills of the year. If the car's mileage has been noted at the time of repair, you can present the bills to the IRS as proof of the numbers of miles you drove through the tax year.

The IRS offers two alternative methods for calculating the amount of automobile expenses:

1) **Standard mileage rate** method provides an umbrella deduction equal to the number of business miles you have driven during the year multiplied by 31.5 cents per mile. The standard mileage rate covers the cost of operating the car, including depreciation, maintenance and repairs, gasoline, oil, insurance and vehicle registration fees. Under this method, those expenditures are not separately deductible, but you can deduct tolls and parking fees in addition to the standard mileage rate calculation.

2) **Actual car expenses** method allows you to deduct the exact costs of each of the above items, as well as tires, garage rental fees, lease payment and even rental car costs. However, you can deduct only the percentage related to the business use of the car. If your records show that you drove 10,000 miles during the year but only 4000 miles were business-related, you can deduct only 40% of actual car expenses.

The IRS lets you choose whichever method will lead to the higher deduction, so it is in your best interest to do both calculations. Remember, if you use a car primarily for business, the actual car expenses method may provide a significantly better deduction.

There are exceptions to the rules, most of which impact the deductibility of your car expenses, including lease payments and depreciation. The first "gotcha" is that if you use the standard mileage rate method the first time you report business use of your car to the Internal Revenue Service, you cannot subsequently depreciate that particular car using the accelerated depreciation method. However, if you calculate your first deduction using the actual expense method, you are allowed to toggle between the two methods in subsequent years.

Under the actual car expenses method, the total amount you can include for depreciation has IRS limitations. These are varying limits based on the year you start using your car for business and on the specific year of the depreciation.

Depreciation deductions apply only to cars you buy outright. If you lease a car, still more rules and exceptions apply. Lease payments are fully deductible if the car is used solely for business. If not, the deductible amount is in proportion to the percentage of miles driven for business. But Section 280F of the IRS code stipulates an add-back, an amount keyed to the value of the car, that you must declare as taxable income. The government's intent is to place a cap on the lease deduction that is equivalent to the ceiling on a depreciation deduction.

It is best to sit down with your accountant while you are shopping for that new car, not after you buy it. The two of you should calculate the tax deductions for both buying and leasing based on the assumed business use percentage including the add-back.

INTEREST ON CAR LOANS

You can deduct interest on the business use portion of a car loan. The nonbusiness use percentage is considered nondeductible interest on a personal loan.

WHO SHOULD LEASE AND WHO SHOULD BUY?

Consider leasing a car if you:

- like having a new car every 2-3 years
- want to drive a more expensive car and still have lower monthly payments
- like having the option of not making a down payment
- like having a car that's always in warranty in case something goes wrong
- hate having to sell or trade your old cars
- don't like tying up your money in depreciating assets

Consider buying a car if you:

- typically drive your cars for several years or until they fall apart
- drive more than 15,000 miles a year on average
- usually sell or trade your cars before they are fully paid for
- drive your cars hard or under rough conditions
- typically buy fad cars that quickly lose their resale value
- like to know you own your car

BUSINESS-RELATED TRAVEL EXPENSES

Whether you travel by air, rail, bus, or personal automobile, expenses associated with travel for business purposes are tax-deductible. Save your ticket stubs, credit card slips and checks to present as evidence of travel expenses.

EDUCATION EXPENSES

An added benefit of joining a professional association is that expenses incurred in attending meetings, including travel expenses, symposium or convention fees, and books can be tax-deductible.

Education expense is deductible if the education improves or maintains a skill required in your business. However, if the education is required to meet minimum education requirements of your present business, or if the education will qualify you for a new trade or business, the expense is not allowed.

Incidentally, any self-employed medical transcriptionist can take a course in bookkeeping, computers or any other course that helps you run your business better and deduct the cost as a business expense.

EXPENSING AND DEPRECIATION

Expensing means taking an income tax deduction for the entire cost of an item in the year it is purchased, up to a current limit of $17,500 per year. *Depreciation* is taking a deduction for business property ratably over its useful life of more than one year — usually at least five years.

Expensing is usually preferable to depreciation because a tax write-off (resulting in cash in your pocket instead of Uncle Sam's pocket) is more valuable earlier than later. However, under certain circumstances, depreciation may be preferable. Remember that the IRS does change depreciation rules periodically, so it might be wise to expense while you can. Again, check with your accountant and refer to IRS Publication 334 for small businesses.

RECORDS NEEDED FOR TAX PURPOSES

Keep all receipts for business expenses and keep all miscellaneous receipts for out-of-pocket purchases, noting what was purchased on the back of the receipt. Use an accordion file for storing all your receipts and checks for the year. This will help tremendously around tax time.

Your business checkbook will also be a valuable resource at tax time to calculate tax-deductible expenditures. The IRS can investigate a return for up to three years after it has been filed, so keep all records for at least three years. In fact, it wouldn't be a bad idea to keep them for seven years or as long as you operate the business.

TAX SHELTERING THROUGH RETIREMENT PLANS

As your business grows and prospers, you should consider tax sheltering as a way to better protect your hard-earned money. A retirement plan tax shelter allows you to reduce taxes by investing a portion of your pretax income in special programs designed to defer payment of tax. Taxes are not avoided but simply postponed until you withdraw money from your fund at a later time, usually in retirement, when presumably you will be in a lower tax bracket.

Popular tax sheltering plans include the Simplified Employee Pension (SEP), Individual Retirement Account (IRA), and Qualified Profit Sharing Plans (Defined Benefit or Defined Contribution).

SIMPLIFIED EMPLOYEE PENSION (SEP)

A Simplified Employee Pension (SEP) is a retirement program whereby an employer makes contributions into employees' IRA accounts. For your one-person business, the pretax contribution is into your IRA. The SEP plan allows a higher contribution than an individual IRA and can be made to owner/employees over 70½ years old. The maximum contribution to a SEP is the lesser of 15% of employee compensation or $22,500. For the owner of a sole proprietorship the maximum contribution is limited to 13.043% of net Schedule C income less one half of self-employment tax percent.

SEPs are attractive for the following reasons:

- They are simple and easy to establish

- They can be established after the close of your business year and after April 15th

- They don't require IRS filing or Form 5500 reporting (which are required in profit sharing plans)

- There are no administration costs

- Contributions are tax deductible and elective (they do not have to be made every year)

- Contribution amount may vary from year to year, from zero to 15%

INDIVIDUAL RETIREMENT ACCOUNT (IRA)

The Individual Retirement Account (IRA) provides an opportunity to establish a personal retirement program using pretax dollars. There are two conditions that must be met to qualify for this plan: 1) You must not participate in any other type of retirement plan (other than social security), and 2) your adjusted gross income must be less than $40,000 in order to have full deductibility.

If you meet the above criteria, the amount saved and earnings generated by an IRA are not currently taxable. The tax-free status continues until you retire. Even if you do not meet the above qualifications, you can put money into an IRA although the money deposited is not fully tax-deductible. However, the income earned on the account's investment is not taxed until withdrawal. The maximum amount you can contribute yearly to an IRA is presently $2000.

Although the IRA is not taxed until payments are received, after age 59½, IRA funds may be withdrawn without a 10% penalty should you become disabled. In the event of your death, the funds are paid to your beneficiary. As of 1997, you can also withdraw IRA funds without penalty in order to pay some medical expenses.

IRA plans are available through banks and savings and loans (certificates of deposit), money market and mutual funds, stockbroker-managed or self-directed IRA accounts, insurance companies annuity plans, and United States minted gold.

HEALTH INSURANCE

If you are a sole proprietor, partner in a partnership, or owner of an S corporation, you are allowed an income tax deduction of 50% of the cost of health insurance in 1997 and 45% for the years 1998 through 2002. According to *Smart Tax Write-offs*, Rayve Productions, there is a way to make your personal health insurance premium 100% deductible. Your business can enroll your employee-spouse as an insured employee in your business's health insurance plan. The insurance premium for this employee is fully deductible, and you can then be covered in the plan as his or her spouse.

SHOULD YOU HIRE AN ACCOUNTANT, BOOKKEEPER OR TAX PREPARER?

Most of us have had experience balancing our own checkbooks and know some basic bookkeeping principles. However, business bookkeeping is much more detailed, and savvy professionals seek the best possible counsel affordable when establishing an accounting system.

We recommend working with an accountant and/or a tax adviser. A knowledgeable bookkeeper may also be capable of setting up a basic system.

An accountant should be consulted a minimum of once or twice a year to analyze the books, prepare and analyze financial statements, and help with tax returns. The accountant can also advise you on financial decisions and help to chart the future course of your business based on an analysis of your financial records.

It is unfortunate, but true, that many businesses fail because of inadequate financial planning and visibility. It is crucial to set up and maintain a system that will be comfortable for you to maintain and use as a tool for running your business smartly.

Do your homework. Review a book such as *Easy Financials for Your Home-based Business* in order to get a basic understanding of your available choices. Then confer with a knowledgeable professional to help you set up your system. It is well worth your investment in time and money to set up a system that will give you the visibility to manage your business successfully. And these professional expenses are tax-deductible.

Beware of hiring a tax preparer instead of an accountant. This could cost you considerable money in the long run. Tax preparers may only be capable of working with the numbers you provide them and may not have the experience to pursue available tax breaks aggressively.

On other hand, an accountant who is knowledgeable about your type of business will be aware of tax advantages, suggesting desirable business actions. It is likely that the accountant will save you more money than his or her fees.

How do you select an accountant or a bookkeeper? Ask professional associates for recommendations. Carefully evaluate training, experience and references.

It is important to find an accountant or bookkeeper who has experience working with small businesses. To prevent any unpleasant surprises, be sure to discuss fees in advance with the bookkeeping or accounting service.

Why Businesses Fail

*"When all is said and done,
there's much more said than done."*

—Anonymous

Businesses fail for a variety of reasons, most of which are not extraordinary. If you plan your business carefully, learn from the wisdom (and mistakes) of others, and consistently and regularly manage well, your chances of business success are greatly increased. From time to time, you should evaluate your business, and if you find weak areas, correct them immediately. Following are basic weaknesses usually found in troubled businesses.

LACK OF PLANNING

Poor planning, or no planning at all, results in hit-or-miss control of your business. Work out a plan of operation, develop measurable goals and objectives, and monitor your progress.

INEXPERIENCE

Managing yourself as an independent requires skill and knowledge. You must devote time to studying good business practices, consult experts frequently for advice and guidance, and follow through with continuing education. This is how professionals succeed.

INSUFFICIENT FINANCIAL RECORDS

Without complete daily figures showing the financial condition of your business, you are working in the dark. With proper financial records you can spot excessive costs, waste, and other drains on your profits. Keep figures current — old figures are worthless. Watch for trends and manage your business accordingly.

INADEQUATE CASH RESERVES

Put money aside regularly into a savings account, even if only a small amount. A cash reserve will provide needed working capital, act as a hedge against unexpected income declines or unexpected emergencies, and enhance your credit rating.

EXCESSIVE OVERHEAD

The steady trend toward higher costs and prices makes control of overhead doubly important. Budget your operating expenses. Carelessness, waste, errors, and general inefficiency may account for 10-20% of your overhead.

OVEREXPANSION

Enthusiasm is a vital ingredient in the growth and progress of a business, but slow, steady growth is safer than rapid, uncontrolled growth. Try not to take on more than you can handle.

COMPLACENCY

Do not allow yourself to become too content with the status quo. To maintain a competitive edge, always look for ways to improve your service and efficiency and reduce overhead costs.

IGNORING COMPETITION

Some of your competitors are more successful than you; others are not. Study their methods and operations and make a conscious decision to avoid known pitfalls while moving forward with successful endeavors. Become a leader, not a follower, and try to understand that there is strength in competition!

POOR SALESMANSHIP, POOR SERVICE

Be aware of new technology and focus on continuing education to provide optimum service. Know how to effectively present yourself and your product, and consistently provide excellent service and follow-up.

What's Ahead?

"Champions keep playing until they get it right."
— Billie Jean King

Throughout this text we have discussed how technology and the new home-based workplace have changed the way we do business. Working from home has been and is still the hot topic of the '90s. Medical transcription is a billion dollar industry that continues to evolve. Telecommunication has had the most influential impact on home-based business success by providing opportunities for service to long-distance clients. Through telecommunication, clients benefit from reduced turnaround time, and medical transcriptionists enjoy increased productivity and more flexible working conditions. It's a winning situation for all.

In recent years there has been a dramatic upswing in the number of people setting up home businesses. This figure had reached just over 12 million in 1992, and two million more than 1989 according to Link Resources. Just under half of those riding the wave are women. The idea of working from home is becoming much more widely accepted now and today 39 million people do at least some of their work from home.

Financial services, computer-related services and consulting services now account for close to 30% of the home-based business market. From 1988 to the present, the self-employed figure for full-time and part-time home workers grew by around 10 percent annually. These home-based businesses are now recognized as serious contenders in the business world. More than 70% of home-based operations are service businesses, according to *BIS Strategic Decisions*.

In a survey of 836 U.S. companies, 46% said they had reduced their work force during the previous year, and many of those companies now outsource work that was once done in-house.

The futurists' previous predictions of incisionless surgery, sketch pads, optical scanners, and voice recognition are now realities.

We predict that at least 50% of the medical transcription industry will be serviced from the home-based office within the next five years. The technology is at our fingertips and the resources are unlimited.

Within the next two decades the number of acute care hospitals, both rural and urban, will be reduced by at least 20%. Hospitals, particularly smaller ones under 200 beds, will increasingly outsource ancillary departments and specialty care units, including their more costly high-tech equipment, to outside contractors in an effort to reduce fixed operating expenses in favor of a more "variable cost management philosophy."

Physicians will continue to consolidate their practices and hospital corporations will form alliances with one another. Hospitals that remain in existence beyond the year 2010 will be run without the current departmentalized system, with less management and more technology. The future will favor managers who can manage resources, particularly human resources.

In the hopes of automating and expediting delivery of transcribed medical documents, some vendors are developing highly automated types of transcription document distribution processes called Automated Document Distribution (ADD). By improving quick document access, patient care will ultimately be augmented by a reduction in the information flow and the time required from the actual moment of dictation until receipt of the document. Transcriptionists will be spending more time typing and less time setting up document shells.

It is up to each of us to determine for ourselves which of the many future employment opportunities we will follow in the years ahead. The era of dedicated word processing systems has come to an end, for these systems can no longer meet the needs of the changing and ever-evolving health care environment.

Within this evolution the health language specialist must stay on the cutting edge of information and technology. Periodically take time to re-evaluate your skills, reposition your career and change your thinking. It is the knowledge of medical language that sets the medical transcriptionist apart from all other health care professionals — that undeniable quality that can turn a health provider's thoughts into clear, concise, legible medical language — and it will be this knowledge, in conjunction with excellent transcription skills, that continues to set us apart in the years to come.

By focusing on the cornerstone of knowledge, we have positioned ourselves to quickly adapt to the dizzying array of new technologies that are either here or in development, including speech recognition, PC technology, digital dictation, guiding-prompting systems, software, and other systems. These systems will only be successful if the medical language they provide is at a very high standard. That standard can only be reached under the judgment and careful eye of the medical language expert.

Will Technology Replace Medical Transcriptionists?

"Destiny is not a matter of chance,
it is a matter of choice;
it is not a thing to be waited for,
it is a thing to be achieved."

—William Jennings Bryan

It is highly unlikely, even with advanced technology and sophisticated software, that medical transcriptionists will become obsolete. The complexity and variety of patients, medical conditions, and physicians will continue to require the human element — especially intelligent, well-trained medical transcriptionists — in medical record quality management.

No two patients are exactly the same. "Routine" procedures and "standard" treatment plans are diverse. Physicians will continue to dictate with accents, rapidity, mumbles, missing and incorrect words, inappropriate comments, sneezes and coughs.

Human intelligence and logical thinking will be necessary to transcribe correct medical terms when dictation isn't clear — "Metatarsal" or "metacarpal?" "Atherosclerosis" or "arteriosclerosis?" Medical transcriptionists have the skills to do this.

Medical technology and treatment will continue to grow rapidly more complex, requiring flexibility and continual updating of information. Computer systems alone will not be able to meet the medical record requirements of the future.

The refinement of voice-activated technology is on the horizon, and the role of the medical transcriptionist will undoubtedly change with the advent of more sophisticated technology. As medical language specialists, transcriptionists will be a vital link in editorial and quality assurance activities, developing or assisting with development of hardware and software, and taking on new career challenges as opportunities arise.

CHALLENGES, CHOICES AND CHANGE

As medical transcriptionists we are a profession of high achievers, obsessive and compulsive about our work. At times we overcommit and can't say "no" and knock ourselves out to be the best that we can be. We are justifiably proud of the service we provide. We like to control our work environment, but our environment is changing. Like many others before it, the medical transcription industry is going global; it is, in fact, now a reality.

Transcription services are sending transcription overseas to countries such as India and the West Indies. The concern, of course, is loss of jobs in the U.S. This is a burning issue. It is creating a division in the medical transcription industry between those who feel threatened and are resisting change and those who realize that changes represent additional resources and opportunities to fill needs on a global scale.

The trend toward globalization of medical transcription, which many are not prepared to face, has created an atmosphere of anger and insecurity in our industry. Each of us wants to have control of his or her destiny. That is why we choose to remain independent. However, sticking our heads in the sand will not make inevitable industry changes disappear. Instead, when we pull our heads out of the sand, we'll discover even greater changes and, because we will have fallen so far behind, we will be lost.

Why are services seeking offshore transcriptionists? Because there have never been enough "qualified" hospital-level medical transcriptionists to fill the need. There are plenty of entry-level transcriptionists and qualified clinical transcriptionists, but training entry-level and hospital-level MTs has always been a problem. Transcription programs and schools can pump out graduates in 12-week to two-year programs, but even after completing a two-year program, MTs have great difficulty finding a hospital that will offer them entry-level positions. Acute-care facilities, which are usually already backlogged and do not have staff available to train new recruits, want "experienced" MTs. It is a catch-22 situation. Unfortunately, as multitudes of health care facilities continue to restructure and downsize, training programs for MTs are simply not viable options within those settings.

Twenty years ago there was no medical transcription industry as we know it today. It was a profession striving to be recognized. There were true pioneers like Bob Seale and Sally Pittman, one who built a transcription service empire and the other with a vision of a professional medical transcription organization that would offer membership and certification and be dedicated to promoting our profession through creativity, resourcefulness and innovation.

Visionaries like Bob Seale and Sally Pittman never promised that the world of medical transcription would remain the same forever; they realized that change is an inevitable fact of life. Their innovations grew and expanded, and there were more that followed. The "profession" became a business and evolved into a multibillion dollar industry in which there have been divisions, reorganizations, mergers and affiliations.

The medical transcription industry playing field is very different today than it was 20 years ago, especially for the independent medical transcriptionist. Twenty years ago there was no such thing as an IMT. We were hidden in the closet, a virtually silent work force, like wine tasting in the Napa Valley used to be. Now it is the rage. We have arrived! Thousands are striving to homebase. This is no cottage industry. It is a revolution into independence. But each day holds a challenge, and there are many changes yet to come. The biggest challenge is to remain competitive in today's marketplace.

POSITIONING YOUR BUSINESS IN THE GLOBAL MARKETPLACE

How do we position ourselves to compete successfully in the global marketplace? We continue to work on our image and our service. Ask yourself these questions:

• What is so special about the service I provide my clients?

375

- What professional image do I reflect? A business image is every bit as critical to your success as your skills.

- What is my strategic plan for providing the best service to my clients?

- What makes my service stand apart from my competitors?

Have you evaluated your business services recently? You should do this at least biannually. Remember, nothing lasts forever! Clients who are here today may be gone tomorrow. What is your strategic plan when you lose a client? How will you market your services to potential clients? Building and operating your business is an ongoing process, just as your processes for improvement should be ongoing. Your goal is to be the best that you can be. Your objectives should include vision, commitment and persistence. Be proactive in your plans for improving your business and your own professional development. Have some processes in place in the event of possible loss of a client/revenue. Constantly seek out and research new industry trends that may affect the way in which you do your work. Have access to technical support in the event of unexpected equipment failure. Keep your technology up-to-date so that your business will remain competitive.

Take responsibility as an independent business owner. Be accountable, consistent, reliable and qualified in the work you are committing to. Follow through with this image in your physical appearance, the physical appearance of your office and how you present yourself to your clients. Your answering machine message should project professionalism, as should your stationery and business cards. Your voice should always be positive and professional.

Be consistent in your project follow-through. When business is slow keep up a positive appearance, even when you're feeling low. Use your downtime to do quality audits of your work and pay attention to details. This can be done by reviewing a number of reports selected randomly within a selected time frame (e.g., 15 days, 30 days). Review the documents and point score errors for punctuation (.25), grammar (.75), dropped letters (.50) typos (1), wrong words (1), etc. Grade yourself. Keep audit logs and quality/productivity reports at designated times during each quarter cycle. Review what can be improved upon. You may find from these self-audits that you can benefit from improving your technical skills and knowledge base. Catch up on reading about industry trends, and attend trade shows and workshops. The more exposure you get the more informed you will become.

Be smart about your business investments. Cost containment is important. Avoid investing in equipment and technology that is just a "fad." Research the market. Don't run out and buy the latest and the greatest just so you can brag about it on the Internet or keep up with the Jones'. Carefully evaluate your options, network with others to what is working for them. It's okay to step back for a time and see which way the tree is going to fall. Products are not always what they are touted to be. The true test is in the hands of the user. Your safest bet is to go with a product that has been established in the marketplace and will suit the needs of your clients. Research technical support and make sure you have a backup for downtime that might occur with equipment failure.

As far as the services you provide your client, the trend is toward service, service, service. Tailor your services to suit your client's needs, not yours. This is an area where you can truly stand out from competing businesses by offering your client the best of the best.

Marketing is still a serious issue for many independent medical transcriptionists. There are those who have only targeted local resources, which is okay, but this could change suddenly. With a change over of office staff, a new office manager, new medical director, or often the chief financial officer, who may make the decision not to use your services and/or to go with a larger service whose bid is lower than what your are charging. Suddenly, with scarcely any notice, you could find yourself without a client. It is never wise to put all of your eggs in one basket. This cannot be emphasized enough.

To remain competitive, you should continually improve your knowledge base, flexibility and diversity. Continuing education is key. You will also benefit by mastering the ability to be flexible and adapt when necessary to changes in the work schedule. Peaks and valleys occur often. Have a backup plan in place. The more diverse your talents as an MT, the more valuable you will be. You should continue to build on your transcription base whenever possible.

If you fear being without a job because transcription work is going offshore, then quit whining and do something about it. Most of those jobs are hospital-level transcription positions. The good old U.S. of A. isn't the only country where there are highly educated and qualified people, and in some countries they are better educated! You still have the choice to be the best that you can be. In our 25-plus years as MTs, we have never ever been without work. More often than not, there is more work than there are qualified MTs. Are you threatened because you are underqualified? Or are you threatened because you do not see the "big picture" and are lacking full awareness of what is going on within the medical transcription industry. You have choices. Do something about it. Think about improving your knowledge base, take that anatomy/physiology course, English grammar course, and advanced terminology course. Attempt to attain a higher level of expertise not only in medical transcription but about technology, because the most technically savvy will merit higher pay. Learning everything you can about telecommuting will improve your position in the market. There are educational opportunities through local, state, regional and national programs. Organizational membership is not required for attendance. If you have no telecommuting experience, network with other telecommuting MTs. This is an area you must pursue. Telecommuting is no longer the future … it is the NOW. Limiting yourself to your little comfort zone may lead to your demise in the current global industry environment.

We still have choices. The future holds many opportunities. Even though medical transcription is just one piece in the very complex health care puzzle, it is a very important piece.

There are many avenues that we independent medical transcriptionists can pursue to expand our horizons and offer greater diversity of services to our clients. Coding and billing services are very viable options, and there are now services and courses that provide training for transcriptionists who wish to pursue these paths.

There are exciting and challenging years ahead. As medical transcriptionists, we need to make wise and healthy choices in our professional and personal lives. We are in an excellent position to thrive and excel as we move into the 21st century. We chose this profession, along with its pleasures and perils. If we are to be players, we must walk the walk and talk the talk. We should embrace change because change is progress. Someone once said, "If you can't change it, change the way you think about it."

Summary

*"Do not delay; Do not delay;
  the golden moments fly!"*
—Henry Wadsworth Longfellow

Lao Tzu is quoted as saying, "The journey of a thousand miles begins with a single step." If after reading this book you find yourself intrigued with the idea of self-employment but are apprehensive about taking the steps necessary to become a home-based medical transcriptionist, take that first experimental step anyway.

Go to a local print shop or desktop publisher and have business cards made. Action always boosts self-esteem; so take action.

You can succeed in anything you attempt by formulating some healthy lifestyle patterns for yourself. Be gentle with yourself and don't be afraid to make mistakes. We have all made them and have learned and grown from each experience.

Don't let fear stand in your way. The key to overcoming fear is knowing our enemy (usually oneself). Take risks, minor ones at the start, and graduate to larger ones. Eat a balanced diet, get enough sleep, exercise regularly, and see how much better you feel about yourself and your environment. Meet each negative situation with a positive response and you will surely become a winner.

Reward yourself at the end of a long day of transcription. Be your own best friend and the type of boss you always wished you had. Take pride in your finished product and be the best you can be.

Our hope is that by reading this book, you will avoid many of the stumbling blocks and pitfalls we have encountered on our journey toward professional freedom.

Problem Solving — Questions and Answers

The following questions are frequently asked at workshops we present. Each subject is covered in more detail elsewhere in this book. Check the index for specific pages.

Q: How do you become a CMT?

A: Call AAMT 800-982-2182. They will send you information regarding certification through the American Association for Medical Transcription.

Q: Can you send brochures/advertising to all doctors without stepping on toes of fellow transcriptionists?

A: Yes, you can. You have the right to make a living just like everyone else. If another transcriptionist is worried, maybe she has reason to be. If clients are happy with the service you provide, they will not shop around.

Q: What turnaround time constitutes "STAT" in regard to charging extra for this type of service?

A: The word "Stat" means different things to different clients. One may consider 24-hours "Stat," another, immediately, and another, 12-hours. The term "Stat" must be clarified with your client. If you are going to charge an additional fee for "Stat" work, you should inform the client of your fee schedule for different types of turnaround.

Q: If you are working in your home as an employee for a service, do you need a business license?

A: No. You are an employee, not a business.

Q: What is the best source for learning about word processing/computer equipment?

A: Others in the field, trade shows, conventions, product suppliers, computer publications, online bulletin boards and networking.

Q: How do you find out the standard rates in your area?

A: Network with others in the field. Approach the subject by asking what is the range (low-high). Do not ask someone directly what they charge as this approach sometimes offends and may put the individual you ask on the defensive.

Q: When working for a service as an independent contractor, how are you paid?

A: The service generally accepts your fee at a rate that is determined by your level of technical expertise. If you are very diversified, you can demand a high rate of pay. If you are limited in your specialties, expect to be paid less for your services.

Q: When working from home, what is the proper disposal method for rough drafts to ensure confidentiality? In other words, can I throw them in the recycling bin?

A: Dispose of drafts by shredding or burning them. **DO NOT** throw them in the recycling bin.

Q: What is the current standard for billing on character count?

A: At the current time, there is no set standard. You will have to network and find out what the standard is in the area you work in. Currently, several industry groups are attempting to standardize character count measurements, but the groups have not yet been able to agree on a standard. Your standard will be what you negotiate with your clients.

Q: How much does the FDA bulletin board cost?

A: The FDA bulletin board is free. You need a computer and modem. Modem settings: Baud 1200, E, 7, 1, N. For more information, call 800-222-0185.

Q: How do I handle a client who requests daily pickup and delivery, yet many times has no work or only one letter on a tape?

A: Perhaps you can renegotiate your agreement/contract with the client and include a clause for a minimum dollar amount for pickup and delivery. Since they insist on daily service, a minimum of $25 would at least compensate you for your time and overhead. The client could go for it, or reconsider whether daily pickup and delivery is really necessary and/or cost-effective.

Q: I was told "no compete clauses" are definitely unenforceable and that it is illegal to deprive anyone the right to do business. Please comment.

A: We would not use the word "definitely." It depends upon the facts and circumstances of the situation. Always remember that you are the negotiator when it comes to the contract. You cannot deprive one of the right to make a living, but if you sign that contract, you are agreeing to what is in it. If it is a reasonable restraint — encompassing a reasonable period of time — it could hold up. **Always** seek legal advice before signing an agreement with this type clause. We have been encouraged by our legal adviser not to sign a contract with a no compete clause. Check with your attorney.

Q: How do you arrange for vacations?

A: This depends on the terms and agreements you maintain with your clients. If they expect coverage from your service whether or not you are the one doing the work, you will have to arrange backup transcriptionists to cover for you. If this is the case, make sure they have the appropriate credentials to be operating a business, and if your backups are your employees, they should also have sufficient skills to manage the client's work. If your client does not expect coverage, they may hold the work until you return (if it's a short vacation). It will take serious planning to arrange vacation plans if you are running a full-time business. For many independents, vacations are few and far between.

Q: What do you do if payments aren't made on time?

A: Assuming that you have set your terms for payment in an agreement with your client, you will have to follow up. Call the accounts payable department and ask if your invoice has been processed. Remember to always include an invoice number at the top of your statement. This expedites processing and tracking for the client, as well as the vendor (you). If your statement has not been processed, kindly ask when it will be. Go from there. You may have to remind them of your payment agreement and make sure that you both had the same understanding of the terms.

Q: How many hours do you work to do 10,000 lines per week?
A: On an average eight-hour day, 2,000 lines per day x 5 days per week.

Q: In what way is a contract binding? If they don't want you anymore, they will simply have no work for you.

A: A contract basically states **how** the work is done. Specify in a contract the volume of work you will be receiving (minimum/maximum), and perhaps a termination or renegotiation date.

Q: Where can I obtain more information about working for outside services? Do they deliver tapes to you? Is there extra cost? Do they pay to deliver and pick up transcription?

A: Check the local yellow pages, also local trade publications. Network with other transcriptionists. Call the service directly and ask them questions. Every service is different and may not provide the same benefit package, etc. If you are considering working for a service, you are looking for employment. Interview them to see if this is the type service you want to work for. If they are a reputable company, the service will interview you and request a resume of your qualifications.

Q: How are you paid when telecommuting? Do you invoice telecommuting clients the same way you invoice clients where you pick up and deliver tapes?

A: Telecommuting offers many advantages in terms of turnaround schedules, confidentiality, and reimbursement. Turnaround is virtually instantaneous. There are no delays with pick up, deliveries and arranging courier schedules. There are fewer people handling documents, which assures confidentiality. Some offices are virtually paperless, and all records are sent via modem. No paper is printed in the transcription office; it is printed out in the client's office. The client can be invoiced via modem or fax, which guarantees delivery to long-distance clients.

Q: I recently heard that the SBA has done a home-based business study. Do you know the results of their findings?

A: The study commissioned by the SBA was titled *Myths and Realities of Working at Home: Characteristics of Homebased Business Owners and Telecommuters.* The research was conducted by Joanne H. Pratt Associates.

The findings of the study included:

- Homebased businesses have a greater net worth than non-homebased businesses.

- There is little difference between the hours working in a homebased business versus a non-homebased business.

- Telecommuters tend to have more positive attitudes towards their jobs than non-telecommuters. They like the kind of work they do, they do not feel isolated from their peers, and they enjoy considerable job stability.

Pratt predicts that home-based businesses will increase in the future. "Because of technology, home-based businesses can contract for what megacorporations, in the process of downsizing, no longer do themselves."

Resources

ASSOCIATIONS, ORGANIZATIONS, NETWORKS

- **American Association of Home-based Businesses**
  P. O. Box 10023
  Rockville, MD 20849
  Voicemail: 202-310-3130

- **American Association for Medical Transcription**
  P.O. Box 576187
  Modesto, CA 95357-6187
  209-551-0883
  Fax: 209-551-9317
  E-mail: aamt@sna.com

- **American Federation of Small Business**
  150 West 20th Avenue
  San Mateo, CA 94403
  415-341-7441

- **American Health Information Management Association**
  (formerly) American Medical Record Association
  919 North Michigan Avenue
  Chicago, Illinois 60611-1683

- **American Home Business Association**
  397 Post Road
  Darien, CT 06820

- **American Medical Writers Association**
  9650 Rockville Pike
  Bethesda, MD 20814
  Phone: 301-493-0003

- **American Woman's Economic Development Corporation**
  60 East 42nd Street
  New York, NY 10165
  212-692-9100

- **Association for Women in Computing, Inc.**
  407 Hillmoor Drive
  Silver Springs, MD 20901

- **Association of Enterprising Mothers**
  914 S. Santa Fe Avenue, Suite 297
  Vista, CA 92084
  619-434-9225

- **Center for Entrepreneurial Management**
  83 Spring Street
  New York, NY 10012
  212-925-7304

- **Council of Smaller Enterprises**
  690 Union Commerce Building
  Cleveland, OH 44115
  216-621-3300

- **The Encyclopedia of Associations**
  Fifteenth edition
  Gale Research Company, 1981

- **Feminist Computer Technology (FCTP)**
  Erin Computer Systems, Inc.
  4412 Jutland Drive
  San Diego, CA 92117

- **Homebased Businesswoman's Network**
  5 Cedar Hill Road
  Salem, MA 01970

- **Home-Workers on the Move to Economic Success**
  (H.O.M.E.S. Guild)
  31255 Cedar Valley Drive
  Westlake Village, CA 91362
  818-707-0008

- **International Information/Word Processing Association**
  1015 North York Road
  Willow Grove, PA 19090
  215-657-6300

- **Keyboard Connection**
  P. O. Box 338, Dept 12
  Glen Carbon, Il 62034

- **Medical Transcription Industry Alliance (MTIA)**
  1-800-543-MTIA
  E-mail: kcameron@ainet.com

- **Medical Transcription Student Network**
  Health Professions Institute
  P. O. Box 801
  Modesto, CA 95353-0801
  209-551-2112
  Fax: 209-551-0404

- **Mother's Home Business Network**
  (A national organization dedicated to helping mothers work at home).
  P. O. Box 423
  East Meadow, NY 11554

- **National Alliance of Home Based Business Women**
  P. O. Box 95
  Norwood, NJ 07648

- **National Association for Public Continuing and Adult Education**
  1201 16th Street, NW
  Washington, D.C. 20036
  202-833-5486

- **The Association of Business Support Services International, Inc. (ABSSI)**
  (Formerly National Association for Secretarial Services—NASS)
  714-282-9398; toll-free 800-237-1462

- **National Association for the Cottage Industry**
  P. O. Box 14460
  Chicago, Illinois 60614
  312-472-8116

- **National Association for the Self-Employed**
  P. O. Box 345749
  Dallas, TX 75234
  800-255-9226 (in Texas 800-442-4733)

- **National Association for the Self-Employed**
  2316 Gravel Road
  Fort Worth, TX 76118

- **National Association of Home-based Businesses**
  1045 Mill Run Circle, Suite 400
  Owings Mill, MD 21117
  410-363-3698

- **National Association of Professional Consultants**
  20121 Ventura Blvd., Suite 227
  Woodland Hills, CA 91364
  213-703-6028

- **National Association of Women Business Owners (NAWBO)**
  200 P Street, NW
  Washington, D.C. 20036
  202-338-8966
      or
  1100 Wayne Avenue, Suite 830
  Silver Spring, MD 20910
  301-608-2590
  Fax 301-608-2596

- **National Business League**
  4324 Georgia Avenue, NW
  Washington, D.C. 20005
  202-638-3411

- **National Computer Security Association**
  10 S. Courthouse Avenue
  Carlisle, PA 17013
  717-258-1816
  FAX 717-243-8642

- **National Federation of Independent Business**
  150 West 20th Avenue
  San Mateo, CA 94403
  415-341-7441

- **National Small Business Association**
  1604 K Street, NW
  Washington, D.C. 20006
  202-296-7400

- **New Families Work Options Network**
  P. O. Box 41108
  Fayetteville, NC 28309

- **Rural Women Cottage Industries**
  505 Linder Street
  Friday Harbor, WA 98250

- **Small Business Administration (SBA)**
  800-827-5722

- **Small Business Administration (SBA) Office of Women's Business Ownership**
  202-205-6673

- **Small Business Development Centers (SBDC)**
  (Every state has one or more SBDC branches.
  Check the telephone directory for your closest SBDC office)

- **Small Business Foundation of America**
  69 Hickory Drive
  Waltham, MA 02154

- **Women in Information Processing, Inc.**
  1000 Connecticut Ave., NW
  Washington, D.C. 20036

UNITED STATES CHAMBERS OF COMMERCE
(Courtesy of World Chamber of Commerce Directory, 970-663-3231)

- **ALABAMA** (Business Council of Ala.)
  William F. O'Connor, Jr., President
  2N. Jackson; P.O. Box 76
  Montgomery, 36101-0076
  334-834-6000; fax 334-262-7371

- **ALASKA** (Alaska State C of C)
  Pamela La Bolle, President
  217 2nd St., #201
  Juneau, 99801-1267
  907-586-2323; fax 907-463-5515
  asccjuno@ptialaska.net

- **ARIZONA** (Arizona C of C)
  Dave O'Neal, Pres./CEO,
  Public Policy & Legislative Issues Only
  1221 E. Osborn Rd., #100
  Phoenix, 85014-5539
  602-248-9172; fax 602-265-1262
  azchamb@primenet.com;
  www.azchamber.com

- **ARKANSAS** (Arkansas C of C)
  Ron Russell, Executive Vice President
  410 S. Cross; P.O. Box 3645
  Little Rock, 72203-3645
  501-374-9225; fax 501-372-2722
  rrussell@ascc-aia.org;
  www.aiea.ualr.edu/dina/statcham/

- **CALIFORNIA** (California State C of C)
  Kirk West, President
  1201 K St., 12th Floor; P.O. Box 1736
  Sacramento, 95812-1736
  916-444-6670; fax 916-444-6685

- **COLORADO** (Col. Assn. of Comm. & Ind.)
  George S. Dibble, Jr., Pres./CEO
  1776 Lincoln St., #1200
  Denver, 80203-1029
  303-831-7411; fax 303-860-1439
  caci@coloradobusiness.com;
  www.coloradobusiness.com

- **CONNECTICUT** (Conn.Bus. & Ind. Assn.)
  Kenneth O. Decko, President
  370 Asylum St.
  Hartford, 06103-2022
  860-244-1900; fax 860-278-8562
  www.cbia.com

- **DELAWARE** (Delaware State C of C)
  John M. Burris, President
  1201 N. Orange St., #200; P.O. Box 671
  Wilmington, 19899-0671
  302-655-7221; fax 302-654-0691

- **DISTRICT OF COLOMBIA**
  (Dist. of Columbia C of C)
  Kwasi Holman, Exec. V.P.
  1301 Pennsylvania Ave. N.W., #309
  Washington, 20004
  202-347-7201; fax 202-347-3537

- **FLORIDA** (Florida C of C)
  Frank M. Ryll, Jr., President
  136 S. Bronough St.; P.O. Box 11309
  Tallahassee, 32302-3309
  904-425-1200; fax 904-425-1260
  fccpolicy@supernet.net;
  www.flchamb.com

- **GEORGIA** (Georgia C of C)
  233 Peachtree St., #200
  Atlanta, 30303-1504
  404-223-2264; fax 404-223-2290

- **GUAM** (Guam C of C)
  Eloise R. Baza, President
  173 Aspinall Ave., #101; P.O. Box 283
  Agana, 96932
  011-671-472-6311; 671-472-8011;
  fax 011-671-472-6202
  gchamber@hasa.net.gu;
  www.gchamber.com.gu

- **HAWAII** (C of C of Hawaii)
  James H. Proctor, Jr., President
  1132 Bishop St., #200
  Honolulu, 96813-2830
  808-545-4300; fax 808-545-4309

- **IDAHO** (No State Chapter)

- **ILLINOIS** (Illinois State C of C)
  Sally A. Jackson, Pres./CEO
  311 S. Wacker Dr., #1500
  Chicago, 60606-6619
  312-983-7100; fax 312-983-7101

- **INDIANA** (Indiana C of C)
  Christopher Lamother, Pres./CEO
  115 W. Washington St., #850S
  Indianapolis, 46204-3407
  317-264-3110; fax 317-264-6855

- **IOWA** (Iowa Dept. of Eco. Dev.)
  David Lyons, Director
  200 E. Grand
  Des Moines, 50309
  515-242-4700; fax 515-242-4749

- **KANSAS** (Kansas C of C & Ind.)
  Ed Bruske, Pres./CEO
  835 S.W. Topeka Blvd.
  Topeka, 66612-1671
  913-357-6321; fax 913-357-4732

- **KENTUCKY** (Kentucky C of C)
  Ken Oilschlager, President
  464 Chenault Rd.; P.O. Box 817
  Frankfort, 40602-0817
  502-695-4700; fax 502-695-6824

- **LOUISIANA** (Louisiana Assn. of
  Business & Industry)
  Daniel Juneau, President
  3113 Valley Creek Dr., P.O. Box 80258
  Baton Rouge, 70898-0258
  504-928-5388; fax 504-929-6054

- **MAINE** (Maine C of C & Business
  Alliance)
  Dana F. Connors, President
  7 Community Drive
  Augusta, 04330-9412
  207-623-4568; fax 207-622-7723
  staff@mainechamber.org;
  www.mainechamber.org

- **MARYLAND** (Maryland C of C)
  Champe C. McCulloch, President
  60 West St., #100
  Annapolis, 21401-2458
  410-269-0642; 301-261-2858; fax 410-269-5247

- **MASSACHUSETTS**
  (Massachusetts C of C)
  Richard Piazza, President
  34 Market St.
  Everett, 02149
  617-389-5221; fax 617-387-0051

- **MICHIGAN** (Michigan C of C)
  James Barrett, President
  600 S. Walnut St.
  Lansing, 48933-2200
  517-371-2100; fax 517-371-7224

- **MINNESOTA** (Minnesota State C of C)
  David Olson, President
  30 E. 7th St., #1700
  Saint Paul, 55101
  612-292-4650; 800-821-2230;
  fax 612-292-4656

- **MISSISSIPPI** (Mississippi Econ. Council)
  Bob W. Pittman, President
  P.O. Box 23276
  Jackson, 39225-3276
  601-969-0022; fax 601-353-0247

- **MISSOURI** (Missouri C of C)
  Mr. Jo Frappier, President
  428 E. Capitol Ave.; P.O. Box 149
  Jefferson City, 65102
  573-634-3511; fax 573-634-8855
  mchamber@computerland.net;
  www.computerland.net/~mchamber

- **MONTANA** (Montana C of C)
  David Owen, President
  2030 11th Ave., P.O. Box 1730
  Helena, 59601
  406-442-2405; fax 406-442-2409

- **NEBRASKA** (Nebraska C of C & Ind.)
  Jack Swartz, CCE, CAE, President
  P.O. Box 95128
  Lincoln, 68509-5128
  402-474-4422; fax 402-474-5681
  nc64456@navix.net

- **NEVADA** (Nevada State C of C)
  David Howard, Legislative Affairs Director
  P.O. Box 3499
  Reno, 89505
  702-686-3030; fax 702-686-3038

- **NEW HAMPSHIRE** (Business and
  Industry Assn. of New Hampshire)
  John D. Crosier, President
  122 N. Main
  Concord, 03301
  603-224-5388; fax 603-224-2872

- **NEW JERSEY** (New Jersey C of C)
  Joan Verplanck, President
  50 W. State St., #1310
  Trenton, 08608-1214
  609-989-7888; fax 609-989-9696

- **NEW MEXICO** (Assn. of Commerce
  & Industry of New Mexico)
  John A. Carey, President
  P.O. Box 9706
  Albuquerque, 87119-9706
  505-842-0644; fax 505-842-0734
  aci@tcchnet.nm.org; www.technet.nm.org/aci

- **NEW YORK** (No State Chapter)

- **NORTH CAROLINA** (North Carolina
  Citizens for Business & Industry)
  Phillip J. Kirk, Jr., President
  225 Hillsborough St.; P.O. Box 2508
  Raleigh, 27602-2508
  919-836-1400; fax 919-836-1425

- **NORTH DAKOTA** (Greater North Dakota
  Assn.)
  Dale O. Anderson, President
  2000 Schafer St.; P.O. Box 2639
  Bismarck, 58502
  701-222-0929; fax 701-222-1611

- **OHIO** (Ohio C of C)
  Andrew E. Doehrel, President
  P.O. Box 15159
  Columbus, 43215-0159
  614-228-4201; fax 614-228-6403

- **OKLAHOMA** (State of Oklahoma Assn.of
  Business & Industry)
  Richard P. Rush, CCE, Pres./CEO
  330 N.E. 10th St.
  Oklahoma City, 73104-3200
  405-235-3669; fax 405-235-3670

- **OREGON** (No State Chapter)

- **PENNSYLVANIA** (Pennsylvania Chamber
  of Business and Industry)
  Floyd W. Warner, President
  One Commerce Square; 417 Walnut St.
  Harrisburg, 17101-1902
  717-255-3252; 800-225-7224; fax 717-255-3298

- **PUERTO RICO** (Puerto Rico C of C)
  Edgardo Bigas, Exec. Vice President
  P.O. Box 9023789
  San Juan, 00902-3789
  787-721-6060; fax 787-723-1891

- **RHODE ISLAND** (No State Chapter)

- **SOUTH CAROLINA** (South Carolina
  State C of C)
  S. Hunter Howard J., Pres./CEO
  1201 Main St., #1810
  Columbia, 29201-3254
  803-799-4601; fax 803-779-6043
  www.sccc.org

- **SOUTH DAKOTA** (Industry &
  Commerce Assn.of South Dakota)
  Ray Trankle, President
  P.O. Box 190
  Pierre, 57501-0190
  605-224-6161; 800-742-8112;
  fax 605-224-7198

- **TENNESSEE** (No State Chamber)

- **TEXAS** (Texas Assn. of Business &
  Chambers of Commerce)
  Dane Harris, President
  1209 Nueces; P.O. Box 2989
  Austin, 78768
  512-447-6721; fax 512-477-0836

- **UTAH** (Utah State C of C)
  Delmar Brewster, President
  2274 S. 1300 E., #G8-147
  Salt Lake City, 84106
  801-467-0844; fax 801-467-6740

- **VERMONT** (Vermont State C of C)
  Christopher G. Barbieri, President
  P.O. Box 37
  Montpelier, 05601
  802-223-3443; fax 802-229-4581
  vtchambr@together.net;
  www.vtchamber.com

- **VIRGIN ISLANDS** (St. Croix C of C)
  Rachel Haines, Exec. Director
  Kings Hill; P.O. Box 4369
  St. Croix, 00851-4369
  809-773-1435; fax 809-773-8172

- **VIRGINIA** (Virginia C of C)
  Hugh D. Keogh, President
  9 S. Fifth St.
  Richmond, 23219
  804-644-1607; fax 804-783-0903

- **WASHINGTON**
  (Assn. of Washington Business)
  Don Brunell, President
  1414 S. Cherry; P.O. Box 658
  Olympia, 98507-0658
  360-943-1600; fax 360-943-5811
  donb@awb.net

- **WEST VIRGINIA** (West Virginia C of C)
  Stephen Roberts, President
  P.O. Box 2789
  Charleston, 25330-2789
  304-342-1115; fax 304-342-1130
  wvchamber@citynet.net; wvweb.com/
  www/cities/wv chamber

- **WISCONSIN**
  (Wisconsin Manufacturers & Commerce)
  James S. Haney, President
  501 E. Washington Ave.; P.O. Box 352
  Madison, 53701-0352
  608-258-3400; fax 608-258-3413

- **WYOMING** (No State Chapter)

OUR FAVORITE REFERENCE BOOKS

To stay on medical transcription's cutting edge, keep your library well stocked with the latest editions of top quality references, especially medical specialty reference books. Our favorites are the following titles:

- *Quick Look Drug Book*, Williams & Wilkins (latest edition)

- *Stedman's Surgical and Medical Equipment Words*, Williams & Wilkins

- *Saunders Pharmaceutical Word Book,* Drake/Drake, W. B. Saunders (latest edition)

- *Mosby's Nursing Drug Reference* (latest edition)

    You can never have too many drug books!

- *The Surgical Word Book*, Tessier, W. B. Saunders Co.

- *Dorland's Medical Speller*, W. B. Saunders Co.

- *Current Medical Terminology*, Pyle, Health Professions Institute

- *Internal Medicine Words*, Minta Danna, MT, edited by Pat Bowen, CMT, Rayve Productions Inc.

- *A Word Book in Pathology and Laboratory Medicine*, Sloan/Dusseau, W. B. Saunders Co.

- *Laboratory Test Handbook*, Williams & Wilkins (latest edition)

- *Medical Transcription Guide — Do's & Don'ts*, W. B. Saunders Co.

Some other essential references for the medical transcription library include grammar and punctuation references such as:

- *Medical Transcription Guide,* Diehl/Fordney, W. B. Saunders Co.

- *Errors in English and Ways to Correct Them*, Shaw, Harper and Row

- *The Elements of Style*, Strunk/White, MacMillan

- *The Manual of Medical Transcription*, Sloan/Fordney, W. B. Saunders Co.

Also necessary are a good collegiate dictionary, medical dictionary, anatomy book, abbreviations, acronyms and symbols book, and the list goes on.
An excellent medical transcription resource list and catalog are available through the American Association for Medical Transcription (AAMT) (see publishers' contact numbers below).

- **AAMT Medical Transcription Resource Library** (latest edition)
  (A comprehensive medical transcription reference list)

- **AAMT Success Catalog**

We have also found the following directory helpful.

- **The Little Blue Book**
  (published by Physician's Telephone Directory)
  302 West Main Street, Suite 206
  Avon, CT 06001-9962
  860-409-7000
  Fax: 860-674-8893

PUBLISHERS SPECIALIZING IN HEALTH CARE BOOKS

In addition to the above, several publishing houses specialize in books for the health care field. To obtain a list of available titles, contact the following publishers.

- **American Association for Medical Transcription (AAMT)**
  P.O. Box 576187
  Modesto, CA 95355 2
  209-551-0883
  Fax: 209-551-9317
  E-mail: aamt@sna.com

- **Churchill Livingston**
  650 Avenue of the Americas
  New York, NY 10011
  808-553-5426

- **F.A. Davis Co.**
  1915 Arch Street
  Philadelphia, PA 19103
  800-523-4049

- **Facts and Comparisons**
  subs. of Wolters Kluwer U.S. Corp.
  111 West Port Plaza, Ste.423
  St. Louis, MO 63146-3098
  800-223-0554

- **Health Professions Institute**
  P.O. Box 801
  Modesto, CA 95353
  209-551-2112

- **Houghton Mifflin Company**
  Two Park Street & One Beacon Street
  Boston, MA 02107
  800-725-5000

- **J.B. Lippincott**
  227 East Washington Square
  Philadelphia, PA 19106
  800-638-3030 (orders);
  800-441-4526 (office)

- **Merriam-Webster, Inc.**
  47 Federal Street
  Springfield, MA 01102
  413-734-3134

- **Physicians' Desk Reference**
  Division of Medical Economics Data
  Five Paragon Drive
  Montvale, NJ 07645
  800-232-7379

- **PMIC**
  625 Plainfield Road, Ste.220
  Willowbrook, IL 60521
  800-633-7467

  or

  4727 Wilshire Blvd., Suite 300
  Los Angeles, CA 90010
  800-MED-SHOP

- **Rayve Productions Inc.**
  P.O. Box 726
  Windsor, CA 95492
  800-852-4890

- **Rittenhouse**
  P.O. Box 1565
  511 Feheley Street
  King of Prussia, PA 19406
  or
  P.O. Box 458
  Sterling Rd.
  S. Lancaster, MA 01561

- **W. B. Saunders Company**
  Curtis Center, Independence Square West
  Philadelphia, PA 19106
  215-238-7800

- **William Kaufmann, Inc.**
  P.O. Box 50490
  Palo Alto, CA 94303
  415-965-4081

- **Williams & Wilkins**
  428 East Preston Street
  Baltimore, Maryland 21202
  800-638-0672

> *"Wear the old coat and buy the new book."*
>
> —Austin Phelps, 1881

OTHER RESOURCES FOR HEALTH CARE BOOKS

Other helpful resources for health care reference books include the following:

- **J.A. Majors Books**
  1851 Diplomat Drive
  Dallas, TX 75234-9014
  972-247-2929

  or

  1220 W. Walnut
  Compton, CA 90220
  310-608-2358

- **L&M Bookstore**
  1716 N. Main Avenue
  San Antonio, TX 78212
  210-222-1323
  Fax: 210-222-1580
  800-285-1323

PRODUCTS & SERVICES

- **BCB Technology Group, Inc.**
  418 Hanlan Road, Unit 4
  Woodbridge, Ontario, Canada L4L4Z

  or

  908 Niagara Falls Blvd.
  North Tonawanda, N.Y. 14120-2060
  Phone: 800-263-9942
  416-850-8266
  (Ask for: Daryl Duda, Vice President
  of Sales or Leo Halpern,
  Director of Customer Support)

- **C.H.A.R.T.S**
  (Cassettes, headsets and related
  transcription supplies)
  P. O. Box 3284
  Springfield, MO 65808
  800-994-3210
  Fax: 417-881-1872

- **Compuserve**
  800-524-3388

- **Creative Impressions**
  (Promotional material)
  P. O. Box 3493
  Fairfield, CA 94533
  707-428-4289

- **Curtis Computer Products**
  (call for a catalog or brochure)
  800-272-2366
  Fax: 800-272-2382

- **DataCal or DataComm**
  800-545-1058
  (resource for WP 5.1)
  800-453-7937

- **Dictaphone Corporation**
  3191 Broadbridge Avenue
  Stratford, CT 06497-2559
  203-381-7124
  Fax: 203-386-8597

- **The Dictionary of Eye Terminology, 1992 edition**
Triad Publishing Company
1110 North West 8th Avenue
Gainesville, Florida 32601

- **Digital Voice, Inc**

- **DM News** (Free marketing publication)
19 West 21st Street
New York, NY 10010
212-741-2095

- **Dragon Systems** (DragonDictate)
888-81DRAGON
Fax: 802-872-3138

- **How Grammar Works, A Self-teaching Guide**
(Review of grammar basics)
Patricia Osborn, published by: John Wiley & Sons
Ask for it at your local book store.

- **Individual Software**
(Audio training cassettes)
Pleasanton, CA
800-822-3522

- **McMillan and Co.**
Professional Organizing
Personal Assets Inventory Workbook
12021 Wilshire Blvd. Suite 670
West Los Angeles, CA 90025
310-478-1870, Fax 310-478-7049

- **MouseMitt International**
800-489-6488
E-mail mousemitt@mousemitt.com

- **Opus Communications**
Resources for Health care Professionals
P. O. Box 1168
Marblehead, MA 01945
800-650-6787
Fax: 800-639-8511

- **Paper Direct**
800-A-PAPERS
205 Chubb Avenue
Lyndhurst, NJ 07071

- **PC-DART Digital Dictation**
BCB Technology Group
418 Hanlan Road, Unit 4
Woodbridge, Ontario, Canada L4L 4Z1
905-850-8266; 905-850-8276
(USA) 800-263-9947; E-mail bcb@io.org

- **Personal Training Systems**
(Audio training cassettes)
800-832-2499 San Jose, CA

- **Phillips Speech Processing**
365 Crossways Park Drive
Woodbury, NY 11797
516-921-9310
Fax: 516-921-9319
E-mail: 104075.3212@compuserve.com

- **PMIC**
800-MED-SHOP
(Medical reference books at a discount)

- **Productive Performance**
31820 N.E. 103rd Street
Carnation, WA 98014-9710
206-788-8300

- **REA's Handbook of English; Grammar, Style and Writing**
Research & Education Association

- **Sea Coast Designs, Inc.**
Chair Technologies
714-542-8644
Fax: 714-542-8734

- **The Survey Research Handbook**
(Marketing Survey)
Alreck, Pamela and Robert Settle
(Provides a good overview of survey research techniques with examples that may point you in the right direction.)

- **Sylvan Software**
  5144 North Academy Blvd., Suite 531
  Colorado Springs, Colorado 80918
  800-235-9455

- **Target Marketing** (marketing publication)
  P. O. Box 12827
  Philadelphia, PA 19108-0827

- **Telecommunications Research and Action Center (TRAC)**
  P. O. Box 12038
  Washington, DC 20005
  202-462-2520
  (Lists least expensive long distance phone carriers. Provides rate comparison chart of five largest national carriers. Mail SASE and check for $2.00 [residential] or $5.00 [small business] to TRAC.)

- **Text Entry Systems, RTT-PC**
  (Real-Time Transcribing, PC)
  Contact Eric Goldwasser
  914-245-2565 or write him at
  Text Entry Systems
  993 Barberry Road
  Yorktown Heights, N.Y. 10598

- **Textware Solutions** (Instant Text)
  83 Cambridge Street
  Burlington, MA 01803-4181
  Tel: 617-272-3200
  Fax: 617-272-1432
  800-355-5251

CATALOGS

- **AAMT Success Catalog**
  AAMT, P.O. Box 576187
  Modesto, CA 95357-6187
  209-551-0883

- **Quill Corporation**
  100 Schelter Road
  Lincolnshire, IL 60069-3621
  312-634-4800

  (Carries a wide variety of office and general business supplies and some computer items. Offers discounts.)

- **Sears**
  800-255-3000
  (Office Essentials for Your Home or Business. Discounted office equipment and furniture.)

- *Computer Shopper*
  Coastal Associates Publishing
  5211 S. Washington Avenue
  Titusville, FL 32780
  800-274-6384

  (Information and merchandise from a variety of suppliers. Good for general reference, money-saving tips on mail order supplies, and sources of supply. If an item exists, it is probably listed here.)

- **Crutchfield Personal Office**
  Crutchfield Corporation
  1 Crutchfield park
  Charlottesville, VA 22906
  800-521-4050

- **Computer Direct, Inc**
  22292 N. Pepper Road
  Barrington, IL 60010
  800-289-9473

- **Fidelity Products Co.**
  5601 International Parkway
  P.O. Box 155
  Minneapolis, MN 55440-0155
  800-328-3034

CONTINUING EDUCATION

- **American Association for Medical Transcription**
  P.O. Box 576187
  Modesto, CA 95357

- **American Health Information Management Association**
  (formerly American Medical Record Association)
  919 North Michigan Avenue
  Chicago, Il 60611-1683

- **Guide to Alternative Colleges and Universities**
  Garrett Park Press
  Garrett Park, MD 20766

- **The Weekend Education Source Book**
  Wilbur Cross/Harper & Row
  153 E. 53rd St.
  New York, NY 10022

- **Directory of Accredited Private Home Study Schools**
  National Home Study Council
  1601 18th Street NW
  Washington, D.C. 29009

> *"I have been blessed by a lifetime of exciting educational adventures.*
> *Everywhere I turn, there is something new*
> *to discover, to learn, to experience."*
> —Beatrice Gage

MAGAZINES AND NEWSPAPER PUBLICATIONS

- *Advance for Health Information Professionals*
  Merion Publications, Inc.
  650 Park Avenue West
  King of Prussia, PA 19406
  Phone: 215-265-7812

- *American Mothers at Home*
  The Association of Enterprising Mothers
  914 S. Santa Fe Avenue, Suite 297
  Vista, CA 92084
  619-434-9225

- *Business Week*
  McGraw-Hill Bldg.
  1221 Avenue of the Americas
  New York, NY 10020

- *California Business*
  6420 Wilshire Blvd., Suite 711
  Los Angeles, CA 90048

- *Changing Times*
  The Kiplinger Washington Editors, Inc.
  Editors Park, MD 20782

- *For the Record*
  Valley Forge, PA 19481

- *The Futurist*
  World Future Society
  P. O. Box 30369
  Bethesda Branch
  Washington, D.C. 20014

- *In Business*
  Box 323
  Emmaus, PA 18049

- *Money*
  3435 Wilshire Blvd.
  Los Angeles, CA 90010

- *Venture*
  35 West 45th Street
  New York, NY 10036

- *Working Woman*
  1180 Avenue of the Americas
  New York, NY 10036

- *Home Office Computing*
  730 Broadway
  New York, NY 10003

Bibliography

ABC'S of WordPerfect 5, The. Alameda, CA: Sybex.

Avila, Donna. *Donna's Home-made Surgical Reference.* 20th ed. St. Helena, CA: Homemade Press, 1991.

Baumback, Lawyer, Kelley. *How To Organize and Operate a Small Business.* 5th ed. New York: Prentice-Hall, Inc., 1973.

Blanchard, Kenneth and Robert Lorber. *Putting the One Minute Manager To Work.* New York: William Morrow Co., 1984.

Bohigian, Valerie. *Real Money From Home. How to Start, Manage, and Profit from a Home-Based Service Business.* New American Library, 1985.

Brody, Herb. "The Body In Question," *PC Computing.* March 1989.

Business Plan for Homebased Businesses, The. #MPl5. Washington D.C.: Small Business Administration.

Business Use of Your Home, #587. Washington, D.C.: Internal Revenue Service.

Calem, Robert E. "When Leasing or Renting Makes Sense," *Home Office Computing.* March 1991.

Danna, Minta, MT, *Internal Medicine Words.* Windsor, CA: Rayve Productions Inc., 1997.

Deken, Joseph. *The Electronic Cottage*. New York: William Morrow Co., 1981.

DeLorenzo, Barbara. *Pharmaceutical Terminology*. 2nd Edition. Slack, Inc., 1988.

Dorland's Medical Dictionary, 27th ed. Philadelphia: W. B. Saunders Co., 1988.

Edwards, Paul and Sarah. *Working From Home - Everything You Need to Know About Living and Working Under the Same Roof*. Los Angeles: Jeremy P. Tarcher, Inc., 1985.

Feldman, E. and Beverly Neuer. *Home Based Businesses*. New York: Ballantine Books, 1982.

Fordney, Marilyn and Marcy Diehl. *Medical Transcription Guide*. Philadelphia: W. B. Saunders Co., 1990.

Frohbieter-Mueller. *Your Home Business Can Make Dollars and Sense*. Radnor, PA: Chilton Book Company, 1990.

Glossbrenner, Alfred. *How to Get Free Software*. New York: St. Martin's Press, 1984.

Gregory, Helen I. *Finding and Keeping Customers. A Small Business Handbook*. Sedro Woolley, WA: Pinstripe Publishing.

Guide to Hiring Independent Contractors. Sacramento: California Chamber of Commerce, 1991.

Health Professions Institute, Modesto, CA:
> *Cardiology Words/Phrases*
> *GI Words/Phrases*
> *Orthopedic Words/Phrases*
> *Psychiatric Words/Phrases*
> *Radiology Words/Phrases*

Holtz, Herman. *The Complete Work-at-Home Companion*. Rocklin, CA: Prima Publishing & Communications, 1990.

Hooper, W.E. *Bookkeeping for Beginners*. Beekman Publishers, Inc., 1970.

Jorgensen, James and Michael G. Rinaldi. *A Clinician's Dictionary of Bacteria and Fungi*. Indianapolis: Eli Lilly & Co., 1986.

Kamoroff, Bernard. *Small-Time Operator*. Laytonville, CA: Bell Springs Publishing, 1990.

Kotler, Phillip and Paul N. Bloom. *Marketing Professional Services*. New York: Prentice-Hall, Inc., 1984.

Lance, Leonard L., Charles Lacy and Warren Flynn. *1991 Quick Look Drug Book*. Baltimore: Williams & Wilkins, 1991.

Lyons, Albert S. and R. Joseph Petrucelli, II. *Medicine. An Illustrated History*. New York: Abradale Press, 1987.

McCann, Ron. *The Joy of Service*. Service Information Source Publications, 1989.

Merck Manual. 14th ed. Robert Berkow, ed. Rahway, NJ: Merck, Sharp & Dohme, 1982.

Milliron, Robert R. *How to Do Your Own Accounting for a Small Business*. Enterprise Del, 1980.

Poynter, Dan. *Word Processors and Information Processing*. Santa Barbara, CA: Para Publishing, 1982.

Pricing Your Products and Service Profitability, #FM13. Washington, D.C.: Small Business Administration.

Pyle, Vera. *Current Medical Terminology*. 3rd ed., Modesto, CA: Prima Vera Publications, 1990.

Ray, Norm. *Easy Financials for Your Home-based Business*. Windsor, CA: Rayve Productions Inc., 1993.

Ray, Norm. *Smart Tax Write-offs*. Windsor CA: Rayve Productions Inc., 1996.

Shaw, Harry. *Errors in English and Ways to Correct Them*. 3rd ed. New York: Harper & Row, 1986.

Sloane, Sheila B. *The Medical Word Book*. 3rd ed., Philadelphia: W. B. Saunders Co., 1982.

Sloane, Sheila B. and John L. Dusseau. *A Word Book in Pathology and Laboratory Medicine*. Philadelphia: W. B. Saunders Co., 1984.

Sloane, Sheila B. *Medical Abbreviations and Eponyms*. Philadelphia: W. B. Saunders Co., 1985.

Stedman's Medical Dictionary. 25th ed. Baltimore: Williams & Wilkins, 1990.

Taber's Cyclopedic Medical Dictionary. 15th ed. Edited by Thomas L.Clayton. Philadelphia: F.A. Davis Co., 1988.

Tax Guide for Small Businesses #2334. Internal Revenue Service. Washington, D.C.

Taylor, Donna M. and Patricia A. Collins. *For Your Information*. Santa Ana, CA: FYI Book Co., 1991.

Tennenhouse, Dan J. *California Health Care Law*. Danville, CA: Contemporary Forums, 1985.

Tessier, Claudia and Sally C. Pittman. *Style Guide for Medical Transcription*. Modesto, CA: American Association for Medical Transcription, 1985.

Tessier, Claudia. *The Surgical Word Book*. Philadelphia: W. B. Saunders Co., 1981.

Webster's College Dictionary. New York: Random House, Inc., 1991.

Whitmyer, Claude, Salli Rasberry and Michael Phillips, *Running a One-Person Business*. Berkeley, CA: Ten Speed Press, 1994.

Wookridge, Susan and Keith London. *The Computer Survival Handbook: How to Talk Back to Your Computer*. Educator Books, Inc., 1973.

WordPerfect Workbook. Orem, Utah: WordPerfect Corp., 1989.

Glossary (Terms related to medical transcription)

AAMT — American Association for Medical Transcription, a national professional transcription association.

Accountant — A person who organizes, maintains or audits the financial records of a company or individual.

Accredited — Status of health care organizations that meet the standards of national accrediting organizations, such as the Joint Commission on Accreditation of Healthcare Organizations (JCAHO) and the National Committee for Quality Assurance (NCQA).

Accredited Records Technician (ART) — An individual who has completed a course of instruction, passed an examination, and achieved entry-level certification in medical records management from the American Health Information Management Association (AHIMA).

Admission — The formal process of registering a patient for service. In a hospital, admission usually involves an overnight stay. In an ambulatory care facility, length of stay is immaterial.

ALOS — Average length of stay.

Adaptor — A device for connecting parts having different sizes.

AHA — American Hospital Association.

AHIMA — American Health Information Management Association.

AMA — American Medical Association; Against Medical Advice.

Ambulatory care — All types of health services provided on an outpatient basis, in contrast to services provided in the home or to persons who are inpatients. Many inpatients may be ambulatory, but the term ambulatory care usually refers to patients who travel to locations other than their home to receive services and then depart the same day.

AMLOS — Arithmetic Mean Length of Stay — Average number of days patients within a given DRG stay in the hospital, also referred to as the average length of stay.

Anatomy — The science of the structure of the animal body and the relation of its parts.

Ancillary Services — Inpatient services other than basic room and board and professional services, and hospital outpatient services other than professional services. They include services such as radiology, drug, laboratory, emergency room and home health care.

ANSI — American National Standards Institute.

ASCII — The code used by all personal computers that use a DOS operating system. Provides a common format for saving and importing into various programs.

Authentication (of an entry in a medical record) — The process of confirming the content of a health care entry by such means as written signature, identifiable entry, biometric identifier, or computer key. In practice, authentication usually involves countersigning a verbal or telephone order or signing the typed copy of a dictated document to confirm that it was accurately transcribed.

Authorship (of an entry in a medical record) — The process of identifying a health care practitioner who has released a health care entry for use by writing, dictation, keyboard, or keyless data entry. In practice, authorship usually involves signing — or using some other method besides signing — to indicate authorship and authenticity of a dictated document.

Backlog — An accumulation of unfinished work.

Backup — Copying a computer file from one disk to another disk. A form of insurance in case one of the copies becomes lost.

Billing — A statement of money owed for services rendered.

BIN — Binary.

Bit — Binary digit. The smallest unit of digital information, represented electronically as either 1 (on) or 0 (off).

Blackout — A period of failure of all electric power.

Blanks — A place or space where something is missing or lacking.

Bookkeeper — One who keeps account books or systematic records of business transactions.

Brochure — A pamphlet used for promotional purposes.

Brownout — Any curtailment of electric power, especially a voltage reduction to prevent a blackout.

Business card — A small card containing the business name, name of owner/operator, address, and telephone number.

Business license — A governmental certificate of permission to operate a business.

Byte — A unit of digital information (eight consecutive bits). Memory and disk capacity are measured in thousands (K) of bytes. One byte is equivalent to approximately one character of text. If a piece has 2000 characters, it needs 2K (kilobytes) of storage.

Call-in-line — A private telephone line and dictating unit specifically used for call-in dictation.

Canned reports or **normals** — A body of a report that can repeatedly be called out and listened to. Although changes can be made to the original, the body of the report need not be redictated each time it is used.

Capital — The net worth of a business; assets minus liabilities of a business.

Capital gain — Profit from the sale of capital assets.

Capitation — The provider receives a fixed payment per member, per month, for which the provider must provide specific services. Though capitation involves less administrative cost than other payment methods, providers must assume the risk that the fixed payment will cover the costs of patient care needs.

Cardiology — The study of the heart and its functions.

Carpal tunnel syndrome — Entrapment of the median nerve at the wrist, caused by accumulative trauma.

Case management — A process through which a single health care professional has the responsibility of monitoring the location and coordination of a patient's overall care to maximize effectiveness, reduce waste of resources, and reduce patient discomfort.

Case mix — The diagnosis-specific makeup of a hospital's work load, which directly influences the lengths of stay and the intensity, cost, and scope of services provided by the hospital.

Cassette — A compact case enclosing audio tape that runs between two reels. It is recordable or playable by inserting it into a recorder or player.

CC — Complication; Comorbid Condition.

CEO — Chief Executive Officer.

CFO — Chief Financial Officer.

Character — In typing, any letter, number or symbol.

Character count — A method of determining transcription productivity by counting letters, numbers or symbols.

Client — A person who engages the services of a professional.

Clinic — A facility or portion thereof used for diagnosis and treatment of outpatients. Also may be loosely defined to include physicians' offices.

Clip art — Copyright-free art, available in books and on diskettes, that can be used and modified without permission.

Closed-end lease — A contract whereby you rent equipment for a specific period of time, and which allows you to purchase the equipment after the last installment has been paid.

CMI — Case-Mix Index — The sum of all DRG relative weights, divided by the number of Medicare cases.

Cold calling — Marketing technique for procuring new clients. Telephoning potential clients directly or visiting their businesses to solicit work.

COMPRO — **C**ompetency **Pro**file. An AAMT description of competencies necessary for a medical transcriptionist.

Concurrent review — Case review conducted while a patient is in treatment, as opposed to **retrospective review**, which occurs after treatment and, therefore, cannot affect treatment.

Continuation — In the insurance context, when a covered person who would otherwise lose insurance coverage due to termination of employment, divorce, etc., is allowed to "continue" his or her coverage under conditions specified in the plan, as opposed to under any law. Health care providers must be aware of "continuation" limits.

Confidential — Communicated in confidence.

Contract — An agreement, especially one enforceable by law.

Copiers — Duplicating machines.

Corporation — An association of individuals, created by law and existing as an entity with powers and liabilities independent of those of its members.

CPR — **C**omputer-based **P**atient **R**ecord.

CPRI — **C**omputer-based **P**atient **R**ecord **I**ndex.

CPU — **C**entral **P**rocessing **U**nit.

CQI — **C**ontinuing **Q**uality **I**mprovement.

412

Credentialing — The two-pronged process that involves establishing requirements and evaluating individual qualifications for entry into a particular status, such as medical staff membership. First, credentialing considers and establishes the professional training, experience and other requirements for medical staff membership. Second, credentialing obtains and evaluates evidence of the qualifications of individual applicants. Most frequently, credentialing applies to medical staff membership; however, it also applies to the process hospital personnel departments use to evaluate applicants for other positions.

Curriculum vitae — A brief summary of a person's schooling and specialty training. For a physician, this information is required for board certification.

Daisy wheel — A letter quality, impact printer which acts much like a typewriter.

Decipher — To make out the meaning of; to decode.

Delivery — To carry transcription to the recipient.

Department — In a hospital, a major unit of the medical staff, headed by a chair, director or chief, usually devoted to providing clinical service in one specialty area.

Departmental QA (or departmental QA/I) — The quality-related activities that, before 1994, the JCAHO required to be carried out by each major medical staff department. This is no longer a JCAHO requirement.

Depreciating — Lessening of price or value due to wear and tear or obsolescence.

Diagnostic related groups (DRGs) — Classification system developed at Yale University using 383 major diagnostic categories (based on the ICD-9 codes) that assigns patients into case types. Designed to facilitate the utilization review process, DRGs are also used to analyze the patient case mix in hospitals and determine their reimbursement policies.

Dictation — Voice recordings to be transcribed.

Digital — A system in which data are stored and transmitted electronically in 1's and 0's for speed and efficiency.

Direct contracting — Individual or groups of employers contract directly with providers for health care services with no managed care intermediary (ie., HMO, PPO, EPO) to customize services for employees.

Discharge days — For each patient, the total number of inpatient days between admission and discharge dates. In calculating total inpatient days, the day of admission is included in the count, but not the day of discharge.

Discharge summary — Synopsis of a patient's stay in the hospital.

Disk — The storage medium for programs and files. A "hard" disk is generally not removable; a "floppy" disk is removable.

Disk drive — The computer device that holds a disk, gets information from it, and saves information on it.

DOS — Date of Service.

Dot matrix printer — A printer which creates characters or graphics in dots through the use of a print head that contains varying numbers of pins. An impact printer.

Download — To receive a computer file electronically.

Downloadable font — A set of instructions defining a family of letter (a font) that is stored in a computer and sent (downloaded) to an output device such as a printer.

dpi — **d**ots **p**er **i**nch — The more dpi, the sharper the image (the higher the resolution).

DRG — **D**iagnosis **R**elated **G**roup — A classification system used to categorize patients according to clinical coherence and expected resource intensity, as indicated by their diagnoses, procedures, age, sex, and disposition. The system was established and is revised annually by the U.S. Health Care Financing Administration.

E-Codes — Supplementary classification of ICD-9-CM, containing external causes of injury and poisoning.

EDI — Electronic Data Interchange.

Editing — The art of preparing and arranging materials for the medical record or for publication.

EIN — Employer Identification Number. Needed for tax purposes.

Electronic books — Books that are read and experienced on a computer, with or without an interactive element.

Electronic mailbox — The address on a computer network where people pick up messages sent by other computer users.

Entrepreneur — A person who organizes, manages and assumes responsibility for a business or other enterprise.

Ergonomics — The study of movement.

Errors and Omissions Policy — An insurance policy, much like malpractice coverage, for the medical transcriptionist.

ES — Electronic Signature.

Esophagus — The musculomembranous passage extending from the pharynx to the stomach.

Ethics — A system of moral standards or values; essential quality; conforming to the standards of a given group or profession.

Facility — Buildings, including the physical plant, equipment and supplies used in providing health services. Major types of health facilities include hospitals and nursing homes.

FAX (Facsimile transmission) — Graphic images or printed matter that are scanned and sent electronically via telephone wires.

FAX machine — A duplicating machine that electronically transmits printed matter or graphic images via telephone wires.

Fee-for-Service (FFS) — A traditional payment system in which the physician or hospital bills the patient or insurer for each visit and service provided.

Fictitious name statement — Required by law for businesses using a name other than that of the business owner.

Floppy disk — A removable diskette, either 3-1/2", 5-1/4", or 8", used to store approximately one megabyte of computer information.

Flier / flyer — A small handbill used in procuring business accounts.

Format — The overall style of a printed document including paper type, size, layout, type, margins, and other document requirements.

Freelancer — A self-employed medical transcriptionist.

Freestanding — Not part of a hospital (neither structurally connected to nor organizationally considered part of a hospital); not hospital-based.

Gastroenterology — The study of the stomach and intestines and their diseases.

Gateway — A device that connects different types of networks and performs protocol translation.

Going rate — The usual and customary fee charged for a particular service in a specific area or locale.

Grouper — Software program that assigns DRGs.

Hard copy — The paper version of what's been generated on a computer.

Hard disk — The rigid disk in a computer used for storing programs and large amounts of data.

Hardware — The physical components of a computer system, such as a computer, monitor, disk drive, and printer.

HCFA — Health Care Financing Administration. A division of the Department of Health and Human Services that administers Medicare and certain aspects of Medicaid. HCFA is responsible for determining which facilities meet federal quality standards for providing health care to beneficiaries.

HCPCS, HCFA — Health Care Common Procedural Coding System; Health Care Financing Administration.

HCQIA — Health Care Quality Improvement Act.

HCWS — Healthcare workers.

HFMA — Healthcare Financial Management Association.

HIS — Hospital Information System.

HMO — Health Maintenance Organization — A legal entity or organized health care system that provides directly or arranges for a comprehensive range of basic and supplemental health care services to a voluntarily enrolled population in a geographic area on a primarily prepaid and fixed periodic basis. This term is defined by federal law in the Health Maintenance Organization Act of 1973 (Public Law 93-222).

Home Health Services — Home medical services.

Hospice — A facility that cares for terminally ill patients, with more emphasis on meeting the psychosocial needs of patients and families.

Hospital — Generally, an institution with an organized medical staff whose primary function is to provide diagnostic and therapeutic inpatient services for a variety of medical conditions, both surgical and nonsurgical.

ICD-9-CM — International Classification of Diseases — Modification developed in the United States based on the official version of the World Health Organization's International Classification of Diseases, 9th Revision, and designed for classification of morbidity and mortality information for statistical reporting purposes and information retrieval.

Icons — Symbols on a computer screen.

Impact printer — Printers which use either a daisy wheel or print thimble as the typing element. Sometimes called a letter quality printer.

Indemnification — A negotiated contract provision under which one party to the contract agrees to pay any judgments, costs and attorney fees incurred by the other for acts or omissions that are the fault of the first. It is important for providers to insist on "mutual" indemnification provision in any contract with a managed care entity.

Information highway — The network of cable and telephone lines that delivers vast new amounts of information directly to consumers.

Inkjet printer — Nonimpact printer that uses ink sprays to produce legible copy.

Interface — Software designed to communicate specific information between the digital dictation system and the department's information system.

Internet — An enormous international interconnected set of computer networks that links government agencies, universities, corporations and individuals.

IRA — Individual Retirement Account.

IRS — Internal Revenue Service.

JCAHO — Joint Commission on Accreditation of Hospitals Organization.

The Joint — A commonly used, informal term for the Joint Commission on Accreditation of Healthcare Organizations (JCAHO).

Keyboard — A row or set of keys, as on a piano, typewriter or computer terminal used to enter data into a computer.

Kilobyte (1024 bytes) — Common measure of memory capacity (a double-spaced type-written page used about 1.5K).

LAN — Local Area Network.

Laser — A device that produces a very narrow beam of extremely intense light, used in communications and industrial processes.

Laser printer — A high-resolution printer that produces type and graphics of near-typeset quality.

LQ — Letter Quality.

Lift-off tape — A tape used with self-correcting typewriters for correcting errors.

Line count — A method used to determine transcription productivity by counting total lines typed, used for billing purposes.

Log sheet — A record of completed transcription.

LTC — Long Term Care — Skilled nursing/intermediate care.

Maintenance contract — An agreement stipulating terms of equipment repair and cost.

Malpractice — Legal liability against a physician or health care organization resulting from negligent or unprofessional treatment in the practice of a health care profession.

Managed care — A health care plan, such as an HMO-style plan, that attempts to monitor and control the quality, cost effectiveness, and resource utilization of doctors, hospitals, and other health care facilities as they provide service to patients. Also, the organization of various types of health care providers into administrative networks in which they collaborate, refer patients to each other and share funding.

Maximize — Raise to highest degree possible.

Medical staff — The semiautonomous group of physicians, other licensed independent practitioners, and other such health care professionals permitted by state law and a hospital to take responsibility as a group for specified aspects of hospital operation. The medical staff is one of the three key parts of hospital governance. (The other two key parts of hospital governance are the governing board and the hospital administration.)

Medical terminology — The language of medicine.

Megabyte (MB) — Unit of measure of computer memory, equal to 1024 kilobytes or roughly one million bytes.

Mentor — A wise and trusted counselor.

Memory — A computer's information storage site, usually measured in thousands (K) of bytes.

Menu — The lists of options on a computer screen.

Microbiology — The science that deals with the study of microorganisms, including algae, bacteria, fungi, protozoa and viruses.

Microcassette — An audio cassette tape that is smaller than a standard cassette.

Modem — A device for transmitting computer data over telephone lines.

Module — A standard or unit for measuring.

Monitor — A computer display screen.

Mouse — A hand-operated pointing device, usually beside the computer keyboard, that enables a computer user to manipulate what is on the screen.

MT — Medical Transcriptionist.

Multimedia — Electronic products that use various media (text, graphics, animation, audio) to deliver information. Often these products are also interactive, allowing the user to pick and choose from a variety of information options.

NCQA — National Committee on Quality Assurance.

NCR PAPER — Specially treated paper on which an original and two or three copies print simultaneously.

Nerd — A computer fanatic.

Netizens — Internet citizens.

Networking — (1) Technology that connects computers at several different locations and allows communication among them. (2) Communicating with other MTs regarding work practices, standards, and problem solving.

NFIB - National Federation of Independent Business

Nondisclosure statement — In a contract between a medical transcriptionist and her client, the section dealing with confidentiality of the medical record.

Online — A state in which information is accessible electronically, via computers, cable TV or telephone lines.

Open-end lease — A rental agreement allowing the renter the options of purchasing the equipment at a fair market price, renegotiating and extending the lease, or terminating the lease and returning the equipment to lessor.

Operating system — The program that enables you to run the computer.

Optimize — Make the most of; develop or realize to the utmost extent; obtain the most efficient or optimum use of. DRG optimization helps increase Medicare DRG payments and case-mix index, improve coding quality, reduce PRO risks and improve physician documentation.

Ordinance — An authoritative law or rule, especially one enacted by a municipal body.

OTJ — On-the-Job.

Outpatient — A person who receives medical, dental, or other health-related services in a hospital or other health care institution but who is not lodged there.

Outsourcing (subcontracting) — To transcribe for another person or service.

Page rate — A method used to measure productivity of transcription; used for billing purposes.

Partnerships — Two or more persons associated as principals or contributors of capital in a business.

Patient mix — The different types of patients served in a hospital in terms of such characteristics as age, sex, diagnosis, and residence.

PC — Personal Computer.

PCL — **P**rinter **C**ommand **L**anguage — The commands for operating printers.

Peer Review — Evaluation of a physician's performance by other physicians, usually within the same geographic area and medical specialty.

Per case — A method of payment in which a provider receives a payment determined by case mix for a particular patient.

Physical therapy — The study and treatment of the body.

Physiology — The science which treats the functions of the living organism and its parts, and of the physical and chemical factors and processes involved.

Pick up — Obtaining work from a client.

Policies and Procedures — Detailed technical directives and guidance that are outlined in documents. Often times, policies are statements of purpose or objectives and procedures are statements of how purposes or objectives will be attained. They usually appear in the same document.

Port — An access path into the digital system for one of the following purposes: Dictate - Transcribe - Listen.

PPO — **P**referred **P**rovider **O**rganization — A health care organization formed by a hospital or physician group to contract with an insurer for health care provided to a defined population. PPOs are not exclusive providers of care to insured groups, but they usually offer lower charges to the insured groups in return for their influence in channeling patients to providers participating in the PPO. (Also see Preferred Provider Organization below.)

Practice Guidelines — Statements, either narrative or pictorial, describing recommended approaches to diagnosis or treatment of specified diseases, injuries, or conditions.

PRD+ — **P**roductivity **Plus**, a medical terminology abbreviation program for computers.

Preferred Provider Organization (PPO) — A system designed to be an alternative to HMOs. Health care providers define a population to service at an agreed-upon fee schedule. (Also see PPO above.)

Printer — A machine that receives electronic signals from a computer and responds by printing on paper.

Professional — One who is connected with or engaged in a profession. A person who is an expert.

PRO — **P**eer **R**eview **O**rganization — Peer review organization; an organization that reviews appropriateness and quality of care for beneficiaries of the Medicare program.

Profiling — Collection and analysis of an individual practitioner's practice statistics for evaluation purposes.

Program (also, **software, application**) — The coding that tells the computer what to do.

Proofreader — A person employed to detect and mark errors to be corrected.

Programmer — A person adept at developing a systematic plan or set of instructions for the solution of a problem by a computer. One who prepares computer programs or supplies a computer with a program.

Provider — A person or organization that provides health care services (e.g., physician, hospital, home health agency).

Quality — Grade of excellence.

Quality assessment/improvement (QA/I) — The term adopted by the JCAHO in 1993 to describe activities required of hospitals to monitor and maintain quality of patient care.

Quality of care — Evaluation of the performance of medical providers according to the degree to which the process of care increases the probability of outcomes desired by patients.

Quantity — Amount.

Radiology — That branch of the health sciences dealing with radioactive substances and radiant energy, and with the diagnosis and treatment of disease by means of both ionizing and nonionizing radiations.

RAM — **R**andom **A**ccess **M**emory. The amount of computer memory, measured in thousands (K) of bytes. Also, computer memory that stores information temporarily while you are working on it.

Ream — Five hundred sheets of paper.

Registered Record Administrator (RRA) — The recognition awarded by the AHIMA to individuals who possess the required credentials and pass the required examination that demonstrate competence in the management of health information record departments.

Reimbursement — Repayment of money spent; compensation for expenses.

Retrospective review — The determination of medical necessity, coverage, or payment for services that have already been rendered.

RIS — **R**adiology **I**nformation **S**ystem.

Reprint — Reproducing transcribed reports which were previously printed.

Rerecord — The ability to repeat record work onto a cassette central recorder. Some systems need to be monitored as they rerecord.

Risk management — An administrative activity aimed to prevent the loss of hospital resources resulting from actual or alleged accidents, neglect, or incompetence.

Rolodex™ — A file box or wheel for holding business cards, clients' names and telephone numbers. Filed items can be readily added or deleted.

ROM — **R**ead **O**nly **M**emory. Programs or instructions that are permanently stored in a computer.

Router — A device that connects segments of networks that use the same protocols.

RSIs - **R**epetitive **S**train **I**njuries. Caused from cumulative trauma at the computer.

Save — To store information on disk.

Seminar — An educational course or meeting.

Service — Work performed for another or a group.

SNF — **S**killed **N**ursing **F**acility — A health facility or a distinct part of a hospital which provides skilled nursing care and supportive care to patients whose primary need is for skilled nursing care on an extended basis. It provides 24-hour inpatient care and, as a minimum, includes medical, nursing, dietary and pharmaceutical services, as well as activity programs.

Software — Programs, procedures and data used for the operation of a computer system.

Sole proprietor —A one-person business owner.

Standard mileage allowance —Standard set by the IRS to facilitate the determining of car expenses as a tax-deduction.

Standard of care — A legal standard defined as the level of care provided by the majority of physicians in a particular clinical situation.

Subcontract (outsource) — To transcribe for another person or service.

SUM — Home study medical transcription program created by Health Professions Institute.

Surge protector — A device to protect computers from damage due to dramatic changes in electrical currents.

Tampering — To make changes in order to falsify.

TAT — Turnaround time. The time between dictation and completion of transcription.

Tax deduction — An item which can be subtracted from income in calculating taxable income.

Tax preparer — One who is in business to complete and file tax returns.

Tax shelter — Investing a portion of otherwise taxable income in programs designed to defer taxation of income.

Template — A pre-designed pattern or grid for printed items such as letters, medical reports, invoices, brochures, and newsletters.

Thermal printer — A printer that uses heat to imprint paper.

Toner — Laser printer "ink" made of fine plastic particles.

TQM — Total Quality Management.

Trademark — A word or symbol distinguishing the product of one company from those of competitors, usually registered with the government to assure its exclusive use by its owner.

Transcriber — The machine used to listen to dictation in order to transcribe.

Transcription — The art or process of transcribing.

Transcriptionist — Person who transcribes.

Transcription pool — A group of transcriptionists usually working in a specified area.

Turnaround time — The specified time when completed work is to be delivered; the time between dictation and completion of transcription.

UHDDS — Uniform Hospital Discharge Data Set — The hospital discharge data set periodically issued by the U.S. Department of Health and Human Services.

Upload — To electronically send a computer file.

Users — An unfortunate reference to those who use computers.

Utilities program — A specialized computer program used to manage information on computer disks.

Utilization Review (UR) — The examination and evaluation of the efficiency and appropriateness of any health care service.

V-Codes — Supplementary classification of ICD-9-CM, containing factors influencing health states and contact with health services.

Video telephony — Telephones that also broadcast video images.

Video card — A printed circuit board that is installed in a computer to drive the monitor display.

Virtual reality — A computer simulation usually experienced through headgear, goggles and sensory gloves that lets the user feel he or she is present in another place.

Virus — In reference to computers, a corrupting influence, a "bug" in the software program which can cause it to malfunction.

WAN — Wide Area Network.

Windows — In some computer programs, sections of the screen (sometimes overlapping) that enable one to work with multiple applications at once.

WordPerfect™ — A computer software program for word processing.

Wordstar™ — A computer software program used in word processing.

Workers' Compensation —An insurance policy for employees injured while performing their job duties.

WYSIWYG (pronounced wizzy-wig) — **What you see is what you get** — Computer systems in which what you see on the computer screen is as it will appear on the printed (hard) copy.

Zoning — An area divided off or somehow differentiated from adjoining zones. Any specific area or district, as one in a city under certain restrictions, especially with regard to building.

Appendix

- Exhibit A: AAMT Model Job Description: Medical Transcriptionist
  (Reproduced with permission from AAMT.)

- Exhibit B: Budget Worksheet
  You may photocopy this worksheet to use for your budget preparation. You
  can enlarge it to 150% for an 8½x11" page. (Reproduced from the book *Easy
  Financials for Your Home-based Business*).

- Exhibit C: Sample Contract

Exhibit A: AAMT Model Job Description

AMERICAN ASSOCIATION FOR MEDICAL TRANSCRIPTION

AAMT Model Job Description:

MEDICAL TRANSCRIPTIONIST

The *AAMT Model Job Description* is a practical, useful compilation of the basic job responsibilities of a medical transcriptionist. It is designed to assist human resource managers, department managers, supervisors, and others in recruiting, supervising, and evaluating individuals in medical transcription positions.

The *AAMT Model Job Description* is not intended as a complete list of specific duties and responsibilities. Nor is it intended to limit or modify the right of any supervisor to assign, direct, and control the work of employees under supervision. The use of a particular expression or illustration describing duties shall not be held to exclude other duties not mentioned that are of a similar kind or level of difficulty.

Position Summary: Medical language specialist who interprets and transcribes dictation by physicians and other healthcare professionals regarding patient assessment, workup, therapeutic procedures, clinical course, diagnosis, prognosis, etc., in order to document patient care and facilitate delivery of healthcare services.

Knowledge, skills, and abilities:
1. Minimum education level of associate degree or equivalent in work experience and continuing education.
2. Knowledge of medical terminology, anatomy and physiology, clinical medicine, surgery, diagnostic tests, radiology, pathology, pharmacology, and the various medical specialties as required in areas of responsibility.
3. Knowledge of medical transcription guidelines and practices.
4. Excellent written and oral communication skills, including English usage, grammar, punctuation, and style.
5. Ability to understand diverse accents and dialects and varying dictation styles.
6. Ability to use designated reference materials.
7. Ability to operate designated word processing, dictation, and transcription equipment, and other equipment as specified.
8. Ability to work independently with minimal supervision.
9. Ability to work under pressure with time constraints.
10. Ability to concentrate.
11. Excellent listening skills.
12. Excellent eye, hand, and auditory coordination.
13. Certified medical transcriptionist (CMT) status preferred.

Working conditions:
General office environment. Quiet surroundings. Adequate lighting.

Physical demands:
Primarily sedentary work, with continuous use of earphones, keyboard, foot control, and where applicable, video display terminal.

AAMT gratefully acknowledges Lanier Voice Products, Atlanta, Georgia, for funding the development of the *AAMT Model Job Description: Medical Transcriptionist.*

For additional information, contact AAMT, P.O. Box 576187, Modesto, CA 95357-6187. Telephone 209-551-0883 or 800-982-2182. FAX 209-551-9317.

AAMT Model Job Description: Medical Transcriptionist

Job responsibilities:	*Performance standards:*
1. Transcribes medical dictation to provide a permanent record of patient care.	1.1 Applies knowledge of medical terminology, anatomy and physiology, and English language rules to the transcription and proofreading of medical dictation from originators with various accents, dialects, and dictation styles. 1.2 Recognizes, interprets, and evaluates inconsistencies, discrepancies, and inaccuracies in medical dictation, and appropriately edits, revises, and clarifies them without altering the meaning of the dictation or changing the dictator's style. 1.3 Clarifies dictation which is unclear or incomplete, seeking assistance as necessary. 1.4 Flags reports requiring the attention of the supervisor or dictator. 1.5 Uses reference materials appropriately and efficiently to facilitate the accuracy, clarity, and completeness of reports. 1.6 Meets quality and productivity standards and deadlines established by employer. 1.7 Verifies patient information for accuracy and completeness. 1.8 Formats reports according to established guidelines.
2. Demonstrates an understanding of the medicolegal implications and responsibilities related to the transcription of patient records to protect the patient and the business/institution.	2.1 Understands and complies with policies and procedures related to medicolegal matters, including confidentiality, amendment of medical records, release of information, patients' rights, medical records as legal evidence, informed consent, etc. 2.2 Meets standards of professional and ethical conduct. 2.3 Recognizes and reports unusual circumstances and/or information with possible risk factors to appropriate risk management personnel. 2.4 Recognizes and reports problems, errors, and discrepancies in dictation and patient records to appropriate manager. 2.5 Consults appropriate personnel regarding dictation which may be regarded as unprofessional, frivolous, insulting, inflammatory, or inappropriate.
3. Operates designated word processing, dictation, and transcription equipment as directed to complete assignments.	3.1 Uses designated equipment effectively, skillfully, and efficiently. 3.2 Maintains equipment and work area as directed. 3.3 Assesses condition of equipment and furnishings, and reports need for replacement or repair.
4. Follows policies and procedures to contribute to the efficiency of the medical transcription department.	4.1 Demonstrates an understanding of policies, procedures, and priorities, seeking clarification as needed. 4.2 Reports to work on time, as scheduled, and is dependable and cooperative. 4.3 Organizes and prioritizes assigned work, and schedules time to accommodate work demands, turnaround-time requirements, and commitments. 4.4 Maintains required records, providing reports as scheduled and upon request. 4.5 Participates in quality assurance programs. 4.6 Participates in evaluation and selection of equipment and furnishings. 4.7 Provides administrative/clerical/technical support as needed and as assigned.
5. Expands job-related knowledge and skills to improve performance and adjust to change.	5.1 Participates in inservice and continuing education activities. 5.2 Provides documentation of inservice and continuing education activities. 5.3 Reviews trends and developments in medicine, English usage, technology, and transcription practices, and shares knowledge with colleagues. 5.4 Documents new and revised terminology, definitions, styles, and practices for reference and application. 5.5 Participates in the evaluation and selection of books, publications, and other reference materials.
6. Uses interpersonal skills effectively to build and maintain cooperative working relationships.	6.1 Works and communicates in a positive and cooperative manner with management and supervisory staff, medical staff, co-workers and other healthcare personnel, and patients and their families when providing information and services, seeking assistance and clarification, and resolving problems. 6.2 Contributes to team efforts. 6.3 Carries out assignments responsibly. 6.4 Participates in a positive and cooperative manner during staff meetings. 6.5 Handles difficult and sensitive situations tactfully. 6.6 Responds well to supervision. 6.7 Shares information with co-workers. 6.8 Assists with training of new employees as needed.

Exhibit B: Budget Worksheet

Budget

Year: _____

		Jan	Feb	Mar	Apr	May	June	July	Aug	Sept	Oct	Nov	Dec	Total
1	Revenue: source A													
2	Revenue: source B													
3	Revenue: source C													
4	**Total revenue**													
	Operating expenses:													
5	Advertising & promotion													
6	Auto expense													
7	Commissions & fees													
8	Insurance													
9	Legal & accounting fees													
10	Office expense													
11	Rentals & leases													
12	Repairs & maintenance													
13	Supplies													
14	Taxes & licenses													
15	Travel													
16	Meals & entertainment													
17	Salaries expense													
18	Bank service charges													
19	Postage & freight													
20	Telephone													
21	Dues & reference material													
22	Utilities													
23	Independent contractors													
24	Cleaning & maintenance													
25	Conventions & trade shows													
26	Bad debts													
27	Other:													
28	Other:													
29	Other:													
30	Other:													
31	Depreciation													
32	**Total operating expense**													
33	**Operating income [line #4 – #32]**													
34	Interest income -- plus													
35	Interest expense -- minus													
36	**Net income before income tax**													
37	*Provision for income taxes*													
38	*Net income*													

From *Easy Financials for Your Home-based Business*

Exhibit C: Sample Contract

This agreement entered into this date, by and between the subcontractor known as: _____ , herein referred to as Subcontractor, whose address is _____ , telephone is _____ and the Contractor:_____ .

WHEREAS SUBCONTRACTOR desires to contract with CONTRACTOR to perform said work and/or service, and

WHEREAS the parties desire to set forth their contractual and business arrangement(s)

THEREFORE, this agreement constitutes the said contractual and business arrangements, and the parties contract and agree as follows:

THAT THE SUBCONTRACTOR agrees to perform, abide by and follow the stipulations listed in the remainder of this contract.

Equipment

The subcontractor is responsible for providing all equipment and supplies necessary for any work done, other than supplies given by the client (i.e., stationery indigenous to the client). These supplies provided by the Subcontractor include, but are not limited to, office equipment (i.e., typewriter, computer, transcription equipment, etc.), paper, dictionaries and manuals, ribbons, tools, etc. The subcontractor is also responsible for all repairs on her [his] own equipment.

Any supplies that are necessary from the client must be requested well in advance by the Subcontractor and the Subcontractor is responsible for keeping an adequate supply on hand at all times. This supply must be returned to the Contractor should this contract ever cease.

Any equipment or supplies loaned by the Contractor to the Subcontractor must be returned to the Contractor at the termination of this contract, or final payment of any payment due will be withheld until said items are returned.

Pricing and Payment

Each client's pricing is set separately, according to the individual client. Pricing is by each piece and/or line as set forth in the Work Scope.

Payment for services rendered is on a twice monthly basis. The Subcontractor is responsible for issuing a billing to the Contractor on the 1st of each month for the 16th through the 31st of the previous month, and on the 16th of each month for the 1st through the 15th of that same month. Payment to the Subcontractor from the Contractor is due on the 5th of each month for the pay period of the 16th through the 31st, and on the 20th of each month for the pay period of the 1st through the 15th. If the pay date falls on a weekend or holiday, the Contractor reserves the right to pay on the first working day following the weekend or holiday. If the Subcontractor does not turn in invoices by the dates specified, the Contractor is not responsible to pay by any set date and pay may be late.

A separate billing for each client must be given to the Contractor by the Subcontractor. Each billing must be typewritten and include the name of the client, the dates of the billing, the pages and specific dates of work completed and, if applicable, a description of each piece of work completed, and individual pricing, as well as a total. The Subcontractor must be prepared to back up each billing with copies of work completed should the Contractor or client request any information regarding any services rendered.

Contractor will pay for any work containing errors. Subcontractor is responsible to redo all work containing errors without charge to the client or Agency. If the client should request a redo of typing with minor editing changes that were not the fault of the typist or Agency, then the Subcontractor will provide redo at one-half of the original cost.

Contractor is not responsible to pay for redo work in the case of power outages or faulty equipment. It is the responsibility of the Subcontractor to keep equipment in working order and to provide backup emergency services should a technical problem occur.

Communication with Clients

Subcontractor may not communicate with client directly regarding billing or pricing structure or anything other than a question directly applying to the typing or work procedure, such as terminology, spelling, etc. When communicating with client on the above matters, Subcontractor must identify herself [himself] as being from the agency of the Contractor and in no way represent herself [himself] as her [his] own agency or business.

Noncompete Clause

The clients of the Contractor will remain the clients of the Contractor. At no time in the future may the Subcontractor do any work for the clients in any way, contract or draw business or clients or accounts from anybody in any way connected with any of the clients' relatives, friends, contacts or anybody associated with the client in any way. All referrals are the express property of the Contractor.

Work Scope

The Subcontractor is responsible for keeping a complete Work Scope on each client assigned by the Contractor. This Work Scope is to be given to the Contractor upon termination originated either by the Subcontractor or the Contractor. The Work Scope must be typewritten, include the client's name, address, telephone number, names of contact personnel, list of specific terminology used by that client, and any specialized instructions for that client.

The Subcontractor is responsible for keeping one month of work for each client on file for reference for billing purposes, termination or request of the client for any particular piece of work.

The Subcontractor is responsible to either pick up and drop off the work load of the client(s) at the office or the Contractor, at the office of the client directly according to the times specified, or make specific arrangements with the management of the Contractor.

All completed work dropped off at the office of the Contractor or given directly to the client's office by the Subcontractor must be in individual folders supplied by _____ with _____ logo on them, separated according to each client, neatly labeled and with any necessary instructions for the daily driver.

The Subcontractor is responsible for providing services for the assigned client at all times during the duration of this contract. The Subcontractor is responsible for providing her [his] own backup service in case of illness, vacation, emergency or any possible occurrence that would render the Subcontractor unable to perform. The Subcontractor is responsible for providing all payment arrangements to backup personnel and it is the responsibility of the Subcontractor to ensure that the backup personnel comply with all stipulations contained within this contract. The Subcontractor is held directly responsible for anything her [his] backup may or may not do.

The Subcontractor is responsible for providing liability insurance of at least $500,000 if any kind of bookkeeping services are contracted for by the Contractor with the Subcontractor.

The Contractor expects loyalty, enthusiasm and total support verbally, in action, and in deed from the Subcontractor at all times.

Miscellaneous

The logo, name, promotional material, and advertising associated with the Contractor are exclusively the property of the Contractor. Unauthorized usage of any stationery or materials or unauthorized representation of the Agency of the Contractor or the Contractor itself is strictly prohibited. The Subcontractor cannot use any name similar to or resembling in any way, shape or form the name, advertising methods and appearances or practices of the Contractor.

The Subcontractor gives her [his] permission for her [his] name, picture, and information to be included in any advertising for the Contractor at any time during this contract or after this contract is terminated.

Termination of this Contract

The Subcontractor must give no less than a 7-day notice to the Contractor in writing for termination of this contract. Anything less than a 7-day notice will result in a 50% penalty fee payable to the Contractor and subtracted from the final payment due to the Subcontractor.

Before the termination is effective, Subcontractor must return all supplies and/or equipment belonging to or loaned by or borrowed from the Contractor. The Subcontractor is also responsible for supplying the Contractor with a copy of all work done for any client(s) within the previous two-week period, as well as a complete and detailed work scope as specified previously in this contract. Failure to comply with any portion of this termination stipulation or any portion of this contract may result in withholding of final payment.

Violation of any part of this contract can result in immediate termination by the Contractor without notice. All termination terms other than the 7-day notice would then be applicable for the Subcontractor and final check would be held until terms are complied with.

Contractor reserves the right to remove a client from the Subcontractor without any notice and give to another Subcontractor. Subcontractor also agrees that clients can be dropped at any time due to termination from the client.

The Subcontractor hereby agrees to abide by all of the terms and stipulations set forth in pages one through five of this contract and understand each item fully, as signified by signing below.

_____

Subcontractor   Date

_____

Social Security Number of Subcontractor

_____

Contractor   Date

Index

ABOUT RAYVE PRODUCTIONS

Rayve Productions is an award-winning small publisher of books and music. Current publications are primarily in the following categories:

(1) Business guidebooks for home-based businesses and other entrepreneurs
(2) Quality children's books and music
(3) History books about America and her regions, and an heirloom-quality journal for creating personal histories.

Rayve Productions' mail-order catalog offers the above items plus business books, software, music, and other enjoyable items produced by others.

Our eclectic collection of business resources and gift items has something to please everyone.

A FREE catalog is available upon request.

Come visit us at www.spannet.org/rayve.

BUSINESS & CAREER

☆*Smart Tax Write-offs: Hundreds of tax deduction ideas for home-based businesses, independent contractors, all entrepreneurs*   by Norm Ray, CPA
ISBN 1-877810-20-7, softcover, $12.95, 1996 pub.
Fun-to-read, easy-to-use guidebook that encourages entrepreneurs to be aggressive and creative in taking legitimate tax deductions. Includes valuable checklist of over 600 write-off ideas. Every small business owner's "must read."
(Recommended by *Home Office Computing, Small Business Opportunities, Spare Time, Independent Business Magazine*).

☆*The Independent Medical Transcriptionist, 3rd edition: The comprehensive guidebook for career success in a home-based medical transcription business*
by Donna Avila-Weil, CMT and Mary Glaccum, CMT
ISBN 1-877810-23-1, softcover, $34.95, 1998 pub.
The industry's premier reference book for medical transcription entrepreneurs.
(Recommended by *Journal of the American Association for Medical Transcription, Entrepreneur, Small Business Opportunities)*

☆*Independent Medical Coding: The comprehensive guidebook for career success as a home-based medical coder*
by Donna Avila-Weil, CMT and Rhonda Regan, CCS
ISBN 1-877810-17-7, softcover, $34.95, 1998 pub.
How to start and successfully run your own professional independent medical coding business. Step-by-step instructions.

☆*Easy Financials for Your Home-based Business*   by Norm Ray, CPA
ISBN 1-877810-92-4, softcover, $19.95, 1992 pub.
Small business & home-based business expert helps you save time by making your work easier, and save money by nailing down your tax deductions.
(Recommended by *Wilson Library Bulletin, The Business Journal, National Home Business Report)*

☆*Internal Medicine Words*   by Minta Danna
ISBN 1-877810-68-1, softcover, $29.95, 1997 pub.
Over 8,000 words and terms related to internal medicine. A valuable spelling and terminology usage resource for medical transcriptionists, medical writers and editors, court reporters, medical records personnel, and others working with medical documentation.

☆*Shrinking the Globe into Your Company's Hands: The step-by-step international trade guide for small businesses*   by Sidney R. Lawrence, PE
ISBN 1-877810-46-0, softcover, $24.95, 1997 pub.
An expert in foreign trade shows U.S. small business owners how to market and export products and services safely and profitably.

HISTORY

☆ 20 Tales of California: A rare collection of western stories by Hector Lee
ISBN 1-877810-63-0, hardcover, $16.95
ISBN 1-877810-62-2, softcover, $9.95, 1998 pub.
Mysterious and romantic tales: real life and folklore set in various California locations. Includes ideas for family outings and classroom field trips.

☆ Link Across America: A story of the historic Lincoln Highway — see Children's Books

☆ Windsor, The Birth of a City by Gabriel A. Fraire
ISBN 1-877810-91-6, hardcover, $21.95, 1991 pub.
Fascinating case study of political and social issues surrounding city incorporation of Windsor, California, 1978—1991. LAFCO impact.

☆ LifeTimes, The Life Experiences Journal
ISBN 1-877810-34-7, hardcover, $49.95
World's easiest, most fun and useful personal journal. Handsome heirloom quality with gilt-edged pages. Over 150 information categories to record your life experiences. Winner of national award for excellence.

GENERAL

☆ Nancy's Candy Cookbook: How to make candy at home the easy way
by Nancy Shipman
ISBN 1-877810-65-7, softcover, $14.95, 1996 pub.
Have fun and save money by making candy at home at a fraction of candy store prices. More than 100 excellent candy recipes — from Grandma's delicious old-fashioned fudge to modern gourmet truffles. Includes many children's favorites, too.

☆ Joy of Reading: One family's fun-filled guide to reading success
by Debbie Duncan
ISBN 1-877810-45-2, softcover, $14.95, 1998 pub.
A dynamic author and mother, and an expert on children's literature, shares her family's personal reading success stories. You'll be inspired and entertained by this lighthearted, candid glimpse into one family's daily experiences as they cope with the ups and downs of life. Through it all, there is love, and an abundance of wonderful books. *More than 600 children's books featured. Learn how to inspire your children to read for pleasure and much more.*

CHILDREN'S BOOKS & MUSIC

☆ Link Across America: A story of the historic Lincoln Highway

by Mary Elizabeth Anderson

ISBN 1-877810-97-5, hardcover, $14.95, 1997 pub.

It began with a long-ago dream . . . a road that would run clear across America! The dream became reality in 1914 as the Lincoln Highway began to take form, to eventually run from New York City to San Francisco. Venture from past to present experiencing transportation history. Topics include Abraham Lincoln, teams of horses, seedling miles, small towns, making concrete, auto courts, Burma Shave signs, classic cars and road rallies. Color photos along today's Lincoln Highway remnants, b/w historical photos, map and list of cities along the old Lincoln Highway. (Ages 7-13 & their parents, grandparents & great-grandparents)

☆ The Perfect Orange: A tale from Ethiopia

by Frank P. Araujo, PhD; illustrated by Xiao Jun Li

ISBN 1-877810-94-0, hardcover, $16.95, 1994 pub., Toucan Tales volume 2

Inspiring gentle folktale. Breathtaking watercolors dramatize ancient Ethiopia's contrasting pastoral charm and majesty. Illustrations are rich with Ethiopian details. Story reinforces values of generosity and selflessness over greed and self-centeredness. Glossary of Ethiopian terms and pronunciation key.

(PBS *Storytime* Selection; Recommended by *School Library Journal, Faces, MultiCultural Review, Small Press Magazine, The Five Owls, Wilson Library Bulletin*)

☆ Nekane, the Lamiña & the Bear: A tale of the Basque Pyrenees

by Frank P. Araujo, PhD; illustrated by Xiao Jun Li

ISBN 1-877810-01-0, hardcover, $16.95, 1993 pub., Toucan Tales volume 1

Delightful Basque folktale pits appealing, quick-witted young heroine against mysterious villain. Lively, imaginative narrative, sprinkled with Basque phrases. Vibrant watercolor images. Glossary of Basque terms and pronunciation key.

(Recommended by School Library Journal, Publishers Weekly, Kirkus Reviews, Booklist, Wilson Library Bulletin, The Basque Studies Program Newsletter: University of Nevada, BCCB, The Five Owls)

☆ The Laughing River: A folktale for peace

by Elizabeth Haze Vega; illustrated by Ashley Smith

ISBN 1-877810-35-5   hardcover book, $16.95, 1995 pub.
ISBN 1-877810-36-3   companion musical audiotape, $9.95
ISBN 1-877810-37-1   book & musical audiotape combo, $23.95
Drum kit, $9.95
Book, musical audiotape & drum kit combo, $29.95

Two fanciful African tribes are in conflict until the laughing river bubbles melodiously into their lives, bringing fun, friendship, peace. Lyrical fanciful folktale of conflict resolution. Mesmerizing music. Dancing, singing and drumming instructions. Orff approach. (Recommended by *School Library Journal*)